PICTORIAL GLOSSARY of ROOTS

(on back papers)

Illustrations by
Lee Allen Peterson

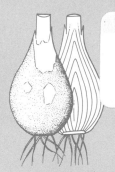

BULB

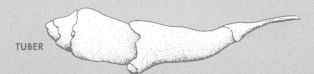

D0927949

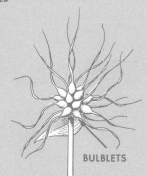

BULBLETS

TAPROOT

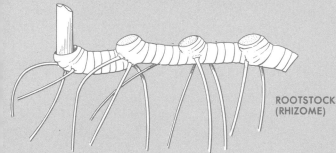

ROOTSTOCK
(RHIZOME)

TUBER

THE PETERSON FIELD GUIDE SERIES®

Edited by Roger Tory Peterson

THE PETERSON FIELD GUIDE SERIES®

A Field Guide to Medicinal Plants

Eastern and Central
North America

Text by
STEVEN FOSTER
and JAMES A. DUKE

Line Drawings by
ROGER TORY PETERSON,
JIM BLACKFEATHER ROSE,
and
LEE ALLEN PETERSON

Photographs by
STEVEN FOSTER

*Sponsored by the National Audubon Society,
the National Wildlife Federation,
and the Roger Tory Peterson Institute*

HOUGHTON MIFFLIN COMPANY · BOSTON

For information about permission to reproduce selections from this book,
write to Permissions, Houghton Mifflin Company, 215 Park Avenue South,
New York, New York 10003

PETERSON FIELD GUIDES and PETERSON FIELD GUIDE SERIES
are registered trademarks of Houghton Mifflin Company.

Library of Congress Cataloging-in-Publication Data

Foster, Steven, date.
  A field guide to medicinal plants : eastern and central North
America / text by Steven Foster and James A. Duke ; line drawings
by Roger Tory Peterson, Jim Rose, and Lee Allen Peterson ; photographs by Steven Foster.
      p. cm. — (The Peterson field guide series ; 40)
  "Sponsored by the National Audubon Society, the National Wild-
life Federation, and the Roger Tory Peterson Institute."
  Includes bibliographical references.
  ISBN 0-395-35309-2. — ISBN 0-395-46722-5 (pbk.)
  1. Medicinal plants — East (U.S.) — Identification.   2. Medicinal
plants — Middle West — Identification.   3. Medicinal plants —
Canada, Eastern — Identification.   I. Duke, James A., date.   II. National Audubon Society.   III. National Wildlife Federation.   IV.
Roger Tory Peterson Institute.   V. Title.   VI. Series.
QK99.U6F68   1990
581.6'34'0973 — dc20   89-71688
                                                        CIP

Printed in the United States of America

VB   10   9   8   7   6   5   4

EDITOR'S NOTE

When Europeans first arrived in North America, one of their observations was of a rich native flora, a wealth of new species, some of which were potentially useful to humans. Early settlements, such as the Plymouth colonies, were financed in part through speculation on the export of Sassafras to Europe. At that time, Sassafras was considered a sort of cure-all, a medicine chest locked in the bark of a single plant.

Many of the early explorers and travel writers, as well as botanists, had noted with a great deal of interest the medicinal uses of plants by the indigenous Indians of North America. At that point, Western medicine relied heavily on medicinal plants. Whereas many of us think that medicinal use of plants ended with the evolution of synthetic drugs, you may be surprised to learn that even today over forty percent of prescription drugs sold in the U.S. contain ingredients derived from nature, and a full twenty-five percent of drugs contain at least one component derived directly, or through chemical modeling, from flowering plants. Plants have always served as important sources of medicine, whether as folk remedies or as pure chemical compounds.

This book by Steven Foster and Jim Duke provides the first survey of medicinal plants of eastern and central North America in a field-guide format. It illustrates and describes nearly 500 medicinal herbs—and tells how to identify them using the "Peterson System," a practical approach based on visual impressions. Many of the drawings have been adapted from my *Field Guide to Wildflowers of Northeastern and North-central North America*, and my son Lee Peterson's *Field Guide to Edible Wild Plants of Eastern and Central North America*. The remainder of the illustrations were drawn by Jim Rose. In addition, Steven Foster has traveled widely throughout North America, photographing medicinal plants, and over 200 plants are illustrated by his color photographs.

Knowing the name of a plant gives us a reference point for beginning to explore the relationship with the rest of the natural world—including humans. Knowing that a plant may provide medical workers with the cure for a previously incurable disease gives us a new perspective on biological diversity and nature as a whole. We learn that the Mayapple (*Podophyllum peltatum*) provides a chemical compound now used in the treatment of small-cell lung cancer, and that Annual Wormwood (*Artemisia*) offers the most promising new malaria treatment in a century, and that Common St. Johnswort (*Hypericum perforatum*) is of interest to medical workers who are fighting against AIDS. Even the lowly Dandelion and the pernicious Japanese Honeysuckle have unexpected potential. Perhaps a good way to accept the "weeds" that have displaced so much of our native flora is to find ways to use them.

The authors survey the medicinal uses of each plants, past and present: historical uses by American Indians and nineteenth-century physicians, folk remedies, and modern scientific rationales that often vindicate past use while investigating leads for the future. They also provide a strong conservation message: appreciate the medicinal value of plants, and be sure to preserve these finite resources in their native habitats. Wild plants contain a storehouse of genetic information that may lead to new treatments for disease. According to the World Health Organization, as much as eighty percent of the world's population still relies on traditional forms of medicine such as herbs. We must make an effort to conserve all native plants, many of which may provide treatment or cures for cancer, heart disease, warts, the common cold, or even AIDS.

This field guide will help you see many familiar plants in an entirely new way. Take it into the field and you may learn that the beauty of a Black-eyed Susan is more than meets the eye.

ROGER TORY PETERSON

PREFACE

Why a field guide to American medicinal plants? Didn't the use of plants as medicine dissolve into obscurity after the Dark Ages? Aren't folk remedies just old wives' tales, and the stuff of witches' brew? The answer is an unequivocal no. Over 40 percent of prescription drugs sold in the U.S. contain at least one ingredient derived from nature. As many as 25 percent of prescription drugs contain an ingredient derived from higher (flowering) plants. Periwinkle (*Catharanthus roseus*, also called Myrtle or *Vinca rosea*) is a common ornamental in the U.S., often planted as a ground cover outside homes or city high-rises. Few people who pass by the plant realize that preparations derived from Periwinkle are used in chemotherapy for leukemia and more than a dozen other types of cancer. Alkaloids derived from the fungus ergot, which grows on Rye Grass and Giant Cane (see p. 312) are used as uterine-contracting drugs. The many cardiac glycosides from Foxglove *(Digitalis)*, commonly planted as an ornamental flower, are used in a variety of products for the management of several phases of heart disease. The primary source of material for the biosynthesis of steroid hormones is the plant kingdom. The social, economic, and political impact of oral contraceptives alone illustrates the importance of this group of plant-derived drugs. The manufacture of progesterone was made commercially feasible by the use of chemicals from Mexican yams, which were then converted to progesterone. With all the advances of modern medicine, there is still nothing to replace morphine, derived from the Opium Poppy, as a pain reliever for major trauma. The fact is, herbs — plant drugs — are a very important and integral part of modern medicine.

We believe that safer natural compounds could be found to replace the synthetic compounds that occur in about 75 percent of our prescription drugs, and that evolution has better equipped us to deal with rational doses of preparations from medicinal plants. But since it costs, in our litigious American society, $125 million to prove a new drug safe and efficacious, we may need to wait for the Japanese to develop these natural medicines for us. Based on a survey in *Phytotherapy Research* in 1987, the Japanese held more than half of the new patents on natural products. Unfortunately, most American medicinal plants have yet to be thoroughly investigated in terms of pharmacology and chemistry, much less through clinical trials in humans. Those that have been extensively studied in recent years have mostly been probed by European or Asian researchers. Little work is performed on American medicinal plants by American researchers, while virtually all other industrialized, technologically advanced societies intensively investigate their native medicinal flora. Much scientific research has also been conducted in developing countries where traditional medicine systems, some thousands of years old, are still an integral part of health care systems. China and India are prime examples. Although these countries may be called "developing" countries in terms of their economic and technical systems, the more than 5,000-year-old traditions of Traditional Chinese Medicine, and of Ayurveda in India, represent highly developed medical systems that are constantly being vindicated and enhanced by modern research. Their experience and research is valuable to our study of American medical botany.

One intention of this book is to further an awareness of the need for plant conservation by recognizing the economic or beneficial history of plants that could provide potential future economic and medicinal benefits for humans. Conservation and preservation are necessary on both the micro and macro levels. Visiting European and Chinese medical botanists on collecting trips to our fields and forests are struck by the abundance of our wild herbs, and they caution that we should conserve them. We should make an effort to conserve native medicinal plants that may provide treatment or cures for cancer, heart disease, warts, the common cold, or even AIDS. The notion that American fields and forests are an endless fountain of animal, plant, or mineral resources is a 19th-century idea, not appropriate to the dwindling natural resources of the 20th century.

Unfortunately, a number of medicinal plants are now being extirpated without regard to preservation and the continued ecological success of the species. While the Endangered Species Act and Lacey Act have helped regulate the harvest of a few medicinals, notably Ginseng, the public consciousness is still swayed more toward protecting animals than plants. Commenting on dramatic declines in Kansas populations of *Echinacea* (Purple Coneflower) in recent years, one frustrated researcher remarked that if *Echinacea* had a little fur and cute little black eyes, it could elicit a little attention!

We hope this little volume will help the reader gain a deeper appreciation of the plants around us. Understanding the traditional medicinal uses of so many of our wildflowers, woody plants, and weeds can help us to gain a deeper sense of our relationship to the natural world. Knowing that a wildflower was a folk remedy for cancer, and that that knowledge may eventually produce the lead that helps researchers develop a new cancer treatment, adds a new dimension, a human element to conservation. Enjoy and be cautious.

STEVEN FOSTER AND JAMES A. DUKE

Symbols:

 = **Poisonous.** Dangerous or deadly to ingest, or perhaps even to touch.

 = **Caution.** See warning in text.

 = Known to cause **allergic reactions** in some individuals.

 = Known to cause **dermatitis** in some individuals.

 = Used in **modern medicine** in the U.S.

ACKNOWLEDGMENTS

The authors would like to thank the Threshold Foundation for partial support of Steven Foster's work in 1987 through a grant to the Ozark Beneficial Plant Project of the Ozark Resources Center, Brixey, Missouri. A note of thanks to Vinnie McKinney, Sally Goodwin, Ella Alford, and Nancy Ward for support of the work. A special thanks to Les Eastman for encouragement and for tracking down photos and plants for the color plates. Phillip P. Keenan provided several photos for the color section. Thanks, too, to all the members of the Josselyn Botanical Society; many of the photos in the color section were taken during field trips sponsored by the Society. The authors deeply appreciate the help, support, and friendship of Mark Blumenthal and other people at the American Botanical Council, Hart Brent-Collins, Dr. Ed Croom, Christopher Hobbs, Kelly Kindscher, Loren Israelsen, Dr. Paul Lee, Bob Liebert, Portia Meares, Ken Murdock, and the members of the Sabbathday Lake Shaker Community.

Peggy Duke and Jude Farar are thanked for their behind-the-scenes contributions, without which this work could not have materialized.

A special note of thanks to Roger Tory Peterson and Lee Peterson for permission to use so many of their line drawings in this volume and for their support of the project.

The contributions of Professor Yue Chongxi, at the Institute of Chinese Materia Medica, Academy of Traditional Chinese Medicine, Beijing, and Dr. Shiu Ying Hu, at Arnold Arboretum, Harvard University, are gratefully acknowledged, for information they provided on Chinese uses of closely related plant species of China and North America.

The authors are grateful for the good work of Harry Foster, Barbara Stratton, Anne Chalmers, Lisa Diercks, and the rest of the staff of Houghton Mifflin for all the thankless details associated with book production.

Rebecca Perry and the staff of the Lloyd Library provided

many useful and obscure research materials. The American
Botanist, Keith Crotz, filled missing gaps in the literature, as
did Patricia Ledlie, Elisabeth Woodburn, and Gary Wayner.
The authors gratefully acknowledge the helpful comments of
Dr. John Kartez at the Botanical Garden, University of North
Carolina at Chapel Hill, and Dr. Arthur O. Tucker at Dela-
ware State College.

Billy Joe Tatum is gratefully acknowledged for her gracious
contribution.

Credit must also be given to the dozens of botanists, medical botanists, pharmacognosists, toxicologists, ethnobotan-
ists, physicians, and researchers in all disciplines touching
upon medicinal plants for their hundreds of published works,
which have been frequently and repeatedly consulted. If this
book cited references in the style of a scientific publication,
the bibliography would be half the length of the book. A few
of the most pertinent works for further references are listed
on pp. 323–324.

Tribute must be paid to the 1,100 to 5,000 generations of
native Americans whose experience and evolution with the
indigenous medicinal flora ultimately made this book, and a
scant two centuries of literature, possible.

Finally, Steven Foster would like to thank his parents,
Herb and Hope Foster, for all they have given, and dedicate
his work on this volume to them.

CONTENTS

A Field Guide to
Medicinal Plants

HOW TO USE THIS BOOK

This book is not a prescriptor, just a field guide to medicinal plants of the eastern and central portion of the North American continent. The purpose of this guide is to help you to identify these plants safely and accurately, and to help you avoid similar-looking plants that could be dangerous or even fatally poisonous.

General Organization

Species covered: There are more than 800 species of plants growing in the eastern U.S. that can be documented as having at least some medicinal use. This book includes 500 of the more significant medicinal plant species of the eastern U.S. with important historical uses, present use, or future potential. We have not attempted to cover all of the alien plants found here that are used medicinally in their native lands. For example, of the hundreds of ornamentals originating from east Asia in American horticulture, over 1,000 species can be documented as being used in Traditional Chinese Medicine. Nearly all common weeds naturalized from Europe have been used as medicinal plants in their native lands. We have included many naturalized weeds, but not all of them.

Area covered: This field guide covers all states east of, but excluding, Colorado, Montana, and New Mexico. It does not fully cover the southern half of Florida or the southern and western halves of Texas. Adjacent regions of Canadian provinces are included. Toward the southern, western, and extreme northern extensions of the range, our coverage is less comprehensive.

Botanical and Medical Terms: Since this book is intended as a guide for the lay person, we have used as few technical terms as possible. Nevertheless, the use of some specific terms relative to plant identification or the medicinal use of plants has been inevitable. We define those terms in the Glossary. Although we have defined terms relative to medicinal effects, we have not attempted to define each disease, condition, or ailment included in this book. We have kept disease terminology as simple as possible. For further explanations, should they be necessary, the reader is referred to any good English dictionary or medical dictionary.

Illustrations: In addition to drawings by Jim Rose, many drawings have been borrowed from the work of Roger Tory Peterson *(A Field Guide to Wildflowers)* and Lee Allen Peterson *(A Field Guide to Edible Wild Plants of Eastern and Central North America)*. Both, of course, are titles in the Peterson Field Guide series. The drawings emphasize the basic outline of the plant and characteristic diagnostic features, with the key features highlighted by arrows on the line drawings. Corresponding details are italicized in the adjacent text.

The color photo section is arranged by habitat and growth habit (tree, shrub, wildflower, etc.). Representative species to be found in each area are included. The photos were taken with a Nikon FE body with a 55 mm Micro-Nikkor, 135 mm Nikkor telephoto, or a 28 mm Nikkor wide-angle lens, on Kodachrome 64 film. All photos are by Steven Foster, except those otherwise noted.

Identifying Plants

Plants are arranged by visual features, based on flower color, number of petals, habitat, leaf arrangement, and so on. These obvious similarities help the reader to thumb quickly through the pages and find an illustration that corresponds with a plant in hand. Once you have matched a plant with an illustration, read all details in the descriptive text, making sure that all characteristics correspond — key *italicized* details, range, habitat, flowering time, color, and the flower or leaf structure (see headings at top of pages facing the plates). *Never, never ingest a plant that has not been positively identified. (Read the sections on warnings on pp. 7 and 10.)*

The first part of the book covers wildflowers, which are arranged by flower color (white, yellow, pink to red, blue-violet, green) and other visual similarities. Please note that there is tremendous variation in flower color in the plant world. If a plant may have white or blue flowers, for example, we have attempted to include the plant in both sections of this guide. Sometimes your interpretation of "pink to red" may be viewed as "violet to blue" by others. Be aware of these subtle differences. Flowering shrubs, trees, and woody vines are in separate sections following the wildflowers. Flowering woody plants are generally not included in the wildflower section. Ferns and related plants follow the woody plant section. Last is a section on grasses or grasslike plants.

Common names: One or two common names are listed at the beginning of each entry. Though some plants have only one common name, others may have many. Common names of wildflowers generally conform to those used in Peterson and McKinney's *A Field Guide to Wildflowers.* Sometimes, in an herbal context, a plant is better known by another common name. In these instances we have used the most commonly known name for the herb. For trees, shrubs, vines, grasses, and ferns, we have used the names we felt were best known.

Part used: The plant part(s) used for medicinal purposes are listed in boldface type opposite the common name. In descriptions of woody plants, the word "bark" almost always refers to the *inner* bark of the tree or shrub, not the rough outer layer. Slippery Elm, for example, has a rough, corky outer bark that is not known to be of medicinal use, though it often is sold as Slippery Elm bark. The tawny white, fibrous, highly mucilaginous (slippery) inner bark can easily be stripped from the branches once the outer bark has been rasped away. Please see the section on "Conservation and Harvesting" (p. 8) for general guidelines on harvesting various plant parts.

Scientific names: Beneath the common name is the scientific or botanical name by which the plant is generally known (in our opinion). Latin names are not set in stone. Although changes in Latin names are annoying, sometimes they must be made according to valid new information developed by botanists with a special interest in taxonomic relationships. Many plant guides in the Peterson Field Guide series have relied on the eighth edition of *Gray's Manual of Botany* (Fernald, 1950), but we have not used it as the final word. Nearly 40 years have passed since its most recent revision, and many changes in nomenclature have since occurred. *Hortus Third* (compiled by the staff of the L. H. Bailey Hortorium, 1976) has been used as an alternative reference when nomenclature was in question. We have provided synonyms in brackets beneath the main botanical name to reflect alternate or obsolete Latin names often encountered in recent botanical manuals, popular field guides, and herbals.

The Latin name is followed by an abbreviation of the name of the botanist, or "species author," who named the plant. This is a useful reference tool for taxonomists and can be a flag for the lay person as well. For example, many old American herbals list the Latin name of the Slippery Elm as *Ulmus fulva* Michx., but all modern botanical works cite this elm as *Ulmus rubra* Muhl. "Michx." is the abbreviation for the name of the French botanist Andre Michaux (1746–1802) who assigned the name *Ulmus fulva* to this species. "Muhl." is the abbreviation for Gotthilf Henry Ernest Muhlenberg (1753–1815), who first proposed the name *Ulmus rubra.* Muhlenberg's *Ulmus rubra* has priority over Michaux's *Ulmus fulva* according to the rules of the *International Code of Botanical Nomenclature,* and *Ulmus rubra* thus becomes the name used by botanists everywhere. Research on medicinal plants requires delving into historical literature, thus it is useful to have the "author citation" as a reference to the Latin name. It is a point of comparison that may help you verify which species is being discussed.

Family names: The Latin name is followed by the common name for the family. Technical names for plant families have not been included.

Description: A brief description of the plant follows. The descriptions are based primarily on visual characteristics, though we have sometimes included scent as an identifying feature. We regret that scratch-and-sniff features cannot be included in the text. The description begins with the growth habit of the plant (annual, perennial, twining vine, tree, shrub, etc.) and height. Characteristic details for leaves, flowers, or fruits follow. Key identifying features of each plant are in *italics,* and those diagnostic characteristics are indicated with arrows on the adjacent illustrations.

The earliest blooming date given is usually the time when the flowering period begins in the South. Blooming time in more northerly areas often begins a month or more later. Though the blooming date may be listed as "April–June," the plant may only bloom for two weeks in any particular location. Take Goldenseal *(Hydrastis canadensis)*, for example. Blooming time is listed as April–May. In northern Arkansas the plant usually blooms around the first week of May. The flowers last only three to five days.

Distribution: Under the heading **"Where found"** the habitat where the plant grows is listed, with notes whether the plant is an introduced alien or is native to the U.S. Many alien (non-native) plants are now naturalized or adventive — well established on their own without being cultivated. Many plants in this category often are still cultivated in herb, kitchen, or flower gardens; others are best known as weeds. Habitat is followed by the plant's range in Canada and the eastern and central U.S. Each plant's range is given from northeast to southeast and from southwest to northwest.

Although many wild plants are common and widespread, others are rare and should not be overcollected. Cautions about plants that are protected by law, or those which should be protected, are also included in this section.

Medicinal Uses

This section presents a brief discussion of the some of the more significant medicinal uses of a plant. Historic or folk uses are described first, generally starting with known uses of the plants by native peoples of North America. In most cases we have chosen to use the term "American Indian," rather than list native groups by their traditional "tribe" names. We sometimes list medicinal uses in India or cite work by Indian researchers, so this helps to avoid confusion. Readers are referred to Daniel Moerman's excellent work *Medicinal Plants of Native America* and Jim Duke's *Handbook of Northeastern Indian Medicinal Plants*, and the original references in their bibliographies, for detailed accounts of uses of native plants by specific indigenous groups of people. (See Bibliography, p. 323.).

The discussion often covers American Indian usage, folk usage by settlers of the North American continent over the past 400 years, historical usage by medical practitioners, and vindication of medicinal uses as suggested by presence of specific chemical components or chemical groups, pharmacological studies (mostly with animals), and, if available, clinical studies or clinical applications.

Often in our discussion we have included notes on the experience of Chinese practitioners with a closely related plant species. For more than 180 years botanists have recognized striking similarities between the floras of eastern Asia and eastern North America. Most plants involved in this pattern of "disjunctions" in plant geography are thought to be remnants of an ancient forest that covered the Northern Hemisphere over 70 million years ago. Many of the more than 140 genera that share ranges in eastern Asia and eastern North America are important medicinal plants on one continent or the other, therefore the Chinese experience is relevant to North American species, and vice versa. Some plants included in this classical pattern of plant disjunctions are the various species of Ginseng (in genus *Panax*), Witch-hazel *(Hamamelis),* Sassafras, Mayapple *(Podophyllum),* Magnolia, Sweetgum *(Liquidambar),* Spicebush *(Lindera),* and dozens of other plant groups included in this book.

In a historical context, we occasionally mention a concept known as the "doctrine of signatures." This refers to an ancient idea that if a plant part was shaped like, or in some other way resembled, a human organ or disease characteristic, then that plant was useful for that particular organ or ailment. With its 3-lobed leaves, Liverleaf (as herbalists referred to the *Hepatica* species), was thought to be useful in treating liver disease. If held to light, the leaves of Common St. Johnswort *(Hypericum perforatum)* appear to have numerous holes pricked through the surface. The resemblance between these holes and the pores in human skin led some people to believe that preparations made from the leaves of this plant were useful for healing cuts. Using this doctrine, one might assume that kidney beans were good for the kidneys, or that the leaves of Broad-leaved Arrowhead *(Sagittaria latifolia)* would be useful for wounds caused by the head of an arrow. This concept has no scientific basis, though sometimes uses conceived centuries ago have persisted and may even have been corroborated by scientific evidence of their efficacy.

Preparations: In the **"Uses"** section we discuss ways in which each plant has traditionally or historically been used. In most instances we have chosen to use the word "tea" to refer to both infusions and decoctions. A simple *infusion* is made by soaking an herb (usually the leaf or flower) in hot water for 10–20 minutes. A cold infusion may be made by soaking the plant material in cold water for a relatively long period of time (varying from 2 hours to overnight), or simply letting the hot infusion sit until it is cool.

A *decoction* is made by simmering the plant material — usually the root, bark, or seed — under low heat. As a general rule of thumb, the word "infusion" is reserved for leaves and flower material and "decoction" for roots, barks, or seeds. Check the plant part used to determine whether a tea should be simmered or "decocted" or simply "infused," based on whether it is made from the bark, root, leaves, flowers, etc.

The term *wash* is often used for the external application of a cooled "tea." A wash is usually applied to the skin over the affected area.

Poultice is another commonly used term for an external application of herbs. A poultice is generally a moist paste made from the plant material, beaten to pulp in a mortar and pestle or with some other instrument if the herbs are fresh, or soaked in warm water if the herbs are dried. The poultice is spread over the affected area. Since some plants, such as Comfrey or Mullein, have leaves with irritating hairs that may adversely affect the skin, a layer of thin cloth such as muslin may be applied to the skin, with the herb material placed on top of the cloth.

A *tincture* is a plant extract dissolved in alcohol. Most tinctures are made with dilute alcohol (100 proof or 50 percent ethanol, 50 percent distilled water). Traditionally a tincture is made simply by soaking a certain percentage of plant material (often 20 percent by weight to the menstruum, or solvent) in the alcohol and water for a period of about two weeks, shaking the material daily, then straining the liquid through cheesecloth or filter paper before bottling. Tinctures are also made by a process known as percolation, in which the menstruum is poured through the plant material, which has been finely ground and then placed in a funnel-shaped container with a receptacle at the bottom to catch the herb-fortified liquid.

Dosage: Since this book is intended to help the reader identify medicinal plants and appreciate their traditional uses, and not to serve as a prescriptor, we have not included dosage except in historical context. See cautions regarding individual sensitivity below.

Warnings: Last but not least we include warnings. *Please be sure to read the warnings under each species account before* *handling the plant,* even for identification purposes; some plants can cause a painful skin rash. Some medicinal plants are very similar to and can be easily confused with a poisonous plant, with unpleasant or even fatal results. *Never eat or taste any part of a wild plant, or use it in any medicinal preparation, unless you are certain of its identification and safety, and that the dosage is correct, and that the plant has been properly prepared.*

Conservation and Harvesting

If you intend to harvest a plant or plant part, *after* you have *properly and positively* identified it, certain rules and values must be observed:

(1) If the plant is unusual or rare in your area, leave it be. Contact your local Audubon Society, native plant societies, botanical gardens, or state conservation agencies for a list of rare or threatened plants in the immediate vicinity. Often plants that are common in one state may be rare in another. Pale Purple Coneflower *(Echinacea pallida)* is common in eastern Kansas, but it is very rare in western North Carolina at the eastern extreme of its range. The plant might be judiciously harvested in Kansas, but in North Carolina it should be left alone. Other plants, like Pink or Yellow lady's-slippers, were historically valuable as medicinal plants, but should be left alone wherever they occur. Once you dig the root the plant is no more. These wild orchids are difficult to propagate and cultivate. Once much more abundant in the wild, they have been historically extirpated as a medicinal plant, and are currently overexploited as plants for wild-flower gardens. We believe their sale should be banned, where appropriate, or carefully regulated. Account books from the 1860s show that one company alone was selling over 300 pounds of dried Lady's-slipper root a month! It takes dozens of plants to get one pound of dried root. Although a number of orchids have traditionally been used in folk medicine, none is abundant enough for harvest.

In China, only a handful of wild harvested Ginseng roots are dug each year. The Oriental Ginseng has been valued as a medicinal plant for over 2,000 years. It has been virtually exterminated from the wild in China. One wild root of Oriental Ginseng can sell for as much as $20,000 on the Hong Kong market. Wild American Ginseng, by comparison, has only been traded as a commodity for a mere 200 years. Tons of wild-harvested American Ginseng are shipped to Oriental markets each year. How long will our plant populations be able to sustain themselves?

Goldenseal *(Hydrastis canadensis)* is one of the best-selling herbs in domestic health food markets. In recent years, supply shortages caused by alleged heavy harvesting of wild populations could threaten the plant's future. Cultivation efforts are now under way for Goldenseal. We strongly encourage the cultivation — rather than harvesting in the wild — of all native medicinal plants that enter commerce.

(2) Never collect all of the specimens of a plant in an area. One fear in publishing a volume such as this is that the interest in harvesting medicinal herbs for profit will outweigh the necessity of conservation. Take only what you need, and no more than ten percent of the individuals in a given population. If you harvest an entire population of most herbs, you will do so only once. Careful consideration and attention to detail are necessary for identification, harvest, usage, *and* conservation.

(3) Find out who owns the property where you intend to harvest a medicinal plant and obtain permission to harvest it *before* going on the property. In Missouri and other areas, state law prohibits the harvest of plant material without the permission of the landowner. Along roadsides, the owner is often the state itself.

(4) Harvest the plant at the correct time of year. Most herbs in which the leaves or whole herb (flowers, leaves, and stem) are used are harvested just before or just as the plant comes into flower. The amount and nature of the biologically active chemical components in a plant varies in quantity and quality according to the stage of the plant's growth, and even the time of day when it is harvested. Flowers are best harvested as they reach their peak bloom. As a general rule, it is best to harvest leaf and above-ground plant materials before noon, on a sunny day after the dew has dried off the leaves.

Seeds should be harvested only when fully ripened, but before they have dispersed.

Roots are usually harvested when the plant is dormant. It is generally better to harvest most roots in autumn rather than spring. In spring, wet weather results in higher moisture content in the roots, which makes them more difficult to dry. Autumn-harvested roots should be dug after the plant's seeds have matured. Federal law prohibits Ginseng from being harvested until after the fruits have ripened. Unfortunately, the practice of harvesting Ginseng roots before the seeds have had a chance to develop is still common. Such practices should be discouraged. Goldenseal is often harvested in the spring, as the plant emerges from the ground and begins flowering, but it *should* be harvested only after it sets seed in late summer. Roots, generally speaking, should not be harvested when the leaves and stem are still growing, in order to avoid affecting both the quality of the plant material and the plant's ability to set seeds.

(5) If you are harvesting bark, always take it from the lateral branches — do not strip it from the main trunk. Harvest only from one side of the branch. Avoid girdling the branches. Bark serves as a protective covering for the plant. The rough outer bark consists mainly of corky cellular tissue that later develops wood cells, especially on the inner surface. The inner bark — the part usually gathered for medicinal purposes — consists mainly of long wood cells, often forming fibers of great strength and toughness. Bark is most easily removed when the sap rises, in spring to early summer. Of course, the bark is the life line from the roots to the top of the tree. Complete girdling (stripping a complete circle of bark around the trunk or branches) will usually kill a tree.

A Word of Caution

We cautiously advise our readers that this field guide is just that, a key to the recognition of medicinal plants. Perhaps we have been overly careful in our warnings, but in fact, there is probably somebody somewhere who is allergic to any given species of plant. All food plants, like medicinal plants, contain greater or lesser amounts of minerals, vitamins, carcinogens, anticarcinogens, oxidants and anti-oxidants, enzyme-agonists and enzyme antagonists, toxins and antitoxins, and other biologically active compounds.

In our excess caution, we have mentioned that dozens of these plants can cause contact dermatitis, although we have handled most of the species treated in this book and have experienced dermatitis only from Stinging Nettles, Poison Ivy, and Rue. Further, we suspect that the pollen of most species, if gathered and forcibly inserted in the nostrils, would induce sneezing and perhaps even allergic rhinitis in some people. And, of course, all plants included in this book contain substances that are poisonous in excess. Dosage and proper preparation are very important. Everyone should be cautious about ingesting any new material, food or medicine. The reaction of one individual may differ from that of another.

Unfortunately, some very innocuous medicinal plants, like Wild Carrot (Queen Anne's Lace), can closely resemble some very poisonous plants, like Poison Hemlock. And some of the Angelicas and Skirret might be confused with poisonous Water-hemlock. We would not trust all botanists, much less all amateurs, to identify them accurately. Even professional botanists have died after misidentifying mushrooms or plants in the unrelated parsley family. In spring it is easy to grab a wild iris among the new cattail shoots. Results might not be fatal, but unpleasant. One elderly couple confused Foxglove for Comfrey, and died shortly thereafter. Father or Mother Nature is not benign: He or She has produced some of our deadlier poisons. If you are imprudent, you may ingest some of Nature's lethal compounds.

In spite of these perils, we lose fewer people to herbal accidents (fewer than 10 per year) than we do to iatrogenic (hospital- or doctor-induced accidents), or intentional ingestion of narcotics derived from plants (6,000 deaths a year in America), alcohol (100,000 deaths a year), or smoking the Indian gift, tobacco (300,000 deaths a year).

Basil, Comfrey, and Sassafras are some herbs that have come under fire lately for containing potential carcinogens. An article published in *Science* (Ames, et. al., "Ranking Possible Carcinogenic Hazards," 17 April 1987, vol. 236, pp. 271–280) puts these carcinogens in proper perspective. A cup of Comfrey leaf tea was stated to be about $\frac{1}{100}$ as carcinogenic for its symphytine as a can of beer was for its ethanol. A gram of basil was $\frac{1}{28}$ as carcinogenic for its estragole as the beer was for its ethanol. A sassafras root beer, now banned by our FDA, was $\frac{1}{14}$ as carcinogenic for its safrole as the can of beer for its ethanol.

We cannot agree with herbalists who say that herbal medicine has no side effects. Probably all natural and synthetic compounds, good and bad, are biologically active in many ways in addition to the one we wish to harness in medication. Moreover, any medicine — herbal, natural, or synthetic — can be toxic in overdoses. We again remind our readers that this field guide is a key to the recognition of medicinal plants, not a prescriptor. Only your doctor or other health-care professional who is licensed to do so can prescribe an herb for you. *We cannot and do not prescribe herbal medication.*

MISCELLANEOUS SHOWY FLOWERS

PRICKLY POPPY   **Stem juice, seeds, leaves**
Argemone albiflora Hornem.   **C. Pl. 39**   Poppy Family
Bluish green herb; 2–3 ft. *Yellow* (or white) *juice. Thistle-like* leaves
and stems with *sharp bristles.* Flowers with 4–6 petals at least 2 in.
wide; May–Sept. **Where found:** Waste places; scattered. Introduced.
Conn. to Fla.; Texas to Mo., Ill.
Uses: Seed tea is emetic, purgative, demulcent. Plant infusion used
for jaundice, skin ailments, colds, colic, wounds. Externally, used for
headaches. Folk remedy for cancers, itching and scabies. **Warning:**
Contains **toxic** alkaloids. Seed oil causes glaucoma and edema.

TURTLEHEAD, BALMONY   **Leaves**
Chelone glabra L.   **C. Pl. 2**   Figwort Family
Smooth perennial; 2–3 ft. Stem somewhat 4-angled. Leaves lance-
shaped to oval, toothed. Flowers white to pink, swollen; in tight clusters atop plant; July–Oct. *Flowers 2-lipped; upper lip arching.* **Where
found:** Moist soils. Nfld. to Ga.; Mo. to Minn., Ont.
Uses: Leaf tea said to stimulate appetite, also a folk remedy for
worms, fever, jaundice; laxative. Ointment used for piles, inflamed
breasts, painful ulcers, herpes.

LILY-OF-THE-VALLEY   **Root, flowers**
Convallaria majalis L.   **C. Pl. 24**   Lily Family
Perennial, spreading by root runners; 4–8 in. Leaves 2–3; basal, oblong-ovate, entire (not toothed); *veins parallel; connecting veins obvious when held to light.* Flowers bell-shaped, white; May–June.
Where found: Europe. Widely escaped from cultivation.
Uses: Tea of flowers and roots traditionally used in valvular heart
disease (Digitalis substitute), fevers; diuretic, heart tonic, sedative,
emetic. Root ointment, folk remedy for burns, to prevent scar tissue.
Russians use for epilepsy. **Warning:** Potentially **toxic.** Leaves can be
a mild skin irritant.

DUTCHMAN'S-BREECHES   **Leaves, root**
Dicentra cucullaria (L.) Bernh.   **C. Pl. 18**   Bleeding-heart Family
Perennial; 5–9 in. Leaves much dissected. Flowers white, yellow-
tipped; appearing upside-down on an arching stalk; April–May. *Each
flower has 2 inflated, "pantlike" spurs.* **Where found:** Rich woods. Se.
Canada to Ga. mountains; Ark., Okla. to N.D.
Uses: Iroquois used leaf ointment to make athlete's legs more limber. Leaf poultice a folk medicine for skin ailments. Root tea diuretic; promotes sweating. Contains alkaloid with CNS-depressant
activity; used for paralysis and tremors. **Warning:** Potentially poisonous; may also cause skin rash.

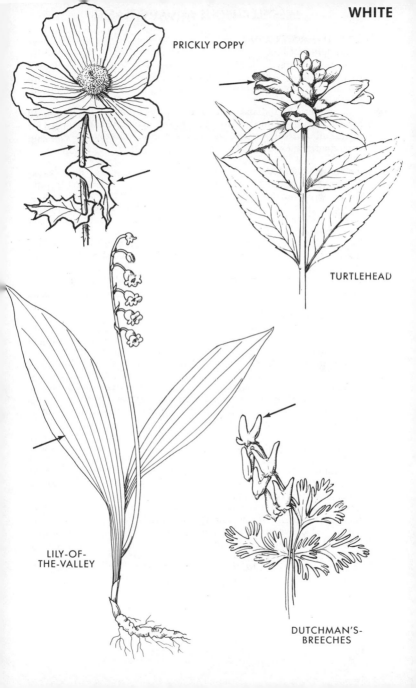

WHITE

PRICKLY POPPY

TURTLEHEAD

LILY-OF-THE-VALLEY

DUTCHMAN'S-BREECHES

MISCELLANEOUS AQUATIC PLANTS

WILD CALLA, WATER-ARUM   **Root**
Calla palustris L.   Arum Family
Note the shining oval, heart-shaped leaves, to 6 in. long. Flower a
white spathe clasping a golden, *clublike* spadix; May–Aug. **Where
found:** Circumpolar. Ponds, mud. Nfld. to N.J.; Ind., Wisc., Minn. to
Alaska.

 Uses: American Indians used dried-root tea for flu, shortness of
breath, bleeding; poultice on swellings and snakebites. **Warning:** Raw
plant contains calcium oxalate; can burn and irritate skin, and mucous membranes, if taken internally.

BUCKBEAN, BOGBEAN   **Root, leaves**
Menyanthes trifoliata L.   Gentian Family
Note the *cloverlike* leaves arising from the root. Flowers 5-parted,
white to pinkish, on a naked raceme; April–July. *Petals with fuzzy
beards.* **Where found:** Bogs, shallow water. Canada south to Md., W.
Va.; Ohio, Ind. to Ill.

Uses: Dried leaf or root tea traditionally a digestive tonic; used for
fevers, rheumatism, liver ailments, dropsy, worms, skin diseases; astringent, stops bleeding. Science confirms phenolic acids may be responsible for bile-secreting, digestive tonic, and bitter qualities.
Warning: Fresh plant causes vomiting.

FRAGRANT WATER-LILY   **Roots**
Nymphaea odorata Ait.   **C. Pl. 1**   Water-lily Family
Aquatic perennial with large, round, floating leaves; leaf notched at
base. Flowers white, to 5 in. across; sweetly fragrant; June–Sept.
Where found: Ponds, slow waters. Nfld. to Fla.; Texas to Neb.

Uses: American Indians used root tea for coughs, tuberculosis, inflamed glands, mouth sores; stops bleeding; poulticed root for swellings. In folk tradition, a mixture of root and lemon juice was used to
remove freckles and pimples. Root tea drunk for bowel complaints.
Warning: Large doses may be **toxic.**

LIZARD'S-TAIL, WATER-DRAGON   **Root, leaves**
Saururus cernuus L.   Lizard-tail Family
Perennial; 2–5 ft. Leaves large, asymmetrically *heart-shaped.* Flowers tiny, white, on a showy, *nodding "tail";* May–Sept. **Where found:**
Shallow water, swamps, R.I. to Fla.; Texas to Minn.
Uses: American Indians used root poultice for wounds, inflamed
breasts (the plant is also known as "Breastweed"), and inflammations. Tea of whole plant a wash for general illness, rheumatism;
internally for stomach ailments.
Related species: Asian counterpart, *S. chinensis,* also used to relieve
inflammation in Traditional Chinese Medicine. Recently shown to
contain a sedative compound with a novel structure.

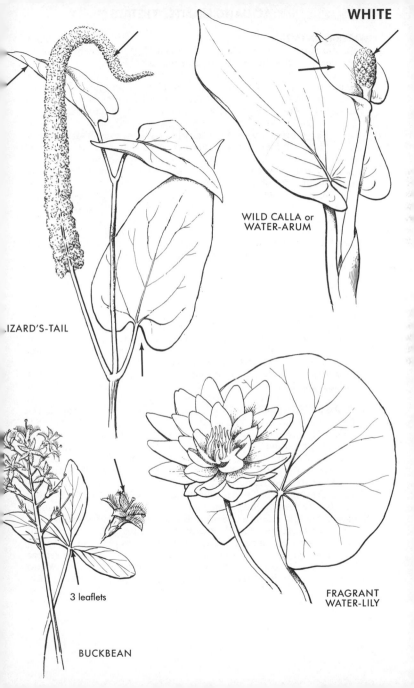

WHITE

WILD CALLA or
WATER-ARUM

LIZARD'S-TAIL

3 leaflets

BUCKBEAN

FRAGRANT
WATER-LILY

WATER-PLANTAIN
Dried leaves, root
Alisma subcordatum Raf.   (not shown)   Arrowhead Family
[*A. plantago-aquatica* var. *parviflorum* (Pursh) Farw.]
Erect or drooping (in deep water) perennial; 1–3 ft. in flower. Long-stemmed, nearly heart-shaped leaves. Flowers tiny (less than ⅛ in. long), in whorls on branched stalks; June–Sept. Petals same length as sepals. **Where found:** Shallow water or mud. N.J. to Ga.; west to Texas, Neb.
Uses: Tea diuretic; used for "gravel" (kidney stones), urinary diseases. Fresh leaves rubefacient — they redden and irritate skin. American Indians used root poultice for bruises, swellings, wounds. An 1899 article by a California physician reported on the use of the root tincture (alcohol extract), mixed with equal parts water and glycerin, as a local application to the nostrils to treat "nasal catarrh."
Related species: The root of the closely related *A. plantago-aquatica* is used in China for diuretic qualities in dysuria, edema, distention, diarrhea, and other ailments. Chinese studies verify the plant's diuretic action. In laboratory experiments with animals, the herb lowers blood pressure, reduces blood glucose levels, and inhibits the storage of fat in the liver.

COMMON WATER-PLANTAIN
Root
Alisima triviale Pursh   Arrowhead Family
[*A. plantago-aquatica* var. *americanum* Schultes & Schultes]
Similar to above species, but leaves are mostly oval, though the base is often slightly heart-shaped; flowers larger, to ¼ in.; June–Sept. Panicle often with fewer branches. **Where found:** Shallow water, ditches. N.S. to Md.; Neb. to Minn. and beyond.
Uses: American Indians used root tea for lung ailments, lame back, and kidney ailments.

BROAD-LEAVED ARROWHEAD
Roots, leaves
Sagittaria latifolia Willd.   **C. Pl. 1**   Arrowhead Family
Aquatic perennial. Leaves *arrow-shaped; lobes ½ as long to as long as* main part of leaf. Flowers white; petals 3, rounded; filaments of stamens smooth. Flowers June–Sept. The bracts beneath the flowers are blunt-tipped, thin, and papery. The beak of the mature fruit (achene) projects at a right angle from the main part of the fruit. **Where found:** Ponds, lakes. Throughout our area. Technical details separate the 15+ species in our range.
Uses: American Indians used the edible tubers in tea for indigestion; poulticed them for wounds and sores. Leaf tea was used for rheumatism and to wash babies with fever. Leaves were poulticed to stop milk production. Roots were eaten like potatoes. **Warning:** Arrowheads (not necessarily this species) *may* cause dermatitis. Do not confuse with Wild Calla or Water-arum (*Calla palustris*); see p. 14.

WHITE

COMMON WATER-
PLANTAIN

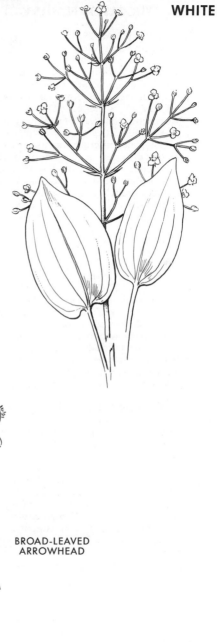

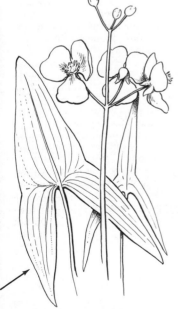

BROAD-LEAVED
ARROWHEAD

YUCCAS OR PLANTS WITH YUCCA-LIKE LEAVES

RATTLESNAKE-MASTER   **Root**
Eryngium yuccifolium Michx.   Parsley Family
Perennial with bluish cast; 1½–4 ft. Leaves mostly basal (reduced on
stem), *yucca-like* (hence the species name), *parallel-veined, spiny-
edged.* Flowers white to whitish green; tiny, covered by bristly
bracts; in tight heads to 1 in. across; Sept–Nov. **Where found:** Prairies, dry soil. S. Conn. to Fla.; Texas to Kans., Minn.
Uses: American Indians used root as poultice for snakebites, toothaches, bladder trouble; for coughs, neuralgia; also an emetic. Traditionally, root tincture was used as a diuretic; also for female reproductive disorders, gleet, gonorrhea, piles, and rheumatism. Chewing
the root increases saliva flow. **Warning:** Do not confuse with False
Aloe or Rattlesnake-master (*Manfreda virginica*, p. 104), which may
produce strongly irritating latex.
Related species: *Eryngium aquaticum* (not shown) has linear leaves
and is found in marshes and bogs.

YUCCA, ADAM'S NEEDLE   **Roots**
Yucca filamentosa L.   Lily Family
Perennial; to 9 ft. in flower. Leaves in a rosette; stiff, spine-tipped,
oblong to lance-shaped, with *fraying, twisted threads on margins.*
Flowers whitish green bells on *smooth* branched stalks; June–Sept.
Where found: Sandy soils. S. N.J. to Ga. Cultivated elsewhere.
Uses: American Indians used root in salves or poultices for sores,
skin diseases, and sprains. Pounded roots were put in water to
stupefy corralled fish so they would float to the surface for easy harvest. Plant yields a strong fiber. Fruits used as food by some people.
Saponins in roots of yucca species possess long-lasting soaping action
and have been used in soaps and shampoos. **Warning:** Root compound (saponins) are **toxic** to lower life forms.

YUCCA, SOAPWEED   **Roots**
Yucca glauca Nutt.   **C. Pl. 39**   Lily Family
Blue-green perennial; 2–4 ft. Leaves in a rosette; stiff, swordlike;
rounded on back, *margins rolled in.* Flowers whitish bells; May–
July. **Where found:** Dry soils. Iowa to Texas; Mo. to N.D.
Uses: American Indians poulticed root on inflammations, used it to
stop bleeding; also in steam bath for sprains and broken limbs; hair
wash for dandruff and baldness. Leaf juice used to make poison arrows. Water extracts have shown antitumor activity against B16 melanoma in mice. One human clinical study suggests that saponin extracts of yucca root were effective in the treatment of arthritis, but
the findings have been disputed. **Warning:** Same as for *Yucca filamentosa.*

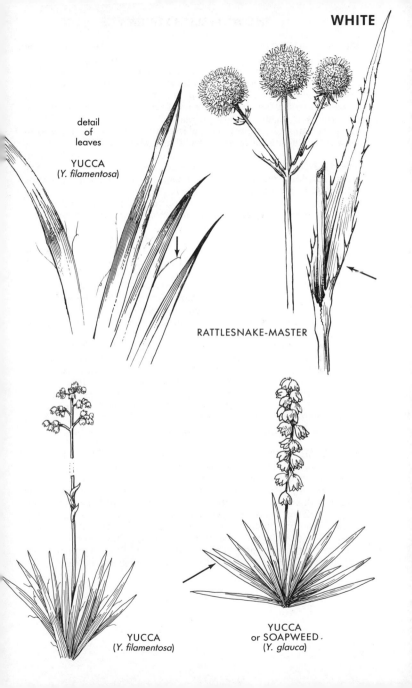

WHITE

detail
of
leaves

YUCCA
(*Y. filamentosa*)

RATTLESNAKE-MASTER

YUCCA
(*Y. filamentosa*)

YUCCA
or SOAPWEED
(*Y. glauca*)

SHOWY BELLS OR TRUMPETS

FIELD BINDWEED
Convolvulus arvensis L.
Leaf, root, flowers
Morning-glory Family
Creeping vine. Leaves arrow-shaped; *lobes sharp, not blunt*; 1–2 in. long. Flowers white (or pink), to 1 in; June–Sept. **Where found:** Fields, waste places. Most of our area. Alien (Europe).
Uses: American Indians used cold leaf tea as a wash on spider bites; internally to reduce profuse menstrual flow. In European folk use, flower, leaf, and root teas considered laxative. Flower tea used for fevers, wounds. Root most active — strongly purgative.

HEDGE BINDWEED
Convolvulus sepium L.
Root
Morning-glory Family
[*Calystegia sepium* (L.) R. Br.]
Trailing vine with white or pink, morning-glory type flowers; May–Sept. Leaves arrow-shaped, with *blunt lobes at base*. **Where found:** Thickets, roadsides. Most of our area.
Uses: Root historically used as a purgative; substitute for the Mexican jalap (*Ipomoea purga*). Traditionally used for jaundice, gall bladder ailments; thought to increase bile flow into intestines.

JIMSONWEED
Datura stramonium L.   **C Pl. 33**
Leaves, root, seed
Nightshade Family
Annual; 2–5 ft. Leaves coarse-toothed. Flowers white to pale violet; 3–5 in., trumpet-shaped; May–Sept. Seedpods spiny, chambered. **Where found:** Waste places. Throughout our area.
Uses: Whole plant contains atropine and other alkaloids, used in eye diseases (atropine dilates pupils); causes dry mouth, depresses bladder muscles, impedes action of parasympathetic nerves; used in Parkinson's disease; also contains scopolamine, used in patches behind ear for vertigo. Leaves were once smoked as an antispasmodic for asthma. Folk cancer remedy. **Warning: Violently toxic.** Causes severe hallucinations. Many fatalities recorded. Those who collect this plant may end up with swollen eyelids.

WILD POTATO-VINE
Ipomoea pandurata (L.) G.F.W. Mey.
Root, whole plant
Morning-glory Family
Twining or climbing, often purple-stemmed vine with a very large tuberous root. Leaves *heart-shaped.* Flowers large (2–3 in.) white, with pink stripes from center; June–Sept. **Where found:** Dry soils. Conn. to Fla.; Texas, Mo., Kans. to Mich.
Uses: American Indians poulticed root for rheumatism, "hard tumors." Root tea used as a diuretic, laxative, and expectorant, for coughs, asthma, beginning stages of tuberculosis; "blood purifier"; powdered plant used in tea for headaches, indigestion.

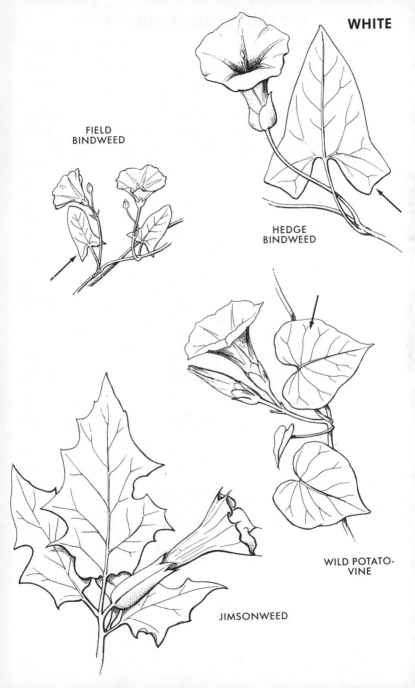

WHITE

FIELD
BINDWEED

HEDGE
BINDWEED

WILD POTATO-
VINE

JIMSONWEED

MISCELLANEOUS NON-WOODY VINES

VIRGIN'S BOWER   Whole flowering plant
Clematis virginiana L.   Buttercup Family
Clambering vine. Leaves divided into 3 *sharp-toothed leaflets*. Flowers white, with *4 petal-like sepals;* in clusters; July–Sept. Feathery plumes attached to seeds. **Where found:** Rich thickets, wood edges. N.S. to Ga.; La., e. Kan. north to Canada.

Uses: Liniment once used by physicians for skin eruptions, itching; weak leaf tea used for insomnia, nervous headaches, nervous twitching, and uterine diseases. **Warning: Toxic;** highly irritating to skin and mucous membranes. Ingestion may cause bloody vomiting, severe diarrhea, and convulsions.

WILD CUCUMBER, BALSAM-APPLE   Root
Echinocystis lobata (Michx.) T. & G.   Cucumber Family
Climbing vine with tendrils. Leaves *maple-shaped; 5-lobed*, toothed along edges. Flowers *6-petaled*, in clusters of leaf axils; June–Oct. Fruits *solitary*, egg-shaped; fleshy, covered with weak *bristles*. **Where found:** Thickets. N.B. to Fla.; Texas to Minn.

Uses: American Indians used the extremely bitter root tea as a bitter tonic for stomach troubles, kidney ailments, rheumatism, chills, fevers, and obstructed menses. Also used in love potions and as a general tonic. Pulverized root poulticed for headaches. **Warning:** Do not confuse this plant with *Momordica balsamina* L., a tropical member of the cucumber family also known as Balsam-apple. Its root is purgative and considered **toxic.** The two plants have been confused in the literature because authors did not carefully compare Latin names of "balsam-apples." Both, as members of the cucumber family, may contain cucurbitacins, which are extremely active as antitumor and cytotoxic agents at levels of less than one part per million.

PASSION-FLOWER, MAYPOP   Whole flowering plant
Passiflora incarnata L.   **C. Pl. 32**   Passion-flower Family
Climbing vine, to 30 ft.; tendrils *springlike*. Leaves *cleft*, with *2–3* slightly toothed lobes. Flowers large, showy, unique; whitish to purplish, with *numerous threads* radiating from center; July–Oct. Fruits fleshy, egg-shaped. **Where found:** Sandy soil. Pa. to Fla.; e. Texas to s. Mo.

Uses: American Indians poulticed root for boils, cuts, earaches, and inflammation. Traditionally used as an antispasmodic, and as a sedative for neuralgia, epilepsy, restlessness, painful menses, insomnia, and tension headaches. Research shows extracts are mildly sedative, slightly reduce blood pressure, increase respiratory rate, and decrease motor activity. Fruits edible, delicious. **Warning:** Potentially harmful in large amounts.

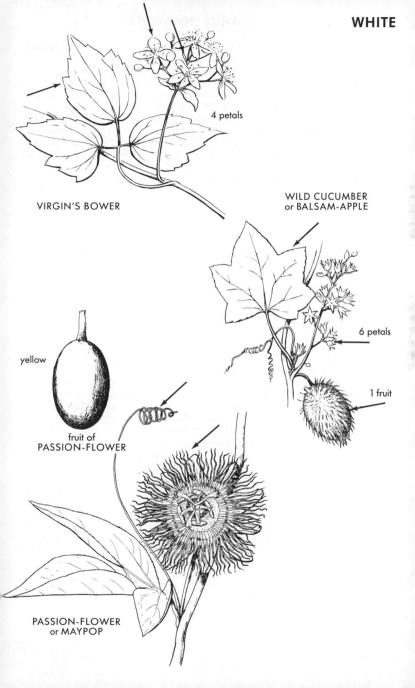

WHITE

4 petals

VIRGIN'S BOWER

WILD CUCUMBER
or BALSAM-APPLE

6 petals

1 fruit

yellow

fruit of
PASSION-FLOWER

PASSION-FLOWER
or MAYPOP

WHITE ORCHIDS

DOWNY RATTLESNAKE-PLANTAIN   Root, leaves
Goodyera pubescens (Willd.) R. Br.   **C. Pl. 18**   Orchid Family
Perennial; to 16 in. (in flower). Leaves essentially basal; oval, with
white veins in a checkered pattern, and white spreading hairs. Whitish flowers on a *dense, woolly raceme*. July–Sept. **Where found:**
Woods. Me. to Fla.; Ala., Ark., Mo. to w. Que. Rare — do not harvest.
Uses: American Indians used root tea for pleurisy, snakebites; leaf
tea taken (with whiskey) to improve appetite, treat colds, kidney ailments, "blood tonic," toothaches. Externally, leaf poultice used to
"cool" burns, treat skin ulcers. Physicians once used fresh leaves
steeped in milk as poultice for tuberculous swelling of lymph nodes
(scrofula). Fresh leaves were applied every 3 hours, while the patient
drank a tea of the leaves at the same time.
Remarks: Of historical interest only. Too scarce to harvest.

NODDING LADIES' TRESSES   Whole plant
Spiranthes cernua (L.) Richard   Orchid Family
Delicate, fleshy-rooted orchid; 4–20 in. Basal leaves firm, thick, pale
green; leaves much reduced on flowering stalk. Tiny, white, *down-
ward-arching* flowers in a double spiral; Aug.–Nov. **Where found:**
Bogs, meadows. Most of our area.
Uses: American Indians used plant tea as a diuretic for urinary dis-
orders, venereal disease; and as a wash to strengthen infants.
Related species: Other N. American, European, and S. American species have also been used as a diuretic and aphrodisiac.

PINK LADY'S-SLIPPER,
MOCCASIN-FLOWER, AMERICAN VALERIAN   Root
Cypripedium acaule Ait.   Orchid Family
Usually pink; *rarely white* in some individual plants or populations.
Perennial; 6–15 in. Leaves 2, *basal.* Flower a strongly veined pouch
with a *deep furrow*; May–June. **Where found:** Acid woods. Nfld. to
Ga.; Ala., Tenn. to Minn. Too rare to harvest.
Uses: This plant, called "American Valerian," was widely used in
19th-century America as a sedative for nervous headaches, hysteria,
insomnia, nervous irritability, mental depression from sexual abuse,
and menstrual irregularities accompanied by despondency (PMS?).
Active compounds are not water-soluble. The Pink Lady's-slipper
was considered a substitute for the more commonly used Yellow
Lady's-slipper (p. 94). Orchids often have swollen, ball-shaped tubers,
suggesting testicles; these roots are widely regarded as aphrodisiacs,
perhaps reflecting the doctrine of signatures (see p. 6). **Warning:** May
cause dermatitis.

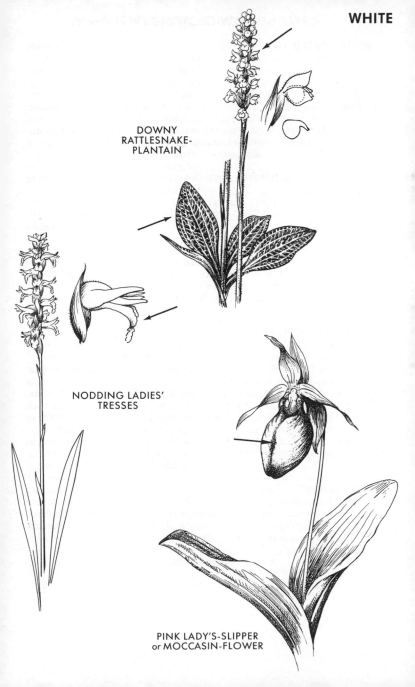

WHITE

DOWNY
RATTLESNAKE-
PLANTAIN

NODDING LADIES'
TRESSES

PINK LADY'S-SLIPPER
or MOCCASIN-FLOWER

CREEPING, LOW-GROWING EVERGREENS

BEARBERRY, UVA-URSI   **Leaves**
Arctostaphylos uva-ursi (L.) Spreng.   **C. Pl. 10**   Heath Family
Trailing shrub; bark fine-hairy. Leaves *shiny-leathery, spatula-shaped*. Flowers white, urn-shaped; May–July. Fruit a dry red berry.
Where found: Sandy soil, rocks. Arctic to n. U.S.

 Uses: Dried leaf tea diuretic, strongly astringent; urinary-tract antiseptic for cystitis (when urine is alkaline), nephritis, urethritis, kidney and gall stones. Also used in bronchitis, gonorrhea, diarrhea, and to stop bleeding. **Warning:** Contains arbutin, which hydrolyzes to the **toxic** urinary antiseptic hydroquinone.

TRAILING ARBUTUS, MAYFLOWER   **Leaves**
Epigaea repens L.   Heath Family
Trailing perennial; to 6 in. Leaves *oval, leathery*. Flowers in clusters, white (or pink), tubular, 5-lobed. March–May. **Where found:** Sandy open woods. Nfld. to Fla.; Miss., Tenn., Ohio to Mich. Protected in some states.

Uses: American Indians used leaf tea for kidney disorders, stomachaches; "blood purifier." Leaf tea a folk remedy for bladder, urethra, and kidney disorders, "gravel" (kidney stones). Shakers sold this plant as "gravel-plant." **Warning:** Contains arbutin; although it is effective as a urinary antiseptic, it hydrolyzes to hydroquinone, which is **toxic.**

WINTERGREEN, TEABERRY   **Leaves**
Gaultheria procumbens L.   **C. Pl. 19**   Heath Family
Wintergreen-scented; to 6 in. Leaves oval, glossy. Flowers waxy, *drooping bells*; July–Aug. Fruit a dry red berry. **Where found:** Woods, openings. Canada to Ga.; Ala. to Wisc., Minn.

Uses: Traditionally, leaf tea used for colds, headaches, stomachaches, fevers, kidney ailments; externally, wash for rheumatism, sore muscles, lumbago. Essential oil (methyl salicylate) in leaves is synthetically produced for "wintergreen" flavor. Experimentally analgesic, carminative, anti-inflammatory, antiseptic. In experiments, small amounts have delayed the onset of tumors. **Warning:** Essential oil is **highly toxic;** absorbed through skin, harms liver and kidneys.

PARTRIDGEBERRY, SQUAW VINE   **Leaves**
Mitchella repens L.   **C. Pl. 11**   Madder Family
Leaves opposite; rounded. Flowers white (or pink); 4-parted, terminal, *paired*; May–July. Fruit a single dry red berry lasting over the winter. **Where found:** Woods. Nfld. to Fla.; Texas to Minn.
Uses: Historically, dried or fresh leaf or berry tea was used for delayed, irregular, or painful menses and childbirth pain; astringent, used for piles, dysentery; diuretic. Externally, used as a wash for swellings, hives, arthritis, rheumatism, and sore nipples, for which it was highly esteemed.

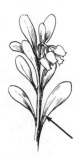

BEARBERRY
or UVA-URSI

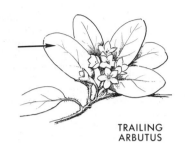

TRAILING
ARBUTUS

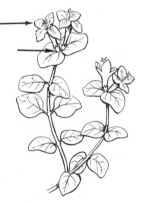

PARTRIDGEBERRY
or SQUAW-VINE

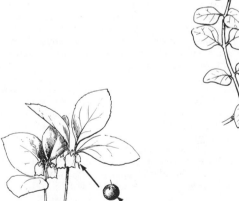

red

WINTERGREEN

CURIOUS FLESHY PLANTS
WITH SPECIALIZED GROWTH HABITS

ROUND-LEAVED SUNDEW
Whole plant

Drosera rotundifolia L.   **C. Pl. 4**   Sundew Family

Small perennial; 4–9 in. Leaves tiny, to ½ in. across; rounded, blade mostly wider than long; *covered with reddish, glandular-tipped hairs exuding sticky "dewdrops."* Flowers white or pinkish, on a 1-sided raceme, opening 1 at a time; June–Aug. **Where found:** Wet acid soil, bogs. Nfld. to Fla.; Ill., Minn.

Uses: Traditionally, tea or tincture used for dry, spasmodic coughs; asthma; arteriosclerosis; chronic bronchitis; also as an aphrodisiac; poultice or plant juice used on corns and warts. Europeans regard the extracts and tinctures as antitussive and spasmolytic. Because of their protein-digesting enzymes, exudates from the leaves have been used to treat warts. Contains proteolytic enzymes and plumbagin, which is antibiotic against certain bacteria.

INDIAN-PIPE
Whole plant, root

Monotropa uniflora L.   **C. Pl. 18**   Indian-pipe Family

Once called "Ice Plant" because it resembles frozen jelly, and "melts" when handled. Also called "Bird's Nest," in reference to the shape of the entangled root fibers. Saprophytic perennial, without chlorophyll; 6–8 in. *Whole plant translucent white.* Scalelike leaves, nearly absent. Flower a *single nodding bell;* June–Oct. **Where found:** Woods. Much of our area. Too scarce for harvest.

 Uses: American Indians used plant juice for inflamed eyes, bunions, warts; drank tea for aches and pains due to colds. Root tea used for convulsions, fits, epilepsy; sedative. Physicians once used tea as antispasmodic, nervine, sedative for restlessness, pains, nervous irritability. As a folk remedy for sore eyes, the plant was soaked in rose water, then a cloth was soaked in the mixture and applied to the eyes. Water extracts are bactericidal. **Warning:** Safety undetermined; possibly **toxic** — contains several glycosides.

GIANT BIRD'S NEST
Stems, fruits

Pterospora andromeda Nutt.   Wintergreen Family

Parasitic perennial; 1–4 ft. Covered with clammy hairs. Stalk purple-brown, leafless; *base scaled.* Flowers small, drooping urns; June–Sept. **Where found:** Pine woods. Local. P.E.I. to Vt., N.Y.; west to Wisc., B.C. Rocky Mts.; south to Mexico.

Uses: American Indians used a cold tea made from the pounded stems and fruits to treat bleeding from the lungs; dry powder used as a snuff for nosebleeds; astringent and hemostatic.

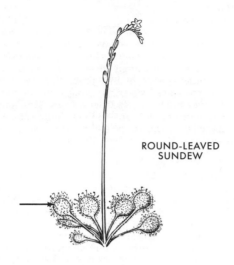

ROUND-LEAVED
SUNDEW

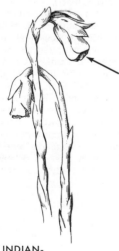

INDIAN-
PIPE

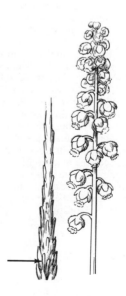

GIANT BIRD'S-
NEST

3–6 PETALS; LEAVES ONION-SCENTED

WILD LEEK, RAMP   **Leaves, root**
Allium tricoccum Ait.   Lily Family
Perennial; 6–18 in. Leaves 2–3, smooth, to 2½ *in. wide;* fleshy,
strongly onion- or leek-scented; leaves wither before whitish to
creamy yellow flowers bloom. Flowers June–July. **Where found:** Rich
moist woods. Localized, but often in abundant populations. N.B.
south to Ga. mountains; west through Tenn., Ill., Iowa.
Uses: Cherokees ate leaves for colds, croup, and as spring tonic.
Warm juice of leaves and bulbs used for earaches. Strong root decoction emetic. Similar to but less potent than Garlic. The wide range
of effects attributed to Garlic (see below) probably accrue to Ramp or
Wild Leek as well.

GARLIC   **Bulb**
Allium sativum L.   Lily Family
To 3 ft. Leaves extend *almost to middle of stem.* Note the 2- to 4-in.
long, *narrow, papery green spathe* around flowers. **Where found:**
Fields, roadsides. Alien. Planted and occasionally escaped from cultivation. N.Y. to Tenn., Ky., Mo.; north to Ind.
Uses: Peeled cloves have been eaten or made into tea, syrup, or tincture to treat colds, fevers, coughs, earaches, bronchitis, shortness of
breath, sinus congestion, headaches, stomachaches, high blood pressure, arteriosclerosis, diarrhea, dysentery, gout, rheumatism, etc. For
external uses, end of Garlic clove is cut, then juice is applied to ringworm, acne (see warning below); folk cancer remedy. Cough syrup
traditionally made by simmering 10 Garlic cloves in 1 pint of milk,
adding honey to taste; syrup taken in 1-tablespoon doses as needed.
In China, Garlic is used for digestive difficulties, diarrhea, dysentery,
colds, whooping cough, pinworms, old ulcers, swellings, and snakebites. Experimentally, it lowers blood pressure and serum cholesterol; antibacterial, antifungal, diuretic. Clinical studies suggest efficacy in gastrointestinal disorders, hypertension, heart ailments,
and arteriosclerosis. According to demographic studies, Garlic is
thought responsible for the low incidence of arteriosclerosis in parts
of Italy and Spain where Garlic consumption is heavy. Allicin, the
substance responsible for Garlic's characteristic odor, is thought to
be responsible for some of the plant's pharmacological qualities. In
experiments with mice, Garlic extracts had an inhibitory effect on
cancer cells. The presence of the trace elements germanium and se-
lenium may have normalized the utilization of oxygen and improved
the immunity of the organism against the cancerous cells. **Warning:**
The essential oil extracted from the bulbs is extremely concentrated
and can be irritating.

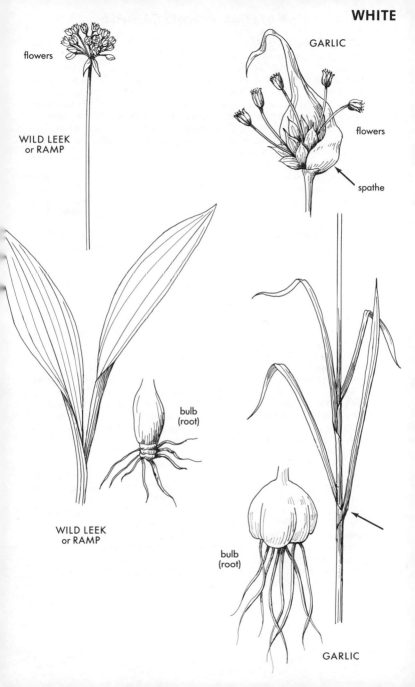

WHITE

flowers

WILD LEEK
or RAMP

GARLIC

flowers

spathe

bulb
(root)

WILD LEEK
or RAMP

bulb
(root)

GARLIC

FALSE SOLOMON'S-SEAL   Root, leaves
Smilacina racemosa (L.) Desf.   Lily Family
Perennial; 1–2 ft. Zigzag stem arched. Leaves oval. Flowers in terminal clusters; May–July. *Stamens longer than petals.* **Where found:**
Rich woods. N.S. to Ga.; Ala., Ark. to Mich. and westward.
Uses: American Indians used root tea for constipation, rheumatism,
stomach tonic, "female tonic"; root smoke inhaled for insanity, and
to quiet a crying child. Leaf tea used as a contraceptive and for
coughs; externally, for bleeding, rashes, and itch. Herbalists used to
induce sweating and urination; "blood purifier."

SOLOMON'S-SEAL   Root
Polygonatum biflorum (Walt.) Ell.   **C. Pl. 14**   Lily Family
Perennial; 1–3 ft. Leaves oval to elliptical; alternate. Flowers tubular,
drooping in pairs from leaf axils; May–June. **Where found:** Rich
woods. Conn. to Fla.; Texas, Neb. to Mich.
Uses: American Indians used root tea for indigestion, profuse menstruation, lung ailments, "general debility"; also to promote sound
sleep, treat coughs; laxative; fresh root poulticed (or root tea used
externally as a wash) for sharp pains, cuts, bruises, sores, and carbuncles. Root tea a folk remedy for piles, rheumatism, arthritis, and skin
irritations.

FALSE LILY-OF-THE-VALLEY,
CANADA MAYFLOWER   Root, whole flowering plant
Maianthemum canadense Desf.   Lily Family
Perennial, often forming large colonies; 3–6 in. Leaves usually 2;
base *strongly cleft (heart-shaped)*. Tiny, *4-pointed* flowers; April–
July. Berries whitish, turning pinkish; speckled. **Where found:**
Woods. Lab. to Ga. mountains; Tenn. to Iowa, Man.
Uses: American Indians used plant tea for headaches, and to "keep
kidneys open during pregnancy." Also a gargle for sore throats. Root
used as a good-luck charm for winning games. Folk expectorant for
coughs, soothing to sore throats.

COLIC-ROOT, STARGRASS   Root
Aletris farinosa L.   Lily Family
Perennial; 1½–3 ft. Leaves in a basal rosette; lance-shaped. Flowers
white, tubular, tightly hugging a tall leafless stalk; May–Aug. Flowers *swollen at base; surface mealy.* **Where found:** Dry or moist peat,
sand. S. Me. to Fla.; west to Texas; north to Wisc., Mich.
Uses: Root decoction used as bitter tonic for indigestion; promotes
appetite; also used for diarrhea, rheumatism, and jaundice. Used for
colic, but small doses may *cause* hypogastric colic. Tincture once
used for rheumatism. Contains diosgenin, which has both anti-inflammatory and estrogenic properties.

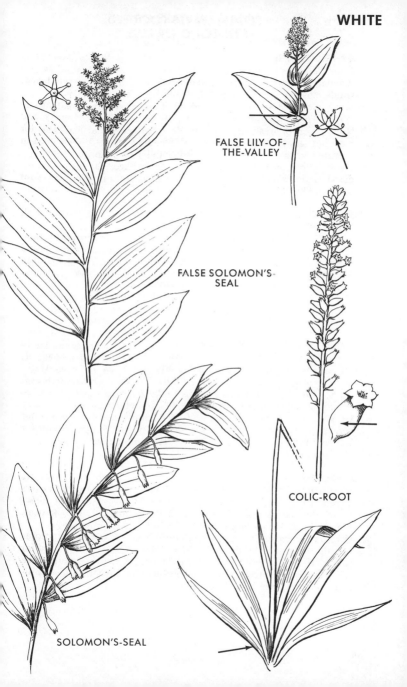

WHITE

FALSE LILY-OF-
THE-VALLEY

FALSE SOLOMON'S-
SEAL

COLIC-ROOT

SOLOMON'S-SEAL

4 PETALS; LEAVES TOOTHED,
6 IN. LONG OR LESS

SHEPHERD'S PURSE   **Whole plant in fruit**
Capsella bursa-pastoris (L.) Medic.   Mustard Family
Annual; 4–23 in. Basal leaves in rosette, *dandelion-like;* stem leaves
small, clasping. Flowers tiny. Seedpods *heart-shaped.* (Pods of *C. rubella,* a related species, have concave sides.) **Where found:** Waste
places. Throughout our area. Alien (Europe).

Uses: Dried or fresh herb tea (made from seeds and leaves) stops
bleeding, allays profuse menstrual bleeding, diuretic. Has proven
uterine-contracting properties; traditionally used during childbirth.
Dried herb a useful styptic against hemorrhage. Tea also used for
diarrhea, dysentery; also externally, as a wash for bruises. **Warning:**
Seeds are known to cause blistering of skin.

TOOTHWORT, TOOTHACHE ROOT,
PEPPER ROOT   **Root**
Dentaria diphylla Michx.   Mustard Family
Perennial; 6–14 in., with creeping rootstock. Stem leaves in opposite
pairs; leaves divided into *3 toothed leaflets,* the middle one largest.
Flowers 4-petaled, in terminal clusters; April–June. **Where found:**
Moist woods. Ont. to S.C. mountains; Ky., Minn.
Uses: Root peppery; used as a folk remedy for toothaches. American
Indians chewed root for colds; poulticed root for headaches. Root tea
gargled for sore throats, hoarseness, and to clear throat.

POOR-MAN'S-PEPPER, PEPPERGRASS   **Seedpods, leaves**
Lepidium virginicum L.   Mustard Family
Smooth or minutely hairy annual or biennial; 6–24 in. Leaves lance-
shaped, sharp-toothed; *stalked at base.* Flowers white, inconspicuous; May–Nov. Petals *as long as or longer* than sepals. Seedpods
roundish. **Where found:** Waste places. Throughout our area.

Uses: American Indians used bruised fresh plant or leaf tea for poison-ivy rash, scurvy; used as a substitute for Shepherd's Purse.
Leaves poulticed on chest for croup. **Warning:** Application may cause
skin irritation, blisters.

WATERCRESS   **Leaves**
Nasturtium officinale R. Br.   **C. Pl. 1**   Mustard Family
Creeping perennial, 4–36 in.; forms large colonies. Mustard-flavored
leaves divided into 3–9 leaflets, or strongly divided. Tiny flowers;
March–June. **Where found:** Widespread in cool running water.
Uses: Fresh leaves are high in vitamins A and C and iodine. Traditionally used as a diuretic, "blood purifier"; also used for lethargy,
rheumatism, heart trouble, bronchitis, scurvy, and goiter. Leaf extracts are used clinically in India to correct vitamin deficiency. **Warning:** Do not harvest leaves from polluted waters.

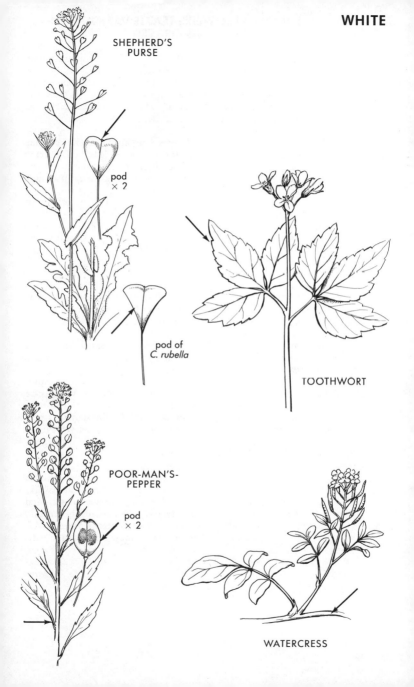

WHITE

SHEPHERD'S PURSE

pod
× 2

pod of
C. rubella

TOOTHWORT

POOR-MAN'S-PEPPER

pod
× 2

WATERCRESS

4-PETALED FLOWERS; LEAVES VARIOUS

HORSERADISH   **Root**
Armoracia rusticana   **C. Pl. 25**   Mustard Family
P. Gaertn., Mey & Scherb. [*A. lapthifolia* Gilib.]
Large-rooted herb; 1–4 ft. Leaves large, broad, lance-shaped (sometimes jagged); *long-stalked.* Leaves much reduced on flowering
stalks. Flowers white, tiny, 4-petaled; May–July. Pods, tiny, egg-
shaped. **Where found:** Most fields. Throughout. Alien (Europe); persists after cultivation.

Uses: Root used as a condiment. Root tea weakly diuretic, antiseptic, and expectorant; used for bronchitis, coughs, bronchial catarrh,
calculus (dental plaque). Root poultice used for rheumatism, respiratory congestion. Few things are better at opening the sinuses than
too large a bite of pungent horseradish sauce. Science confirms plant
is antibiotic against gram-negative and gram-positive bacteria, path-
ogenic fungi. Experimentally, it has antitumor activity, as science
has come to expect from the mustard family. **Warning:** Large
amounts may irritate digestive system. Plant tops are a **fatal poison**
to livestock. External use may cause skin blisters.

BUNCHBERRY   **Leaves, roots**
Cornus canadensis L.   **C. Pl. 19**   Dogwood Family
Perennial; 3–8 in. Leaves in *whorls of 6.* Flowers in clusters;
surrounded by *4 showy, petal-like bracts*; May–July. Fruits scarlet.
Where found: Cool woods. Northern N. America south to W. Va.
mountains; also in n. Calif.
Uses: American Indians used leaf tea for aches and pains, kidney and
lung ailments, coughs, fevers, and as an eye wash. Root tea was used
for infant colic.

CLEAVERS   **Whole plant**
Galium aparine L.   **C. Pl. 7**   Madder Family
Weak-stemmed, often drooping annual; 1–2 ft. Stem *raspy*, with
prominent prickles. Leaves lance-shaped; *usually 8, in whorls.* Inconspicuous whitish flowers on stalks from leaf axils; April–Sept.
Where found: Thickets. Throughout our area. Alien.
Uses: Herbal tea traditionally used as a diuretic, "blood purifier";
used for bladder and kidney inflammation, dropsy, "gravel" (kidney
stones), fevers. Juice of fresh herb used for scurvy. Herb tea used internally and externally as a folk cancer remedy. Juice contains citric
acid, reported to have antitumor activity. Experimentally, extracts
are hypotensive (lower blood pressure). Also contains asperuloside,
which is anti-inflammatory. **Warning:** Juice may cause contact dermatitis.

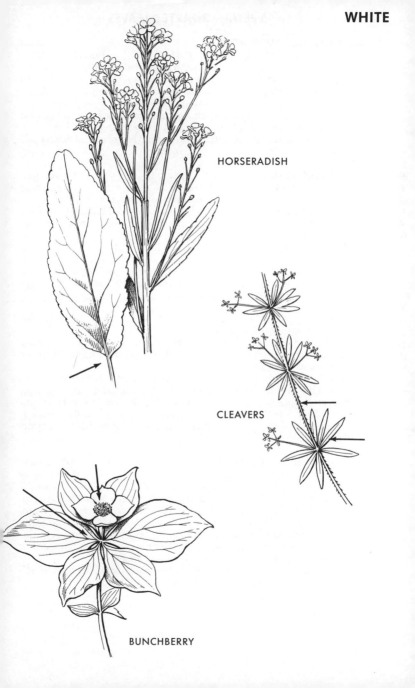

HORSERADISH

CLEAVERS

BUNCHBERRY

5 PETALS; 3-PARTED LEAVES

GOLDTHREAD, CANKER ROOT   Root
Coptis groenlandica L.   **C. Pl. 20**   Buttercup Family
Mat-forming perennial; to 3 in., with *bright yellow, threadlike* roots.
Leaves shiny, evergreen, like strawberry leaves. Flowers with 5 white
showy sepals; May–July. **Where found:** Cool forests. Canada to N.C.
mountains; Tenn. north to n. Ohio, Ind., Iowa.
Uses: Root highly astringent, chewed for canker sores; tea used for
jaundice, induces vomiting. Contains berberine, which has many
properties, including anti-inflammatory and antibacterial effects (see
p. 240).

WOOD STRAWBERRY   Leaves, root
Fragaria vesca L.   **C. Pl. 24**   Rose Family
Perennial, with runners; 3–6 in. Leaves *pointed*, not rounded, at tip.
Flowers white; calyx lobes spreading or recurved. Flowers May–Aug.
Fruits with *seeds on surface*. **Where found:** Woods. Canada to Va.;
Mo. to N.D. Alien (Europe).
Uses: American Indians used root tea for stomach ailments, jaun-
dice, profuse menses. In European folk medicine, leaf tea used as a
"blood purifier" and as a diuretic for "gravel" (kidney stones). Tea
also used as an external wash on sunburn. Root tea diuretic. Root
used as "chewing stick" (toothbrush).

COMMON or VIRGINIA STRAWBERRY   Leaves, root
Fragaria virginiana Duchesne   Rose Family
Generally larger than Wood Strawberry (above); leaves *more
rounded, seeds embedded* in fruits. **Where found:** Fields, openings.
Most of our area. Native.
Uses: American Indians and early settlers used leaf tea as a nerve
tonic; also for bladder and kidney ailments, jaundice, scurvy, diarrhea, stomachaches, gout. Considered slightly astringent. Fresh leaf
tea used for sore throats. Berries eaten for scurvy, gout. Root tea traditionally used to treat gonorrhea, stomach and lung ailments, irregular menses; diuretic.

BOWMAN'S ROOT, INDIAN PHYSIC   Whole plant
Gillenia trifoliata (L.) Moench.   Rose Family
Smooth, slender perennial; 2–3 ft. Leaves alternate; *divided into 3
nearly stalkless*, sharp, unequal, toothed leaflets. Flowers terminal,
in a loose panicle; May–July. Flowers white with a reddish tinge;
petals scraggly. **Where found:** Rich woods. Ont. to Ga.; Ala. to Mich.
Uses: Traditionally, plant tea is strongly laxative and emetic; minute doses used for indigestion, colds, asthma, hepatitis. Poultice or
wash used for rheumatism, bee stings, swellings.
Related species: *G. stipulata* (not shown) has prominent leaflike stipules and is used similarly. **Warning:** Potentially **toxic.**

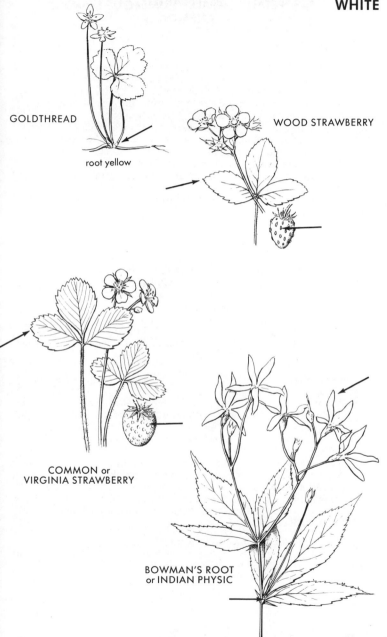

WHITE

GOLDTHREAD

root yellow

WOOD STRAWBERRY

COMMON or
VIRGINIA STRAWBERRY

BOWMAN'S ROOT
or INDIAN PHYSIC

5–7 "PETALS" (SEPALS), NUMEROUS STAMENS; ANEMONES

CANADA ANEMONE Roots, leaves
Anemone canadensis L. Buttercup Family
Perennial; 1–2 ft. Basal leaves on long stalks; stem leaves stalkless, *tightly hugging stem.* Leaves deeply divided with 5–7 lobes. Flowers white. "Petals" (actually 5 showy sepals) 1–1½ in. long. May–July.
Where found: Damp meadows. N.S. south through New England to W. Va.; west to Ill., Mo., Kans.; B.C. south to N.M.

 Uses: Astringent, styptic. American Indians used root or leaf tea (as a wash or poultice) for wounds, sores, nosebleeds. Eye wash used for twitching and to cure cross-eyes. The root was chewed to clear the throat before singing. Among certain Plains Indian groups, the root was highly esteemed as an external medicine for many ailments, and mystical qualities were attributed to the plant. **Warning:** Probably all our anemones contain the caustic irritants so prevalent in the buttercup family.

PASQUEFLOWER Whole plant
Anemone patens L. Buttercup Family
Perennial; 2–16 in. *Silky* leaves arising from root; leaves *dissected into linear segments.* Showy flowers, 1–1½ in. wide; "petals" (sepals) purple or white, in a *cup-shaped receptacle;* March–June. Seeds with *feathery plumes.* **Where found:** Moist meadows, prairies, woods. Iowa to Colo.; north to Wash., Alaska.

Uses: Minute doses diluted in water have been used internally in homeopathic practice for eye ailments, skin eruptions, rheumatism, leukorrhea, obstructed menses, bronchitis, coughs, asthma. **Warning: Poisonous.** Extremely irritating.

THIMBLEWEED Roots, seeds
Anemone virginiana L. Buttercup Family
Perennial; 2–4 ft. Leaves *strongly veined,* with distinct stalks (not sessile). Flowers 2 or more, with greenish white, petal-like sepals (no true petals). Flowers late April–Aug. Fruit thimble-like. Seeds covered in *cottony fluff.* **Where found:** Dry open woods. Me. to Ga.; Ark. to Kans.; north to S.D.
Uses: Expectorant, astringent, emetic. American Indians used root decoction (see p. 7) for whooping cough, tuberculosis, diarrhea. Root poulticed for boils. In order to revive an unconscious patient, the smoke of the seeds was blown into the nostrils. To divine the truth about acts of a "crooked wife," the roots were placed under her pillow, to induce dreams.

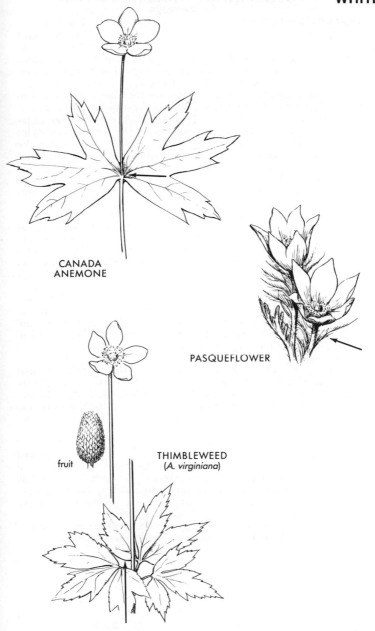

CANADA
ANEMONE

PASQUEFLOWER

fruit

THIMBLEWEED
(*A. virginiana*)

MISCELLANEOUS FLOWERS WITH 5 PETALS

COMMON NIGHTSHADE
Leaves, berries

Solanum nigrum L. — Nightshade Family

Perennial; 1–2½ ft. Leaves broadly triangular; irregularly toothed. Flowers white stars with *protruding yellow stamens*; petals curved back; May–Sept. Fruits black berries. **Where found:** Waste places. N.S. to Fla.; local westward. Alien (Europe).

Uses: Externally, leaf-juice preparations have been used as a folk remedy for tumors, cancer. Berries formerly used as a diuretic; used for eye diseases, fever, rabies. Extracts used in tea in India, China, Europe, Japan, Africa, etc. **Warning:** Some varieties contain solanine, steroids; deaths have been reported from use. In India, some varieties are eaten as vegetables, but similar varieties may be **violently toxic.**

CANADA VIOLET
Root, leaves

Viola canadensis L. — Violet Family

Slightly hairy to smooth perennial; to 10 in. Leaves oval to heart-shaped. Flowers white; April–July. Petals *yellowish at base*, becoming violet-tinged at base, especially when older. **Where found:** Mostly in northern deciduous woods. N.H. to S.C. mountains; Iowa to N.D. **Uses:** American Indians used root tea for pain in bladder region. Root and leaves traditionally used to induce vomiting; poulticed for skin abrasions, boils.

CHICKWEED
Whole plant

Stellaria media (L.) Cyrillo   **C. Pl. 7** — Pink Family

Annual or biennial prostrate weed; 6–15 in. Leaves oval, smooth (*long leafstalks hairy*). Flowers small, white; March–Sept. Petals *2-parted, shorter than sepals.* **Where found:** Waste places. Throughout our area. Alien.

Uses: Tea of this common Eurasian herb is traditionally used as a cooling demulcent and expectorant to relieve coughs; also used externally for skin diseases and to allay itching; anti-inflammatory. Science has not confirmed folk use. Still much used. Said to curb obesity.

FOAMFLOWER
Leaves, root

Tiarella cordifolia L. — Saxifrage Family

Perennial; 6–12 in. Leaves *maple-like.* Flowers white; 5 petals (with claws); stamens long; April–May. **Where found:** Rich woods. N.B. to N.C., S.C., and Ga. mountains; Tenn. mountains to Mich.

Uses: American Indians used leaf tea as a mouthwash for "white-coated tongue," mouth sores, and eye ailments; considered tonic, diuretic. Root tea once used as a diuretic; used for diarrhea; poulticed on wounds. High tannin content may explain traditional uses.

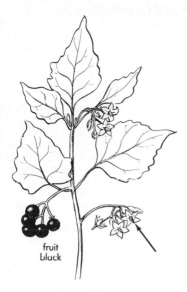

fruit
black

COMMON NIGHTSHADE

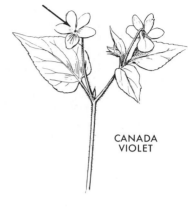

CANADA
VIOLET

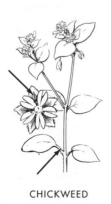

CHICKWEED

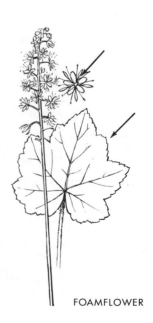

FOAMFLOWER

NODDING WAXY FLOWERS
WITH 5 PETALS

SPOTTED PIPSISSEWA   Leaves
Chimaphila maculata (L.) Pursh   Wintergreen Family
Perennial; 4–10 in. Leaves lance-shaped, in whorls; *midrib broadly white-marked.* Flowers whitish pink; drooping, waxy; June–Aug.
Where found: Rich woods. Me. to Ga.; Ala., Tenn. to Mich.
 Uses: Substitute for *C. umbellata* (below). **Warning:** Said to be a skin irritant.

PIPSISSEWA   Leaves
Chimaphila umbellata (L.) Nutt.   **C. Pl. 20**   Wintergreen Family
Perennial; 6–12 in. Leaves in *whorls;* lance-shaped, toothed, shiny. Flowers whitish pink, with a ring of red anthers; drooping, waxy; June–Aug. **Where found:** Dry woods. N.S. to Ga.; Ohio to Minn.
Uses: American Indians used leaf tea for backaches, coughs, bladder inflammations, stomachaches, kidney ailments; "blood purifier," diuretic, astringent; drops used for sore eyes. Leaves were smoked as a tobacco substitute. Physicians formerly used leaf tea for bladder stones, kidney inflammation (nephritis), prostatitis, and related ailments. Science confirms diuretic, tonic, astringent, urinary antiseptic, and antibacterial activity. Loaded with biologically active compounds — arbutin, sitosterol, ursolic acid. **Warning:** Leaves poulticed on skin may induce redness, blisters, and peeling. Arbutin hydrolyzes to the **toxic** urinary antiseptic hydroquinone.

SHINLEAF   Whole plant
Pyrola elliptica L.   Wintergreen Family
Perennial; 5–10 in. Leaves in a basal rosette; leaves thin, elliptical; top rounded, blade usually longer than stem. Flowers greenish white; style curving; June–Aug. **Where found:** Dry to rich woods. P.E.I. to Md., W. Va.; Neb. and across Canada to Alaska.
Uses: American Indians used tea of whole plant to treat epileptic seizures in babies; leaf tea was gargled for sore throats, canker sores; leaf poulticed for tumors, sores, and cuts. Root tea a tonic.

ROUND-LEAVED PYROLA   Leaves
Pyrola rotundifolia L.   Wintergreen Family
Like Shinleaf but larger; leaves more rounded, shinier, thicker, and more leathery. Leaf *stems as long as blades.* **Where found:** Woods, bogs. Nfld. to N.C. mountains; west to Minn., S.D.
 Uses: Formerly used by physicians as an astringent for skin eruptions, sore throat or mouth; diuretic for urinary infections; antispasmodic for epilepsy, nervous disorders; leaves poulticed on boils, carbuncles, swelling, painful tumors. Bruised plant used as a styptic. Contains arbutin, a proven diuretic and antibacterial agent that breaks down into **toxic** hydroquinone when metabolized.

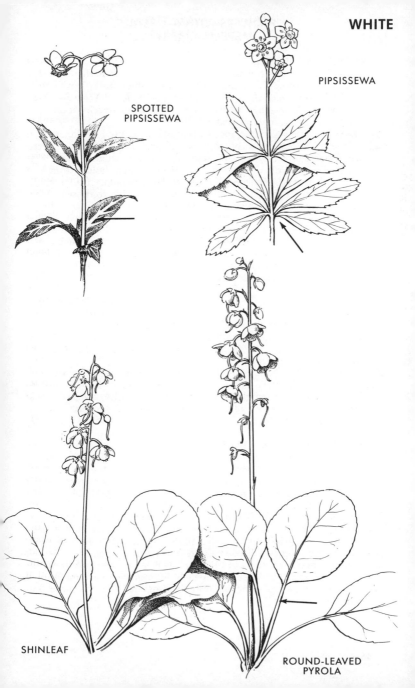

WHITE

SPOTTED PIPSISSEWA

PIPSISSEWA

SHINLEAF

ROUND-LEAVED PYROLA

FLOWERS WITH 6–8 PETALS;
UMBRELLA-LIKE LEAVES

UMBRELLA-LEAF   **Root**
Diphylleia cymosa Michx.   Barberry Family
Smooth perennial; 8–36 in. Leaves 2, on a stout stalk; leaves *cleft, umbrella-like; each division with 5–7 toothed lobes.* Flowers white, in clusters; May–Aug. **Where found:** Rich woods (rare). Mountains. Va. to Ga. Too rare to harvest.

⚠ **Uses:** A related Chinese species (see below) is used in Traditional Chinese Medicine, but the scarcity and narrow range of the American species probably limited interest in medicinal use of this plant. The Cherokees used the root tea of Umbrella-leaf to induce sweating. It was considered diuretic, antiseptic, and useful for smallpox. Physicians thought its effects might be similar to those of Mayapple (see below). **Warning:** Probably **toxic.**
Related species: A closely related Chinese species, *D. sinensis* (not shown), contains the toxic anticancer compound podophyllotoxin. In Traditional Chinese Medicine, *D. sinensis* is used for coughs, malaria, cancerous sores, snakebites, and jaundice, and is considered antiseptic. Historical and modern uses of *D. sinensis* indicate parallels in chemistry and use with Mayapple.

TWINLEAF   **Whole plant, root**
Jeffersonia diphylla (L.) Pers.   Barberry Family
Perennial; 8–16 in. Leaf broadly rounded in outline, but with *2 distinct sinuses (notches).* Flowers white, 8-petaled; April–May. **Where found:** Rich woods. W. N.Y. to Md., W. Va., Va., N.C.; Tenn., Ky. to Wisc. Too rare to harvest.

⚠ **Uses:** American Indians used root tea for cramps, spasms, nervous excitability, diarrhea; diuretic for "gravel" (kidney stones), dropsy, urinary infections; gargle for sore throats; externally, used as a wash for rheumatism, sores, ulcers, inflammation, and cancerous sores. **Warning:** Probably **toxic.**

MAYAPPLE, AMERICAN MANDRAKE   **Roots**
Podophyllum peltatum L.   **C. Pl. 13**   Mayapple Family
Perennial; 12–18 in. Leaves smooth, paired, *umbrella-like; distinctive.* A single waxy white flower, to 2 in. across, droops *from crotch of leaves;* April–June. **Where found:** Woods, clearings. S. Me. to Fla.; Texas to Minn.

☠ **Uses:** American Indians and early settlers used roots as a strong purgative, "liver cleanser," emetic, worm expellent; for jaundice, constipation, hepatitis, fevers, and syphilis. Resin from root, podophyllin (highly allergenic), used to treat venereal warts. Etoposide, a semisynthetic derivative of this plant, is FDA-approved for testicular and small-cell lung cancers. Fruits edible. **Warning:** Tiny amounts of root or leaves are **poisonous.** Powdered root and resin can cause skin and eye problems.

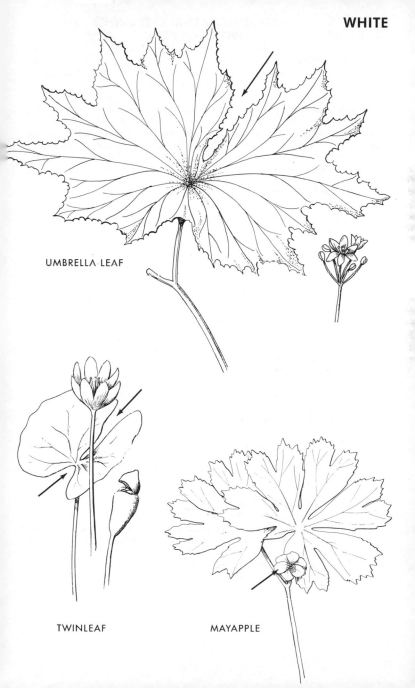

WHITE

UMBRELLA LEAF

TWINLEAF

MAYAPPLE

LOW, SHOWY SPRING FLOWERS
WITH 6–10 PETALS

WINDFLOWER, RUE ANEMONE   Root
Anemonella thalictroides (L.) Spach   **C. Pl. 18**   Buttercup Family
[*Thalictrum thalictroides* (L.) Boivin.]
Delicate perennial; 4–8 in. Leaves *in whorls;* small, *3-lobed.* Flowers
white (or pink), with 5–11 "petals" (sepals); March–May. **Where
found:** Rich woods. Me. to Fla.; Ark. and e. Okla. to Minn.

Uses: American Indians used root tea for diarrhea and vomiting.
Tuberous roots considered edible. Historically, root preparation used
by physicians as an experimental application to treat piles. **Warning:**
Possibly **toxic.**

BLOODROOT   Root
Sanguinaria canadensis L.   **C. Pl. 13**   Poppy Family
Perennial; 6–12 in. Juice *orange.* Leaves distinctly round-lobed.
Flowers white, to 2 in., with 8–10 petals; appearing before or with
leaves; March–June. **Where found:** Rich woods. N.S. to Fla.; e. Texas
to Man.
Uses: The blood-red fresh root was used in minute doses as an appetite stimulant; in larger doses as an arterial sedative. Formerly,
root used as an ingredient in cough medicines. American Indians
used root tea for rheumatism, asthma, bronchitis, lung ailments, laryngitis, fevers; also as an emetic. Root juice applied to warts, also
used as a dye and as a decorative skin stain. A bachelor of the Ponca
tribe would rub a piece of the root as a love charm on the palm of his
hand, then scheme to shake hands with the woman he desired to
marry. After shaking hands, the girl would be found willing to marry
him in 5–6 days. Experimentally, the alkaloid sanguinarine has
shown antiseptic, anesthetic, and anticancer activity. It is used commercially as a plaque-inhibiting agent in toothpaste, mouthwashes,
and rinses. **Warning: Toxic. Do not ingest.** Jim Duke has experienced
tunnel vision from nibbling the root.

SHARP-LOBED HEPATICA, LIVERLEAF   Leaves
Hepatica acutiloba DC.   **C. Pl. 12**   Buttercup Family
Flowers usually bluish lavender or pinkish, though often whitish.
Feb.–early June. See p. 176 and color plate.

ROUND-LOBED HEPATICA   Leaves
Hepatica americana (DC.) Ker.   **C. Pl. 12**   Buttercup Family
Similar to Sharp-lobed Hepatica, but leaf lobes are *rounded.* Flowers
often white; March–June. **Where found:** Dry woods. N.S. to Ga., Ala.;
Mo. to Man.
Uses: Same as for *H. acutiloba* (see above). See p. 176.

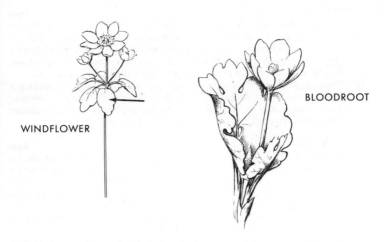

WINDFLOWER

BLOODROOT

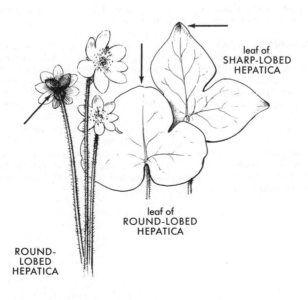

leaf of
SHARP-LOBED
HEPATICA

leaf of
ROUND-LOBED
HEPATICA

ROUND-
LOBED
HEPATICA

FLOWERS IN SINGLE, GLOBE-SHAPED CLUSTERS; FRUITS RED

RED BANEBERRY   Root
Actaea rubra (Ait.) Willd.   **C. Pl. 16**   Buttercup Family
Perennial; 2–3 ft. Similar to White Baneberry (see p. 52), though the
flowerhead is rounder, and the berries are *red* and on less stout stalks.
Fruits; July–Oct. **Where found:** Rich woods. S. Canada to n. N.J., W.
Va.; west through Ohio and Iowa to S.D., Colo., Utah, and Ore.

☠ **Uses:** American Indians used root tea for menstrual irregularity,
postpartum pains, and as a purgative after childbirth; also used to
treat coughs and colds. **Warning:** Plant is **poisonous** — may cause
vomiting, gastroenteritis, irregular breathing, and delirium.

GOLDENSEAL   Root
Hydrastis canadensis L.   **C. Pl. 13**   Buttercup Family
Hairy perennial; 6–12 in. Usually 2 leaves on a forked branch; one
leaf larger than the other; each rounded, with *5–7 lobes; double-
toothed*. Flowers single, with greenish white stamens in clusters;
April–May. Berries like those of raspberry. **Where found:** Rich woods.
Vt. to Ga.; Ala., Ark. to Minn. Goldenseal is becoming less common
in our eastern deciduous forests due to overcollection.

⚠ **Uses:** Root traditionally used in tea or tincture to treat inflamed
mucous membranes of mouth, throat, digestive system, uterus; also
used for jaundice, bronchitis, pharyngitis, gonorrhea. Tea (wash) a
folk remedy for eye infections. Contains berberine, an antibacterial
that increases bile secretion and acts as an anticonvulsant; experimentally lowers blood pressure, acts as mild sedative. **Warning:**
Avoid during pregnancy. Scientists have disproved rumor that Goldenseal masks morphine in urine tests.

AMERICAN GINSENG   Root
Panax quinquefolius L.   **C. Pl. 14**   Ginseng Family
Perennial; 1–2 ft. Root fleshy, sometimes resembling human form.
Leaves *palmately divided* into 4–5 (occasionally 3–7) sharp-toothed,
oblong-lance-shaped leaflets. Flowers whitish, in *round umbels*;
June–July. Fruits *2-seeded red berries*. **Where found:** Rich woods. Me.
to Ga.; Okla. to Minn.

⚠ **Uses:** Root considered demulcent, tonic. Research suggests it may
increase mental efficiency and physical performance, aid in adapting
to high or low temperatures and stress (when taken over an extended
period). Ginseng's effect is called "adaptogenic" — tending to return
the body to normal. **Warning:** Some caution required; large doses are
said to raise blood pressure.

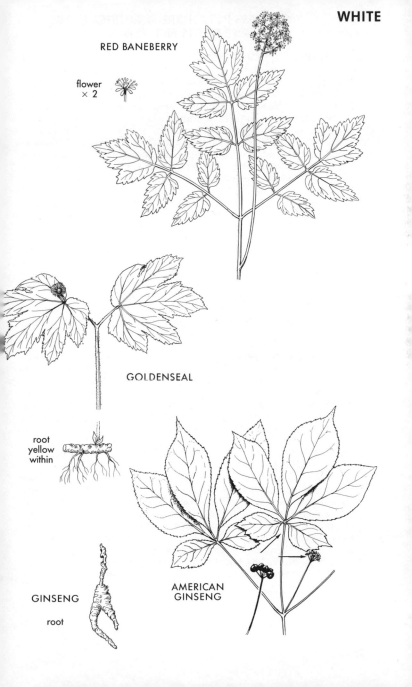

WHITE

RED BANEBERRY

flower
× 2

GOLDENSEAL

root
yellow
within

GINSENG

root

AMERICAN
GINSENG

WHITE BANEBERRY, DOLL'S EYES
Root

Actaea pachypoda L.   **C. Pl. 16**   Buttercup Family

Perennial; 1–2 ft. Leaves twice-divided; leaflets oblong, sharp-toothed. Flowers in oblong clusters *on thick red stalks.* Fleshy *white berries with a dark dot at tip;* July–Oct. **Where found:** Rich woods. S. Canada to Ga., La.; Okla. to Minn.

Uses: Menominees used small amount of root tea to relieve pain of childbirth, headaches due to eye strain. Once used for coughs, menstrual irregularities, colds, and chronic constipation; thought to be beneficial to circulation. **Warning: Poisonous.** All parts may cause severe gastrointestinal inflammation and skin blisters.

INDIAN HEMP
Root, stems, berries, latex

Apocynum cannabinum L.   Dogbane Family

Shrub-like; 1–2 ft. Leaves (except lowermost ones) with *definite stalks,* to ½ in. long. Flowers *terminal, whitish green;* bell-like, 5-sided; June–Aug. Seedpods paired; 4–8 in. long. **Where found:** Much of our area and beyond.

Uses: Used as in *A. androsaemifolium* (p. 152); also, stems used for fiber, cordage. Milky sap a folk remedy for venereal warts. American Indians used berries and root in weak teas for heart ailments; diuretic. **Warning: Poisonous.** Contains toxic cardioactive (heart-affecting) glycosides. Cymarin and apocymarin have shown antitumor activity; the latter also raises blood pressure.

FOUR-LEAVED MILKWEED
Root

Asclepias quadrifolia Jacq.   Milkweed Family

Flowers white or pinkish. Leaves *in whorls of 4.* See p. 154.

VIRGINIA WATERLEAF
Whole plant

Hydrophyllum virginianum L.   Waterleaf Family

Flowers whitish to violet. See p. 178.

DWARF GINSENG
Leaves, root

Panax trifolius L.   Ginseng Family

Globe-rooted perennial; 2–8 in. Leaves divided into 3 (occasionally 5) *toothed, oblong to lance-shaped* leaflets. Flowers white to yellow (or pinkish), in small umbels; April–May. Fruits green or yellow. **Where found:** Rich woods. N.S. to Pa., Ga. mountains; Ind., Iowa to Minn.

Uses: American Indians used tea of whole plant for colic, indigestion, gout, hepatitis, hives, rheumatism, and tuberculosis; root chewed for headaches, short breath, fainting, nervous debility. Little used or researched. Above ground for only 2 months.

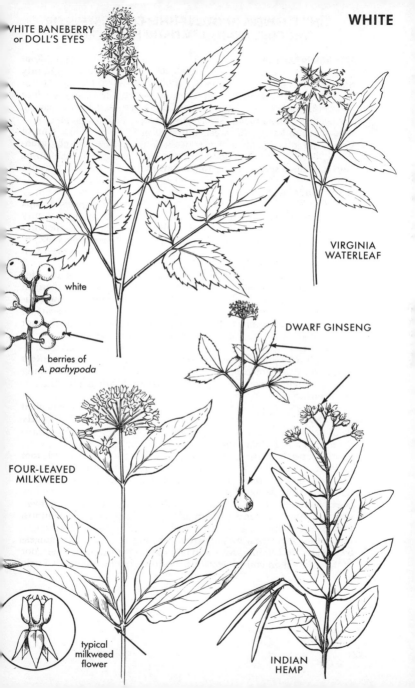

WHITE

WHITE BANEBERRY
or DOLL'S EYES

VIRGINIA
WATERLEAF

white

berries of
A. pachypoda

DWARF GINSENG

FOUR-LEAVED
MILKWEED

INDIAN
HEMP

typical
milkweed
flower

TINY FLOWERS IN GLOBE-SHAPED CLUSTERS OR PANICLES; ARALIAS; MOSTLY HERBACEOUS

HAIRY SARSAPARILLA   **Root, leaves**
Aralia hispida Vent.   **C. Pl. 43**   Ginseng Family
Shrubby; 1–3 ft. Foul-smelling. Stem with *sharp stiff bristles*. Leaves twice-compound; leaflets oval, cut-toothed. Small, greenish white flowers in *globe-shaped umbels*; June–Aug. Fruits dark, foul-smelling berries. **Where found:** Sandy open woods. E. Canada, New England south to Va., W. Va.; west to Ill., Minn.
Uses: Leaf tea promotes sweating. Bark (root bark especially) diuretic, "tonic"; allays kidney irritation and associated lower back pain, increases secretions in dropsy and edema.

WILD SARSAPARILLA   **Root**
Aralia nudicaulis L.   **C. Pl. 19**   Ginseng Family
Smooth perennial; to 2 ft. Leaves twice-divided; each of the 3 divisions has 3–5 toothed, oval leaflets. Flowers in a single umbel on a separate stalk, *below leaves*; May–July. Root long-running, horizontal, fleshy. **Where found:** Moist woods. Nfld. to Ga.; west to n. Mo., Ill., N.D. to Colo. and Idaho.
Uses: American Indians used the pleasant-flavored root tea as a beverage, "blood purifier," tonic; used for lassitude, general debility, stomachaches, and coughs. Externally, the fresh root was poulticed on sores, burns, itching, ulcers, boils, and carbuncles, to reduce swelling, and cure infections. In folk tradition, root tea or tincture was used as a diuretic and "blood purifier"; promotes sweating; used for stomachaches, fevers, coughs. Root poultice used for wounds, ulcers, boils, carbuncles, swelling, infection, rheumatism. Former substitute for true (tropical *Smilax*) sarsaparilla. This plant was widely used in "tonic" and "blood-purifier" patent medicines of the late 19th century.

SPIKENARD   **Root**
Aralia racemosa L.   **C. Pl. 15**   Ginseng Family
Perennial; 3–5 ft. Stem *smooth; dark green or reddish*. Leaves compound, with 6–21 toothed, *weakly heart-shaped* leaflets. Flowers whitish, in small umbels on branching racemes; June–Aug. Root *spicy-aromatic*. **Where found:** Rich woods. Que. to Ga.; west to Kans.; north to Minn.
Uses: Same as for *A. nudicaulis* (above); also used for coughs, asthma, lung ailments, rheumatism, syphilis, kidney troubles. Formerly used in cough syrups. Root tea widely used by American Indians for menstrual irregularities, for lung ailments accompanied by coughs, and to improve the flavor of other medicine. Externally, root poulticed on boils, infections, swellings, and wounds.

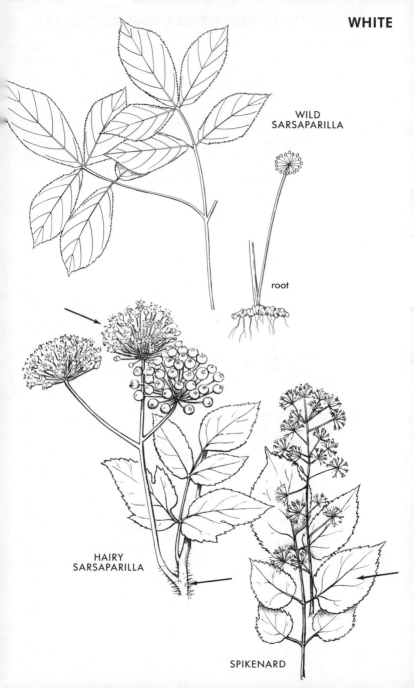

WHITE

WILD
SARSAPARILLA

root

HAIRY
SARSAPARILLA

SPIKENARD

FLOWERS IN LONG, SLENDER, TAPERING CLUSTERS

BLACK COHOSH   **Root**
Cimicifuga racemosa (L.) Nutt.   Buttercup Family
Perennial; 3–8 ft. Leaves thrice-divided; sharply toothed; *terminal leaflet 3-lobed, middle lobe largest.* Flowers white, *in very long spikes;* May–Sept. *Tufts of stamens conspicuous.* **Where found:** Rich woods. S. Ont. to Ga.; Ark., Mo. to Wisc.

⚠ **Uses:** Insoluble in water. Tincture used for bronchitis, chorea, fevers, nervous disorders, lumbago, rheumatism, snakebites, menstrual irregularities, childbirth. Traditionally important for "female ailments." Research has confirmed estrogenic, hypoglycemic, sedative, and anti-inflammatory activity. Root extract strengthens female reproductive organs in rats. **Warning:** Avoid during pregnancy.

POKEWEED, POKE   **Root, fruits, leaves**
Phytolacca americana L.   **C. Pl. 33**   Pokeweed Family
Coarse, large-rooted perennial; 5–10 ft. *Stem often red* at base. Leaves large, entire (toothless), oval. Flowers with greenish white, petal-like sepals; July–Sept. Fruits *purple-black,* in drooping clusters; Aug–Nov. **Where found:** Waste places. Much of our area (except N.D., S.D.).

☠ **Uses:** American Indians used berry tea for rheumatism, arthritis, dysentery, berries poulticed on sore breasts. Root poulticed for rheumatism, neuralgic pains, bruises; wash used for sprains, swellings; leaf preparations once used as an expectorant, emetic, cathartic; poulticed for bleeding, pimples, blackheads. Folk uses similar. **Warning: All parts are poisonous,** though leaves are eaten as a spring green, after cooking through 2 changes of water. (Do not confuse with American White Hellebore, *Veratrum viride,* p. 104, which is **highly toxic.**) Plant juice of Pokeweed can cause dermatitis, even damage chromosomes.

LIZARD'S-TAIL, WATER-DRAGON   **Root, leaves**
Saururus cernuus L.   Lizard-tail Family
Aquatic or wet-ground-loving perennial. See p. 14.

CULVER'S-ROOT   **Root**
Veronicastrum virginicum (L.) Farw.   Figwort Family
[*Leptandra virginica* Nutt.]
Perennial; 2–5 ft. Leaves lance-shaped, toothed; in *whorls of 3–7.* Flowers tiny white (or purple) tubes with 2 projecting stamens; on showy spikes; June–Sept. **Where found:** Moist fields. Mass. to Fla.; e. Texas to Man.

⚠ **Uses:** American Indians used root tea as a strong laxative, to induce sweating, to stimulate liver, to induce vomiting; diuretic. Used similarly by physicians. **Warning:** Traditionally, *dried* root is used; *fresh* root violently laxative. Potentially **toxic.**

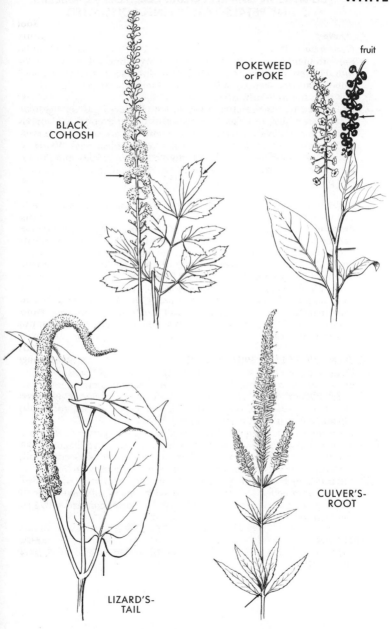

BLACK
COHOSH

POKEWEED
or POKE

fruit

LIZARD'S-
TAIL

CULVER'S-
ROOT

FLOWERS IN UMBRELLA-LIKE CLUSTERS (UMBELS); 5 TINY PETALS; LEAVES FINELY DISSECTED

CARAWAY   **Seeds**
Carum carvi L.   Parsley Family
Smooth biennial; 1–2 ft. Stem hollow. Leaves finely divided, *carrot-like*. Flowers tiny, white (or pink); May–July. Seeds slightly curved, ribbed, caraway-scented. **Where found:** Fields. Scattered throughout our area; not in South. Alien.
Uses: Seed tea carminative, expectorant. Relieves gas in digestive system, soothing to upset stomach; also used for coughs, pleurisy. Thought to relieve menstrual pain, promote milk secretion. Externally, used as a wash for rheumatism. Oil is antibacterial. **Warning:** Young leaves are very similar to those of Fool's Parsley and Poison Hemlock. To identify Fool's Parsley, see *A Field Guide to Wildflowers*, p. 48.

POISON HEMLOCK   **Poison — Identify to avoid**
Conium maculatum L.   Parsley Family
Branched perennial; 2–6 ft. Stems hollow, grooved; *purple-spotted*. Leaves *carrot-like*, but in overall outline more like an equilateral triangle, and with more divisions; leaves *ill-scented when bruised*. Leafstalks *hairless*. Flowers white, in umbels; May–Aug. **Where found:** Waste ground. Most of our area. Alien.
Uses: Whole plant a traditional folk cancer remedy, narcotic, sedative, analgesic, spasmolytic, anti-aphrodisiac. **Warning: Deadly poison. Ingestion can be lethal. Contact can cause dermatitis. Juice highly toxic.** Young Poison Hemlock plant closely resembles the western Osha root.

QUEEN ANNE'S LACE, WILD CARROT   **Root, seeds**
Daucus carota L.   **C. Pl. 27**   Parsley Family
Bristly stemmed biennial; 2–4 ft. Leaves finely dissected. Flowers in a *flat cluster*, with 1 small *deep purple floret* at center; 3-forked bracts beneath; April–Oct. **Where found:** Waste places, roadsides. Throughout our area. Alien (Europe).
Uses: Root tea traditionally used as a diuretic, to prevent and eliminate urinary stones and worms. Science confirms its bactericidal, diuretic, hypotensive, and worm-expelling properties. Seeds a folk "morning-after" contraceptive. Experiments with mice indicate seed extracts may be useful in preventing implantation of fertilized egg. (Not recommended for such uses, but scientists should investigate.) **Warning:** May cause dermatitis and blisters. Do not confuse with Poison Hemlock.

VALERIAN   **Root**
Valeriana officinalis L.   **C. Pl. 25**   Valerian Family
See p. 140.

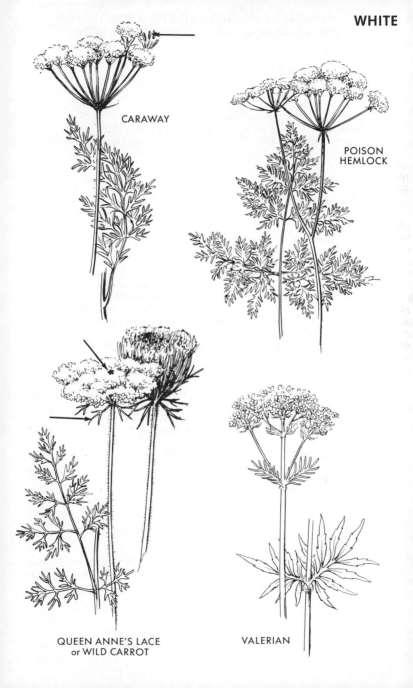

WHITE

CARAWAY

POISON HEMLOCK

QUEEN ANNE'S LACE
or WILD CARROT

VALERIAN

ANGELICA
Leaves, root, seeds

Angelica atropurpurea L.   **C. Pl. 6**   Parsley Family

Smooth, *purple-stemmed* biennial; 4–9 ft. Leaves with 3 leaflets, each *divided again 3–5 times.* Upper leafstalks have *inflated* sheaths. Flowers in large, semiround heads; June–Aug. **Where found:** Rich, wet soil. Nfld. to Del., W. Va.; Ill. to Wisc.

Uses: Leaf tea used for stomachaches, indigestion, gas, anorexia, obstructed menses, fevers, colds, colic, flu, coughs, neuralgia, rheumatism. Roots, seeds strongest; leaves weaker.

Related species: Other Angelicas are famous Chinese drugs for "female ailments."

WATER-HEMLOCK
Poison — Identify to avoid

Cicuta maculata L.   Parsley Family

Biennial; 1–7 ft. *Stems smooth; purple-streaked or spotted.* Leaves divided 2–3 times; leaflets lance-shaped, coarsely toothed. Flowers in loose umbels; May–Sept. *Strong odor.* **Where found:** Wet meadows, swamps. Most of our area.

Uses: Too lethal for use; contains compounds similar to those found in Poison Hemlock (below). **Warning: Highly poisonous.** Do not confuse with harmless members of the parsley family.

POISON HEMLOCK
Poison — Identify to avoid

Conium maculatum L.   Parsley Family

Stems *purple-spotted.* **Warning: Deadly poison.** Ingestion can be lethal. Contact can cause dermatitis. See p. 58.

COW-PARSNIP
Root, leaves, tops

Heracleum lanatum Michx.   Parsley Family
[*Heracleum maximum* Bartr.]

Large, woolly, strong-smelling biennial or perennial; to 6–9 ft. Leaves divided into *3 maple-like segments;* sheath *inflated.* Umbels large — 6–12 in. across; flowers with notched petals; May–Aug. **Where found:** Moist soils. Nfld. to Ga. mountains; west to Mo., Kans., N.D. and westward.

Uses: Root tea was widely used by American Indians for colic, cramps, headaches, sore throats, colds, coughs, flu; externally poulticed on sores, bruises, swellings, rheumatic joints, boils, etc. In folk use, root tea was used for indigestion, gas, asthma, epilepsy. Powdered root (1 teaspoon per day over a long period) was taken, along with a strong tea of the leaves and tops, for epilepsy. Root contains psoralen, under investigation for treatment of psoriasis, leukemia, and AIDS. **Warning:** Foliage is **poisonous** to livestock; roots contain phototoxic compounds, including psoralen. Acrid sap can cause blisters on contact.

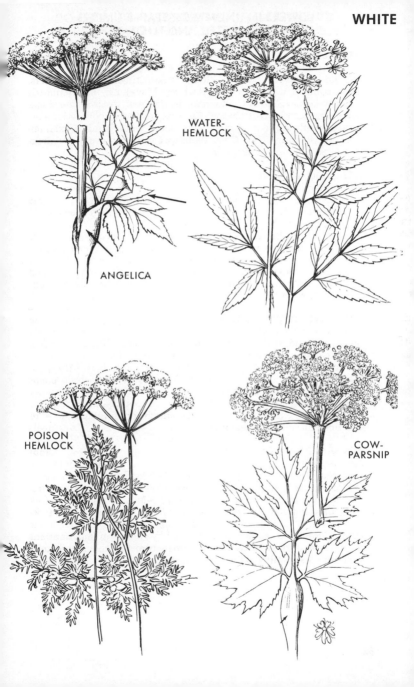

WHITE

ANGELICA

WATER-HEMLOCK

POISON HEMLOCK

COW-PARSNIP

FLOWERS IN UNEVEN OR SPARSE UMBELS; LEAVES PARTED AND TOOTHED

SWEET CICELY   **Root**
Osmorhiza claytonii (Michx.) Clarke   Parsley Family
Soft-hairy perennial; 1–3 ft. Root rank-tasting. Leaves *fernlike*; thrice-compound. Flowers tiny, white; May–June. **Where found:** Moist woods. N.S. to N.C. mountains; Ala., Ark. to Sask.
Uses: American Indians chewed the root or gargled root tea for sore throats; poulticed root on boils, cuts, sores, wounds; tea a wash for sore red eyes, drunk for coughs. **Warning:** Do not confuse with Poison Hemlock (*Conium*) — see p. 58.

SWEET CICELY, ANISE ROOT   **Root**
Osmorhiza longistylis (Torr.) DC.   Parsley Family
A relative of *O. claytoni*, but stouter and nearly smooth; distribution more western. Root *very sweet, aromatic, fleshy.* **Where found:** Ont. to N.C.; Okla. to N.D.
Uses: American Indians used root tea for general debility, panacea, tonic for upset stomach, parturition (childbirth); root poulticed on boils, wounds; root tea an eye wash. In folk medicine, used as an expectorant, tonic for coughs, stomachaches. Root eaten or soaked in brandy. **Warning:** Do not confuse with Poison Hemlock (*Conium*) — see p. 58.

BLACK or CANADIAN SANICLE   **Leaves, root**
Sanicula canadensis L.   Parsley Family
Biennial; to 36 in. Leaves long-stalked; palmate, with *3–5 leaflets* that are double-toothed or deeply incised; upper leaves reduced, becoming bract pairs. Flowers whitish, in uneven umbels; May–July. Fruits *on a small but distinct stalk.* **Where found:** Dry woods, openings. S. N.H. to Fla.; Texas to Neb.
Uses: American Indians used the powdered root as a heart remedy; to stimulate menses; abortive. Leaves, which contain allantoin, were poulticed for bruises, inflammation.

BLACK SANICLE or SNAKEROOT   **Root**
Sanicula marilandica L.   Parsley Family
Perennial; 1–4 ft. Leaves palmate, with *5–7 leaflets*; 2 of the leaflets are deeply cleft, suggesting 7 leaflets. Flowers whitish, in uneven umbels with leaflike bracts beneath; April–July. *Prickled fruits sessile (without stalks); base of bristles bulbous.* **Where found:** Thickets, shores. N.S. to Fla.; Mo. to e. Kans., N.D.
Uses: The thick rhizome (root) was used by American Indians in tea for menstrual irregularities, pain, kidney ailments, rheumatism, fevers; root also poulticed on snakebites.

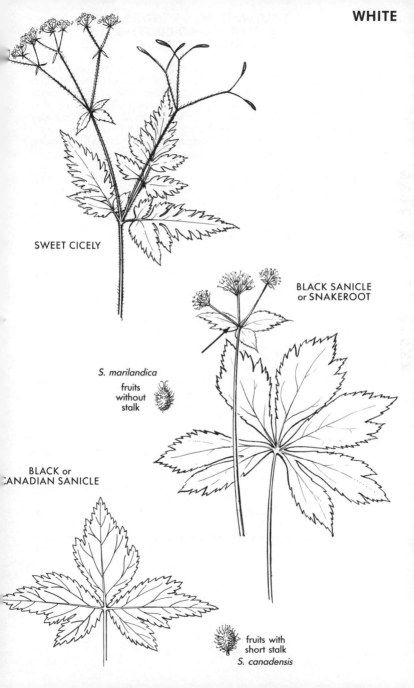

SWEET CICELY

BLACK SANICLE
or SNAKEROOT

S. marilandica
fruits
without
stalk

BLACK or
CANADIAN SANICLE

fruits with
short stalk
S. canadensis

FLOWERS WITH 5 "PETALS," IN FLAT-TOPPED CLUSTERS

YARROW   Whole plant in flower
Achillea millefolium L.   **C. Pl. 26**   Composite Family
Soft, fragrant perennial; 1–3 ft. Leaves lacy, *finely dissected*. Flowers
white (less frequently pink), in flat clusters; May–Oct. Each tiny
flowerhead has 5 petal-like rays that are usually slightly wider than
long; each ray has 3 teeth at tip. **Where found:** Fields, roadsides.
Throughout.

Uses: Herbal tea (made from dried flowering plant) used for colds,
fevers, anorexia, indigestion, gastric inflammations, and internal
bleeding. Fresh herb a styptic poultice. Expectorant, analgesic, and
sweat-inducing qualities of some components may provide relief
from cold and flu symptoms. Used similarly by native cultures
throughout the Northern Hemisphere. Experimentally, extracts are
hemostatic and anti-inflammatory. Over 100 biologically active
compounds have been identified from the plant. **Warning:** May cause
dermatitis. Large or frequent doses taken over a long period may be
potentially harmful. Contains thujone, considered **toxic.**

FLOWERING SPURGE   Leaves, root
Euphorbia corollata L.   Spurge Family
Deep-rooted, milky-juiced, smooth-stemmed perennial; 1–3 ft.
Leaves without stalks, *oval or linear.* Flowers white, in many forked
umbels, rising from *whorl of reduced leaves.* Note the 5 "petals"
(actually bracts) surrounding flowers. Flowers June–Aug. **Where
found:** Fields, roadsides. Ont., N.Y. to Fla.; Texas to Minn.

Uses: American Indians used leaf tea for diabetes; root tea as a
strong laxative, emetic, for pinworms, rheumatism; root poultice
used for snakebites. **Warning:** Extremely strong laxative. Juice may
cause blistering.

TALL CINQUEFOIL   Whole plant, root
Potentilla arguta Pursh   Rose Family
Erect, *glandular-hairy* perennial; 1–3 ft. Pinnate leaves at base of
stem divided into 7–11 oval, sharp-toothed leaflets, downy beneath;
minute, leaflike "folioles" often present between alternating leaflets.
Flowers white to cream, 5-petaled; June–Aug. **Where found:** Rocky
soils, prairies. N.B. to Ind., Mo., Okla.; west to Ore., Alaska.
Uses: As with yellow-flowered members of the genus (and the rose
family in general), the whole plant or root, in tea or as a poultice,
stops bleeding (astringent to capillaries); used for cuts, wounds, diarrhea, dysentery.

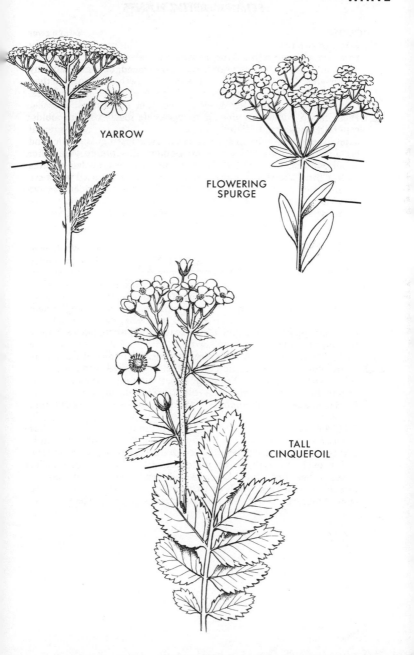

YARROW

FLOWERING SPURGE

TALL CINQUEFOIL

SMALL WHITISH FLOWERS IN LEAF AXILS; PARASITIC OR SEMI-PARASITIC PLANTS

DODDER   Whole plant
Cuscuta species   Morning-glory Family
Parasitic, chlorophyll-lacking, leafless annuals; leaves replaced by a few scales. *Stems yellow or orange.* **Where found:** Low ground. Most of our area. Dodders clamber over other growth and cause serious damage as annual weeds.

⚠ **Uses:** Stems used by Cherokees as a poultice for bruises. **Warning:** Dodders are called love vines and "vegetable spaghetti" but are not generally considered edible.
Related species: About 15 species in our area, distinguished by flowers and fruit details. (1) **Common Dodder** (*C. gronovii* Willd.) has small, whitish, waxy, 5-lobed flowers in loose or crowded clusters. (2) In China, the stems of other *Cuscuta* species are used in lotions for inflamed eyes. The Chinese value the seeds of dodders for urinary-tract ailments. The tea of **Chinese Dodder** (*C. chinensis*) has demonstrated anti-inflammatory, cholinergic, and CNS-depressant activity.

EYEBRIGHT   Whole plant
Euphrasia officinalis L.   **C. Pl. 42**   Figwort Family
[*Euphrasia americana* Wettst.]
Slender, semiparasitic (root is attached to grasses) annual; 4–8 in. Leaves tiny, bristle-toothed. Flowers June–Sept. *3 lower lobes notched*, with purple lines. Highly variable. **Where found:** Thought to have been introduced from Europe at an early date, probably as a medicinal plant. Dry or moist fields, roadsides, waste places. Subarctic south to Que., Me., Mass., N.Y.

⚠ **Uses:** Tea astringent. A folk remedy (wash or poultice) for eye ailments with mucous discharge; coughs, hoarseness, earaches, headaches with congestion. **Warning:** Experimentally, may induce side effects, including dim vision. Avoid use without physician's advice.
Related species: Other *Euphrasia* species have been used similarly.

SEA MILKWORT   Root
Glaux maritima L.   Primrose Family
Light-colored, fleshy perennial; 2–12 in. Leaves opposite, without stalks; oval. Flowers solitary, whitish to pink; 5-parted, in axils just above leaves; June–July. **Where found:** Sandy shores, salt marshes; mostly coastal. Que. south to Va.
Uses: American Indians ate the boiled roots to induce sleep.

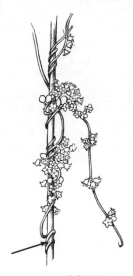

DODDER

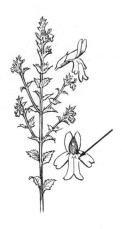

EYEBRIGHT

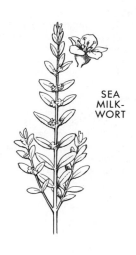

SEA
MILK-
WORT

SQUARE-STEMMED AROMATIC HERBS (MINTS); FLOWERS IN AXILS OR TERMINAL

LEMON BALM, MELISSA
Leaves
Melissa officinalis L.　　　　**C. Pl. 30**　　　Mint Family

Perennial; 1–2 ft. Leaves opposite; oval, round-toothed; *strongly lemon-scented.* Flowers whitish, inconspicuous, in whorls; May–Aug. **Where found:** Barnyards, old house sites, open woods. Scattered over much of our area. Alien (Europe).

Uses: Dried or fresh leaf tea a folk remedy for fevers, painful menstruation, headaches, colds, insomnia; mild sedative, carminative; leaves poulticed for sores, tumors, insect bites. Experimentally, hot-water extracts have been shown strongly antiviral for Newcastle disease, herpes, mumps; also antibacterial, antihistaminic, antispasmodic, and anti-oxidant. Sold in commercial antiviral preparations in Germany.

WILD MINT
Leaves
Mentha canadensis L.　　　　　　　　　Mint Family
[*Mentha arvensis* L.]

Perennial; 6–25 in. Fine, backward-bending hairs, at least on stem angles. Flowers tiny, whitish or pale lilac; in small axillary clusters; June–Oct. **Where found:** Damp soil. Canada, Northern U.S. Our only native mint plant; a highly variable species.

Uses: American Indians used leaf tea for colds, fevers, sore throats, gas, colic, indigestion, headaches, diarrhea; in short, same medicinal uses as for Peppermint and Spearmint in Western folk medicine.

HOARY MOUNTAIN MINT
Leaves
Pycnanthemum incanum (L.) Michx.　　　　Mint Family

Perennial; 2–6 ft. Leaves oval to lance-shaped, *stalked, toothed; hoary beneath (upper ones white-haired on both sides).* Flowers pale lilac; July–Sept. Calyx lobes apparently 2-lobed; lobes lance-shaped. **Where found:** Dry thickets. N.H. to Fla.; north to Tenn., s. Ill.

Uses: Leaf tea once used for fevers, colds, coughs, colic, stomach cramps; said to induce sweating, relieve gas. American Indians poulticed leaves for headaches; washed inflamed penis with tea.

VIRGINIA MOUNTAIN MINT
Leaves
Pycnanthemum virginianum (L.) Pers.　　　　Mint Family

Perennial; 2–4 ft. Leaves lance-shaped, *without stalks; base rounded.* Flowers whitish lilac, in dense terminal clusters; July–Sept. **Where found:** Dry thickets. Me. to N.C.; Mo., e. Kans. to N.D.

Uses: Same as for *P. incanum* (above); also used for amenorrhea, dysmenorrhea. Other Mountain Mints are used similarly.

WHITE

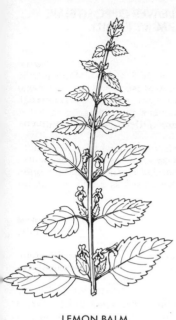

LEMON BALM
or MELISSA

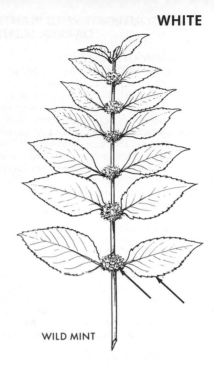

WILD MINT

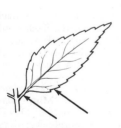

HOARY
MOUNTAIN-
MINT

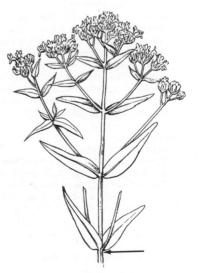

VIRGINIA
MOUNTAIN-MINT

SQUARE-STEMMED PLANTS; LEAVES OPPOSITE; WEAK OR RANK SCENTS; MINT FAMILY

AMERICAN BUGLEWEED,
CUT-LEAVED WATER HOREHOUND — Whole plant
Lycopus americanus Muhl.   **C. Pl. 5**   Mint Family
Perennial; 1–2 ft. Grows from edible, whitish, screwlike horizontal root. Leaves deeply cut; *lower ones suggest oak leaves.* Flowers in whorls of leaf axils; June–Sept. Stamens protruding; calyx lobes sharply pointed, longer than mature nutlets. **Where found:** Wet places. Throughout our area.
Uses: Thought to be the same as for *L. virginicus* (below).
Remarks: The bugleweeds (*Lycopus* species) are known as water-horehounds in some books. Like the true Horehound (*Marrubium vulgare,* below), these plants have been used as a folk remedy for coughs.

BUGLEWEED — Whole plant
Lycopus virginicus L.   Mint Family
Perennial; 6–40 in. Leaves lance-shaped, *strongly toothed;* lower ones with long, narrow bases. Flowers *in axils,* with broadly triangular calyx lobes, shorter than nutlets; July–Oct. **Where found:** Wet places. N.S. to Ga.; Ark. to Okla., Neb. to Minn.
Uses: Traditionally, used as a mild sedative, astringent; especially for heart diseases, chronic lung ailments, coughs, fast pulse, thyroid disease, diabetes. Science has confirmed the potential value of this plant in treating hyperthyroidism.

HOREHOUND — Leaves
Marrubium vulgare L.   **C. Pl. 29**   Mint Family
White-woolly, rank-scented perennial; 12–20 in. Leaves round-oval; toothed, *strongly wrinkled.* Flowers in whorls; May–Sept. White calyx with 10 bristly, curved teeth. **Where found:** Waste places; escaped. Scattered over much of our area. Alien.
Uses: Famous folk remedy for coughs, bronchitis, sore throats, stomach and gall bladder disorders, jaundice, hepatitis; fresh leaves poulticed on cuts, wounds. Experimentally, marrubiin is an expectorant and increases liver bile flow. Volatile oil is an expectorant, acts as a vasodilator. **Warning:** Plant juice may cause dermatitis.

CATNIP — Leaves, flowering tops
Nepeta cataria L.   **C. Pl. 29**   Mint Family
Perennial; 12–24 in. Leaves *stalked,* ovate; *strongly toothed.* Flowers in crowded clusters; June–Sept. Flowers whitish, purple-dotted; *calyx soft-hairy.* **Where found:** Much of our area. Alien.
Uses: Tea made from leaves and flowering tops a folk remedy for bronchitis, colds, diarrhea, fevers, chicken pox, colic, headaches, irregular menses; said to induce sleep, promote sweating, alleviate restlessness in children; leaves chewed for toothaches. Experimentally, nepetalactone, a mild sedative compound in Catnip, also possesses herbicidal and insect-repellant properties.

WHITE

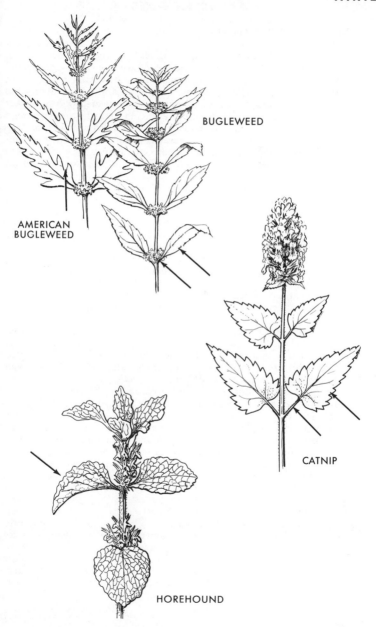

BUGLEWEED

AMERICAN
BUGLEWEED

CATNIP

HOREHOUND

DELICATE TINY FLOWERS LESS THAN ¼ IN. LONG, IN DENSE SPIKES

NARROW-LEAVED PLANTAIN   Leaves, seeds
Plantago lanceolata L.   Plantain Family
Annual; 10–23 in. Leaves *lance-shaped; 3-ribbed.* Flowers tiny, whitish, in a *short cylindrical* head on a grooved stalk; April–Nov.
Where found: Waste places. Throughout our area. Alien weed.
Uses: Traditionally, leaf tea used for coughs, diarrhea, dysentery, bloody urine. Leaves applied to blisters, sores, ulcers, swelling, insect stings; also used for earaches, eye ailments; thought to reduce heat and pain of inflammation. Science has vindicated utility in healing sores. The mucilage from any plantain seed may lower cholesterol levels. **Warning:** Some plantains may cause dermatitis.
Related species: *P. asiatica* is used clinically in China to reduce blood pressure (50 percent success rate). Seeds of *P. ovata* and *P. psyllium* (not shown) are widely used in bulk laxatives; also reduce rate of coronary ailments.

COMMON PLANTAIN   Leaves, seeds
Plantago major L.   **C. Pl. 23**   Plantain Family
Perennial; 6–18 in. Leaves *broad-oval; wavy-margined* or toothed, ribbed; stalk grooved. Flowers in a slender, elongate head; May–Oct.
Where found: Waste places. Throughout our area. Alien.
Uses: Same as for *P. lanceolata* (above). Prominent folk cancer remedy in Latin America. Used widely in folk medicine throughout the world. Confirmed antimicrobial; stimulates healing process.

SENECA SNAKEROOT   Root
Polygala senega L.   Milkwort Family
Perennial; 6–18 in. Leaves alternate; lance-shaped, small. Small, pea-like, white flowers in a terminal spike; May–July. **Where found:** Rocky woods. N.B. to Ga.; Ark. to S.D.
Uses: American Indians used root tea as emetic, expectorant, cathartic, diuretic, antispasmodic, sweat inducer; used to regulate menses; also for cold, croup, pleurisy, rheumatism, heart troubles, convulsions, coughs; poulticed root for swellings. Historically, root tea used similarly, also in pneumonia, chronic bronchitis, asthma; thought to "relax respiratory mucous membranes." Research suggests use for pulmonary conditions. Reported occurrence of methyl salicylate (see Wintergreen, p. 26) in root suggests a rationale behind use of this plant's root to relieve pain, rheumatism, etc.

DEVIL'S-BIT   Root
⚠ *Chamaelirium luteum* (L.) Gray   Lily Family
Flowers whitish at first, then turning yellow. See p. 104.

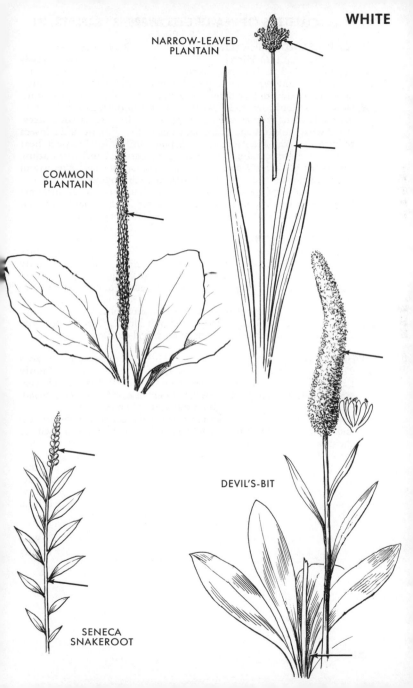

WHITE

NARROW-LEAVED
PLANTAIN

COMMON
PLANTAIN

DEVIL'S-BIT

SENECA
SNAKEROOT

CLUSTERS OF PEA-LIKE FLOWERS; 3 LEAFLETS

ROUND-HEADED BUSH-CLOVER   **Root, stem, whole plant**
Lespedeza capitata Michx.   Pea Family
Perennial; 2–5 ft. Leaves cloverlike, with 3 lance-shaped leaflets.
Flowers creamy white (base pink), in crowded, bristly heads; July–
Sept. **Where found:** Dry fields. New England to Fla.; Texas to Minn.
Uses: Moxa (burning sticks) were used by American Indians to treat
neuralgia and rheumatism. Small pieces of dried stem were mois-
tened with saliva on one end, then stuck to the skin, lit, and allowed
to burn the skin. Plant extract of disputed utility in chronic kidney
disease. Experimentally, extract has demonstrated antitumor activity against Walker-256 carcinosarcoma, and is reportedly effective in
lowering blood cholesterol levels. Also thought to lower blood levels
of nitrogen compounds in persons with high nitrogen levels in urine.
Contains several biologically active compounds. Pharmaceutical
preparations are manufactured in Europe from this plant.

WHITE SWEET-CLOVER   **Flowering plant**
Melilotus alba Desr.   **C. Pl. 22**   Pea Family
Biennial; 1–9 ft. Leaves cloverlike; leaflets elongate, slightly
toothed. Small, white, pea-like flowers in long, tapering spikes;
April–Oct. **Where found:** Roadsides. Throughout our area. Alien (Eu-
rope).
Uses: Dried flowering plant once used in ointments for external ul-
cers. In animal studies, components lower blood pressure. **Warning:**
Coumarins in this clover may decrease blood clotting.

WHITE CLOVER   **Whole plant, flowers**
Trifolium repens L.   **C. Pl. 24**   Pea Family
Perennial; 4–10 in. Leaves 3-parted, often with "V" marks. Flowers
stalked, white (often pink-tinged); in round heads; April–Sept. **Where
found:** Fields, lawns. Throughout our area. Alien (Europe).
Uses: American Indians adopted leaf tea for colds, coughs, fevers,
and leukorrhea. In European folk medicine, flower tea is used for
rheumatism and gout.

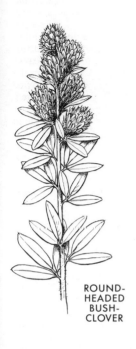

ROUND-
HEADED
BUSH-
CLOVER

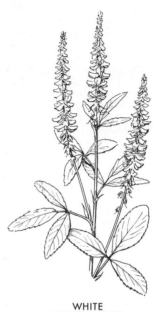

WHITE
SWEET-CLOVER

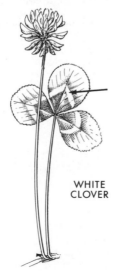

WHITE
CLOVER

STIFF-STEMMED LEGUMES
WITH 15 OR MORE LEAFLETS

PRAIRIE MIMOSA   Leaves, seeds
Desmanthus illinoensis (Michx.) MacM.   Pea Family
Smooth-stemmed, erect perennial; 1–4 ft. Leaves twice-divided; *leaflets 20–30, tiny.* Flowers greenish white, in *globular heads;* June–Aug. Pods curved, in loose globular heads. **Where found:** Prairies, fields. Ohio to Ala.; Texas, Colo. to N.D.
Uses: Pawnees used leaf tea as a wash for itching. A single report states that a Paiute Indian placed 5 seeds in the eye at night (washed out in morning) for chronic conjunctivitis. The leaves are reportedly high in protein.

WILD LICORICE   Root, leaves
Glycyrrhiza lepidota (Nutt.) Pursh   Pea Family
Shrubby perennial; 5–9 ft. Leaves compound; *leaflets 15–19,* oblong to lance-shaped, *glandular-dotted* (use lens). Flowers whitish, on short spikes. Fruits oblong, with *curved prickles;* June–Aug. **Where found:** Prairies, fields. W. Ont. to Texas; Mo. west to Wash.
Uses: American Indians applied a poultice of leaves infused in hot water to ears to treat earaches. The fresh root was chewed to treat toothaches. Root tea was used to reduce fevers in children.
Related species: This American species is similar to the Eurasian **Licorice Root** (*G. glabra*) and the Chinese species (*G. uralensis*), both extensively used in European and Asian herbal medicine. Sweet to musty-flavored roots of these related species were traditionally used for soothing irritated mucous membranes, inflamed stomach, ulcers, asthma, bronchitis, coughs, bladder infections, etc. *G. glabra* and *G. uralensis* have been extensively investigated; considered estrogenic, anti-inflammatory, anti-allergenic, anticonvulsive, and antibacterial. Chinese studies indicate antitussive effects of these plants are equal to and longer-lasting than codeine. Clinically useful against gastric and duodenal ulcers, bronchial asthma, coughs. Licorice root is one of the most extensively used drugs in Chinese herbal prescriptions. In combinations, the Chinese believe that it helps to detoxify potentially poisonous drugs, weakening their effects. Our Wild Licorice (little studied) contains the active component glycyrrhizin.
Warning: Wild Licorice can raise blood pressure.

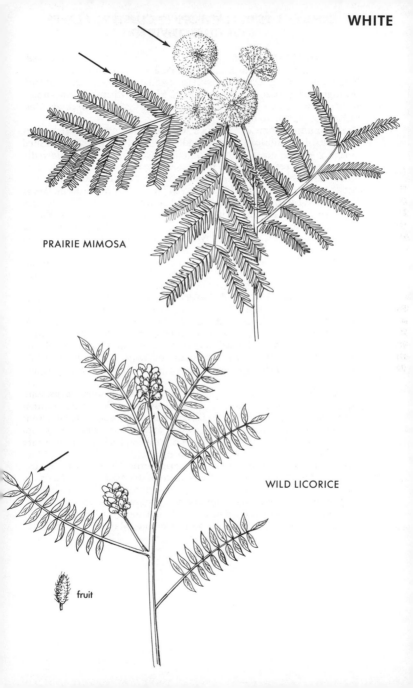

WHITE

PRAIRIE MIMOSA

WILD LICORICE

fruit

COMPOSITES IN FLAT-TOPPED CLUSTERS; LEAVES NOT FINELY DIVIDED

BONESET, THOROUGHWORT   Leaves
Eupatorium perfoliatum L.   **C. Pl. 3**   Composite Family
Perennial; 1–4 ft. Leaves *perfoliate* (stem appears to be inserted
through middle of leaf pairs), *wrinkled*. Flowers white to pale purple,
in flat clusters; July–Oct. **Where found:** Moist ground, thickets. N.S.
to Fla.; La., Texas to N.D.

 Uses: Common home remedy of 19th-century America, extensively
employed by American Indians and early settlers. Widely used, reportedly with success, during flu epidemics in 19th and early 20th
century. Leaf tea once used to induce sweating in fevers, flu, and
colds; also used for malaria, rheumatism, muscular pains, spasms,
pneumonia, pleurisy, gout, etc. Leaves poulticed onto tumors. West
German research suggests nonspecific immune system-stimulating
properties, perhaps vindicating historical use in flu epidemics. **Warning:** Emetic and laxative in large doses. May contain controversial
and potentially liver-harming pyrrolizidine alkaloids.

WHITE SNAKEROOT   Root, leaves
Eupatorium rugosum Houtt.   Composite Family
Variable perennial; 2–5 ft. Leaves opposite, on slender stalks; some-
what heart-shaped, toothed. Flowers white, in branched clusters;
July–Oct. **Where found:** Thickets. Que. to Ga.; Texas to Sask.

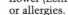 **Uses:** American Indians used root tea for ague, diarrhea, painful ur-
ination, fevers, "gravel" (kidney stones); poultice for snakebites.
Smoke of burning herb used to revive unconscious patients. **Warning:** "Milk sickness," with weakness and nausea, may result from
consuming the milk of cows that have grazed on this plant.

WILD QUININE   Root, leaves, tops
Parthenium integrifolium L.   **C. Pl. 40**   Composite Family
Large-rooted perennial; 2–5 ft. Large, oval, lance-shaped leaves, *to 1
ft. long*; rough, blunt-toothed. Flowerheads to ¼ in. wide; white, in
loose umbels; May–July. **Where found:** Prairies, rock outcrops, roadsides. Mass. to Ga.; e. Texas to Minn.
Uses: Catawbas poulticed fresh leaves on burns. Flowering tops were
once used for "intermittent fevers" (like malaria). Root used as a diuretic for kidney and bladder ailments, gonorrhea. One study suggests Wild Quinine may stimulate the immune system. Common
adulterant — historically and in modern times — to Purple Coneflower (*Echinacea purpurea*, p. 200). **Warning:** May cause dermatitis
or allergies.

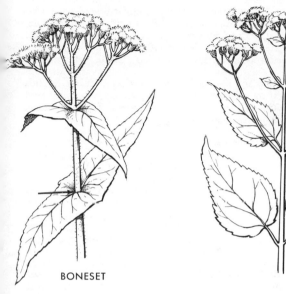

BONESET

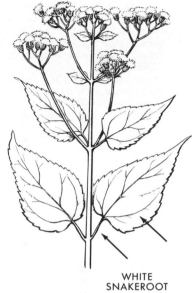

WHITE
SNAKEROOT

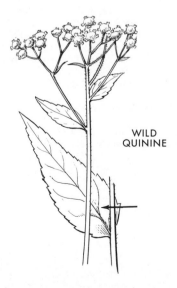

WILD
QUININE

FLOWERHEADS LONG, CYLINDRICAL; COMPOSITES WITH WEEDY GROWTH HABITS

PALE INDIAN PLANTAIN
Cacalia atriplicifolia L.

Leaves
Composite Family

Large perennial; 4–9 ft. Stems smooth or slightly striated. Leaves broadly rounded to triangular, with irregular rounded teeth; glaucous beneath, *palmately veined.* Flowers in flat clusters; July–Sept. Each tubular head has 5 flowers, apparently without rays (petals minute).
Where found: Dry woods, openings. N.J. to Ga.; Okla., Neb. to Mich., Minn.
Uses: American Indians used the leaves as a poultice for cancers, cuts, and bruises, and to draw out blood or poisonous material.
Related species: *Cacalia muhlenbergii* (not shown) is similar, but its leaves are green on both sides; stems grooved.

PILEWORT, FIREWEED
Erechtities hieracifolia (L.) Raf.

Whole plant
Composite Family

Annual; 1–9 ft. Leaves lance-shaped to oblong, 2–8 in. long; toothed, often lacerated. Flowers white, with no rays; flowers are enveloped in a *swollen group of leafy bracts.* **Where found:** Thickets, burns, waste places. Me. to Fla.; Texas, Okla., S.D. to Minn.
Uses: Tea or tincture of whole plant formerly used as an astringent and tonic in mucous-tissue ailments of lungs, bowels, stomach; also used externally for muscular rheumatism, sciatica. Used in diarrhea, cystitis, dropsy, etc. Neglected by scientific investigators.

WHITE LETTUCE, RATTLESNAKE ROOT
Prenanthes alba L.

Whole plant
Composite Family

Perennial; 2–5 ft. Stem smooth, purple, with whitish bloom. Leaves triangular or deeply lobed; toothed. Flowers white, in *drooping clusters;* July–Sept. "Seed" (technically fruit) fuzz a *deep rust color.*
Where found: Rich woods, thickets. Me. to Ga.; Mo. to N.D.
Uses: American Indians put powdered root in food to stimulate milk flow after childbirth. Root tea used as a wash for "weakness." Stem latex used as a diuretic in "female" diseases; boiled in milk, taken internally for snakebites. Leaves poulticed on snakebites. Roots poulticed on dog bites and snakebites. Tea drunk for dysentery.

HORSEWEED, CANADA FLEABANE
Erigeron canadensis L.

Whole plant
Composite Family

Bristly annual or biennial weed; 1–7 ft. Leaves numerous, lance-shaped. Flowers greenish white. See p. 210.

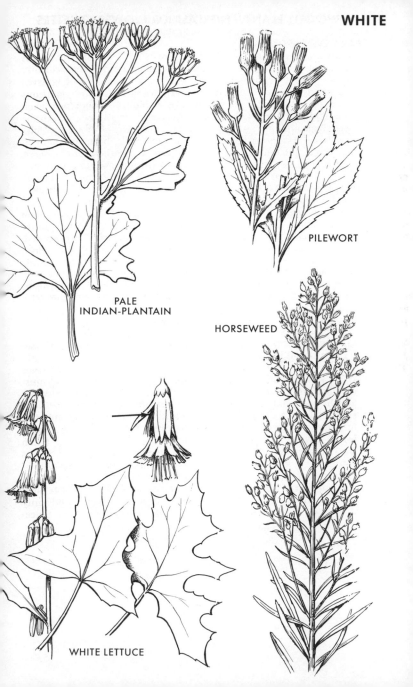

WHITE

PILEWORT

PALE
INDIAN-PLANTAIN

HORSEWEED

WHITE LETTUCE

WOOLLY PLANTS; EVERLASTING FLOWER CLUSTERS

PEARLY EVERLASTING
Whole plant

Anaphalis margaritacea (L.) C.B. Clarke Composite Family

Perennial; 1–3 ft. Highly variable. Stem and leaf undersides *cottony.* Leaves linear; gray-green above. Flowers in a cluster of globular heads; July–Sept. Heads with several rows of *white, dry, petal-like* bracts (male flowers have yellow tufts in center). **Where found:** Dry soil, fields. Nfld. to N.C.; Calif. to Alaska.

Uses: Expectorant, astringent, anodyne, sedative. Used for diarrhea, dysentery. American Indians used tea for colds, bronchial coughs, and throat infections. Poultice used for rheumatism, burns, sores, bruises, and swellings. Leaves smoked for throat and lung ailments.

PLANTAIN-LEAVED PUSSYTOES
Whole plant

Antennaria plantaginifolia (L.) Hook. Composite Family

Highly variable, *woolly-stemmed* perennial; 3–16 in. Basal leaves spoon-shaped, *silky*, with *3–5 nerves* (veins); more woolly on lower surface than above. Stem leaves small, lance-shaped. Flowers white, in several flowerheads; April–June. **Where found:** Dry woods, fields. Me. to Ga.; Okla. to N.D.

Uses: Boiled in milk, this plant was a folk remedy for diarrhea, dysentery. Tea drunk for lung ailments. Leaves poulticed on bruises, sprains, boils, and swellings. One of the multitude of snakebite remedies.

Related species: (1) **Field Pussytoes** (*A. neglecta*, not shown) is smaller, and its leaves have 1 prominent nerve or midvein. (2) **Solitary Pussytoes** (*A. solitaria*, not shown) differs from *A. plantaginifolia* in that it has only 1 flowerhead.

SWEET EVERLASTING, RABBIT TOBACCO
Leaves

Gnaphalium obtusifolium L. Composite Family

Soft-hairy biennial; 1–2 ft. Leaves alternate; lance-shaped, without stalks. Flowers dirty white *globular heads* in *spreading* clusters; July–Nov. Flowerheads enclosed by dry, petal-like bracts. **Where found:** Dry soil, fields. Much of our area.

Uses: Leaves and flowers (chewed or in tea) traditionally used for sore throats, pneumonia, colds, fevers, upset stomach, abdominal cramps, asthma, flu, coughs, rheumatism, leukorrhea, bowel disorders, mouth ulcers, hemorrhage, tumors; mild nerve sedative, diuretic, and antispasmodic. Fresh juice considered aphrodisiac.

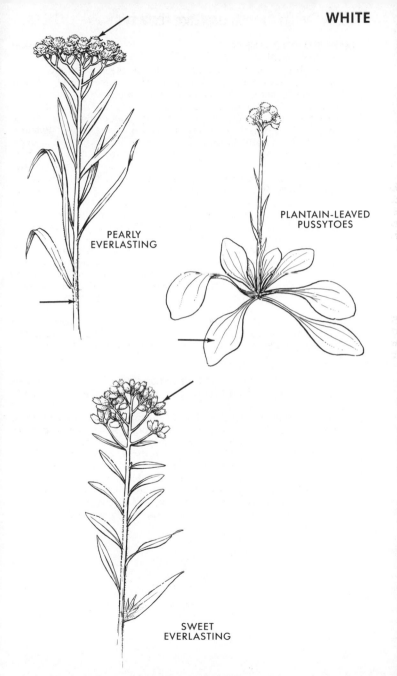

PEARLY
EVERLASTING

PLANTAIN-LEAVED
PUSSYTOES

SWEET
EVERLASTING

MAYWEED, DOG FENNEL
Whole plant

Anthemis cotula L.
Composite Family

Bad-smelling annual; 8–20 in. Leaves finely (thrice-) dissected. Flowers white; May–Nov. Disk flowers studded with *stiff chaff*. **Where found:** Waste places. Throughout our area. Alien.

Uses: Tea used to induce sweating, vomiting; astringent, diuretic. Used for fevers, colds, diarrhea, dropsy, rheumatism, obstructed menses, and headaches. Leaves rubbed on insect stings. **Warning:** Touching or ingesting plant may cause allergies.

FEVERFEW
Leaves

Chrysanthemum parthenium (L.) Bernh.
Composite Family
[*Tanacetum parthenium* (L.) Shultz-Bip.]

Bushy perennial; 1–3 ft. Leaves *pinnately divided into ovate divisions*; coarsely toothed. Flowers daisy-like (but smaller), with a *large disk* and *stubby white rays*; June–Sept. **Where found:** Roadsides. Alien; escaped from cultivation.

Uses: Tea of whole plant a folk remedy for arthritis, colds, fevers, cramps, worms; regulates menses; sedative. Proven effective (1–4 fresh leaves chewed per day) against some migraine headaches, and is antiseptic. **Warning:** May cause dermatitis or allergic reactions. Mouth sores common.

CHICORY
Roots, leaves

Cichorium intybus L.
Composite Family

Flowers usually blue (rarely white or pink). See also p. 198 and C. Pl. 22.

GERMAN, HUNGARIAN, or WILD CHAMOMILE
Flowers

Chamomilla recutita (L.) Rauschert
Composite Family
[*Matricaria chamomilla* L.]   **C. Pl. 35**

Smooth, *apple-scented* annual; 6–24 in. Leaves *finely divided*. Flowers daisy-like, ¾ in. across; receptacle hollow within. Flowers May–Oct. **Where found:** Locally abundant. Much of our area. Alien.

Uses: Dried flowers make a famous beverage tea, traditionally used for colic, diarrhea, insomnia, indigestion, gout, sciatica, headaches, colds, fevers, flu, cramps, and arthritis. Flowers also a folk cancer remedy. Experimentally, essential oil is antifungal, antibacterial, anodyne, antispasmodic, anti-inflammatory, and anti-allergenic. **Warning:** Ragweed allergy sufferers may react to Chamomile, too.

MAYWEED

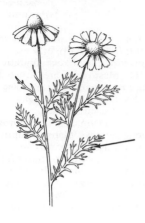

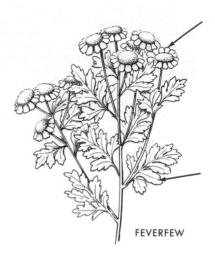

FEVERFEW

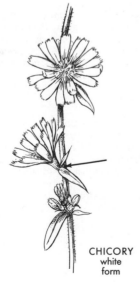

CHICORY
white
form

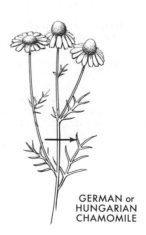

GERMAN or
HUNGARIAN
CHAMOMILE

GRASSLIKE OR LINEAR LEAVES; MOIST SOILS

SWEETFLAG, CALAMUS   Rootstock
Acorus americanus (Raf.) Raf.   **C. Pl. 5**   Arum Family
[*Acorus calamus* L.]
Strongly aromatic, colony-forming perennial; 1–4 ft. *Root jointed.*
Cattail-like leaves, with a *vertical midrib.* Flowers tightly packed
on a fingerlike spadix, jutting *at an angle* from leaflike stalk; May–
Aug. **Where found:** Pond edges, wet fields. Most of our area.
Uses: Dried-root tea (or chewed root) used as aromatic bitter for gas,
stomachaches, indigestion, heartburn, fevers, colds, and coughs; antispasmodic, anticonvulsant, and CNS-depressant. In India, used as
aphrodisiac. American Indians nibbled root for stomach ailments, to
assuage thirst, and as a stimulant on long journeys. German studies
show that for maximum efficacy and safety against spasms, diploid
American strains, devoid of beta-asarone, should be used. Oils devoid
of beta-asarone showed spasmolytic properties comparable to those
of standard antihistaminic drugs. Controlled dosage of root helped
lower serum cholesterol levels in rabbit studies. **Warning:** Some
strains said to contain the carcinogen beta-asarone. Vapors from
roots repel some insects.

ASPARAGUS   Root, shoots, seeds
Asparagus officinalis L.   Lily Family
Perennial; 6 ft. or more. Leaves *finely fernlike* (actually branches
functioning as leaves). Flowers seldom noticed. Fruits reddish. June.
Where found: Garden escape. Throughout our area. Alien.
Uses: Spring shoots a popular vegetable. Asian Indians report aspar-
agine (in shoots) is a good diuretic in dropsy and gout. Japanese report
green asparagus aids protein conversion into amino acids. Roots considered diuretic, laxative (due to fiber content), induce sweating.
Chinese report roots can lower blood pressure. Seeds possess antibiotic activity. **Warning:** May cause dermatitis.

YELLOW-EYED GRASS   Root
Xyris caroliniana Walt.   Lily Family
Perennial; 6–36 in., in flower. Leaves *grasslike,* about ⅛ in. wide, ⅓
as long as flower scape. Flowers yellow, 3-petaled, above a *conelike
head* of leathery scales. Differs from about 15 other species in our
range in that flower stalks are 2-ribbed, opposite, sheathed. Flowers
June–Sept. Seeds 13-ribbed. Variable. **Where found:** Moist sandy soil.
Cen. Me. to Fla.; La. to Wisc.
Uses: American Indians used root tea for diarrhea.

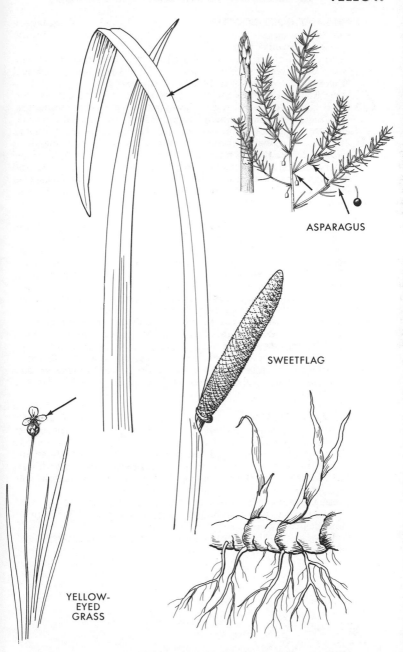

YELLOW

ASPARAGUS

SWEETFLAG

YELLOW-
EYED
GRASS

CUPLIKE FLOWERS (AT LEAST WHEN YOUNG)

MARSH-MARIGOLD, COWSLIP   **Root, leaves**
Caltha palustris L.   Buttercup Family
Aquatic perennial with a *succulent hollow* stem. Leaves *glossy,
heart- or kidney-shaped*. Flowers like a large buttercup (to 1½ in.
wide); deep yellow, with 5–9 "petals" (actually sepals); April–June.
Where found: Swamps, wet ditches. Most of our area.

Uses: Root tea induces sweating, emetic, expectorant. Leaf tea diuretic, laxative. Ojibwas mixed tea with maple sugar to make a
cough syrup that was popular with colonists. Syrup used as a folk
antidote to snake venom. Contains anemonin and protoanemonin,
both with marginal antitumor activity. **Warning:** All parts may irritate and blister skin or mucous membranes. Sniffing bruised stems
induces sneezing. Intoxication has resulted from the use of the raw
leaves in salads or using the raw flower buds as substitutes for capers.
Do not confuse with American White or False Hellebore, which is
toxic (see p. 104).

SPATTERDOCK, YELLOW POND LILY   **Root**
Nuphar luteum (L.) Sibthorp and Smith   Water-lily Family
Aquatic perennial. Leaves round-oval; *base V-notched*; leaves sub-
mersed or erect above water. Flowers yellow, cuplike; stigma disk-
like; May–Sept. **Where found:** Ponds, slow-moving water. Canada
south to S.C.; west to Ill., Iowa.

Uses: American Indians used root tea for "sexual irritability," blood
diseases, chills with fever, heart trouble; poulticed on swellings, inflammations, wounds, contusions, boils. Elsewhere, roots used for
gum, skin, and stomach inflammations. Folk remedy for impotence;
rhizome contains steroids. Alkaloids reportedly hypotensive, antispasmodic, cardioactive, tonic; vasoconstrictor. Like many other species, this plant contains antagonistic alkaloids, one hypotensive, one
hypertensive. Can the human body select the one it needs? **Warning:**
Large doses of root potentially **toxic.**

PRICKLY-PEAR CACTUS   **Pads, fruits**
Opuntia humifusa (Raf.) Raf.   **C. Pl. 37**   Cactus Family
[*O. compressa* (Salisbury) McBride]
Cactus; to 1 ft. Jointed pads have tufts of bristles, usually sharp-
spined. Large, showy yellow flowers; May–Aug. **Where found:** Dry
soils. Mass. to Fla.; Texas to Minn. Our most common eastern cactus.
Uses: American Indians poulticed peeled pads on wounds; applied
juice of fruits to warts; drank pad tea for lung ailments. In folk medicine, peeled pads poulticed for rheumatism; juice used for "gravel"
(kidney stones); baked pads used for gout, chronic ulcers, and
wounds.

YELLOW

MARSH-MARIGOLD

SPATTERDOCK

PRICKLY-PEAR
CACTUS

FOUR-PETALED FLOWERS IN TERMINAL CLUSTERS; MUSTARDS

WINTER CRESS   **Leaves**
Barbarea vulgaris R. Brown   **C. Pl. 7**   Mustard Family
Highly variable, smooth-stemmed mustard; 1–2 ft. Lower leaves
with 4–8 lateral, *earlike* lobes; uppermost leaves *clasping, cut,
toothed.* Flowers deep yellow; April–Aug. Seedpods (silique) mostly
erect, *short-beaked;* fruit stalks more slender than the pods. **Where
found:** Wet fields. Ont. to S.C.; Ark., Okla. to Ill. Alien.
Uses: Cherokees ate greens as a "blood purifier." The leaf tea was
taken once every half hour to suppress coughs. Tea thought to stimulate appetite; diuretic, used against scurvy. Europeans poulticed
leaves on wounds. **Warning:** Although this plant has been described
as an edible wild food, studies indicate it may cause kidney mal-
functions. Internal use should be avoided.

BLACK MUSTARD   **Seed, leaves, oil**
Brassica nigra (L.) Koch   Mustard Family
Annual; 2–3 ft. Lower leaves bristly, coarsely lobed; upper leaves
lance-shaped, with no hairs. Flowers yellow; June–Oct. Pods *hug
stem.* **Where found:** Waste places. Throughout our area. Alien.
Uses: Leaves and seeds irritant, emetic. Leaf poultice used for rheumatism, chilblains, toothaches, headaches. Seeds eaten as a tonic
and appetite stimulant, for fevers, croup, asthma, bronchial conditions. Ground seeds used as a snuff for headaches. **Warning:** Allyl
isothiocyanate (responsible for mustard flavor) is a strong irritant.
May blister skin. Eating large quantities may cause red, burnlike skin
blotches, sometimes developing into ulcers.

FIELD or WILD MUSTARD   **Seeds**
Brassica rapa L.   Mustard Family
Succulent, gray-green, annual herb; 24–32 in. Lower leaves sparsely
toothed or divided. Differs from other *Brassica* species in that the
upper leaves *clasp the stem,* with *earlike lobes.* Flowers pale yellow;
June–Oct. Pods erect, slender-beaked. **Where found:** Fields. Throughout our area. Alien (Eurasia).
Uses: Crushed ripe seeds poulticed on burns. Like some other mustard family members, it contains factors that the National Cancer
Institute has suggested may prevent certain cancers. Leafy vegetables
of many wild and cultivated Brassicas (cabbage, cauliflowers, broc-
coli, collards, kale, kohlrabi, mustard, rape, turnips, etc.) are rich in
vitamins A and C, fiber, and isothiocyanates, all cited by the National Cancer Institute as having some cancer-preventing activity.

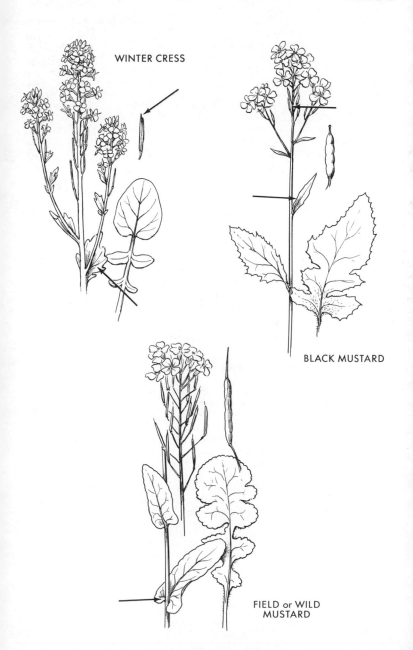

WINTER CRESS

BLACK MUSTARD

FIELD or WILD
MUSTARD

CELANDINE
Stem juice, roots, leaves

Chelidonium majus L.   **C. Pl. 7**   Poppy Family
Smooth-stemmed biennial; 1–2 ft. Stems brittle; *yellow juice within.* Leaves divided; *round-toothed or lobed.* Flowers yellow, 4-petaled; to ¾ in. across; April–Aug. Seedpods *smooth, linear, 2-valved.* **Where found:** Waste places. Much of our area. Alien (Europe). **Uses:** Fresh stem juice a folk remedy (used externally) for warts, eczema, ringworm, corns. Root tincture once used by physicians for inflammations, hemorrhoids; taken internally for jaundice, lung ailments, diuretic. Fresh leaves once used for amenorrhea; poulticed for wounds. Folk cancer remedy in China. **Warning: Toxic.** Stem juice highly irritating, allergenic, may cause paralysis.

ST. ANDREW'S CROSS
Root, leaves

Hypericum hypericoides (L.) Crantz.   St. Johnswort Family
Variable, smooth subshrub (somewhat woody); 1–2½ ft. Leaves linear-oblong; in pairs. Flowers terminal, solitary, with 4 sepals; *1 pair of sepals large and leaflike,* the other pair *tiny or lacking; narrow* yellow petals form a cross. Flowers July–Aug. **Where found:** Sandy soil. Mass. to Fla.; e. Texas to Ill.
Uses: American Indians chewed the root for snakebites; root tea used for colic, fevers, pain, toothaches, diarrhea, dysentery; externally, as a wash for ulcerated breasts. Leaf tea used for bladder and kidney ailments, skin problems, and children's diarrhea. **Warning:** May cause photodermatitis (see *H. perforatum,* p. 114).

COMMON EVENING-PRIMROSE
Seeds, root, leaves

Oenothera biennis L.   **C. Pl. 24**   Evening-primrose Family
Biennial; 1–8 ft. Leaves *numerous,* lance-shaped. Flowers yellow, with 4 broad petals; June–Sept. *Sepals drooping, stigma X-shaped.* Flowers bloom after sunset, unfolding before the eyes of those who watch them open, hence the common name. **Where found:** Roadsides, fields. Throughout our area.
Uses: American Indians used root tea for obesity, bowel pains; poulticed root for piles, bruises; rubbed root on muscles to give athletes strength. Recent research suggests seed oil may be useful for atopic eczema, allergy-induced eczema, asthma, migraines, inflammations, premenstrual syndrome, breast problems, metabolic disorders, diabetes, arthritis, and alcoholism. Research has demonstrated that extracts of this plant can alleviate imbalances and abnormalities of essential fatty acids in prostaglandin production. Evening-primrose oil is a natural source of gamma-linolenic acid.

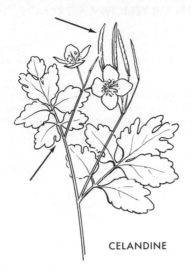

CELANDINE

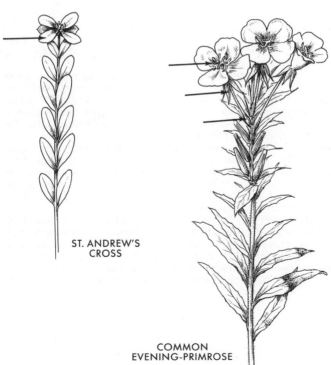

ST. ANDREW'S
CROSS

COMMON
EVENING-PRIMROSE

YELLOW OR YELLOWISH ORCHIDS

ADAM-AND-EVE ROOT, PUTTYROOT   Root
Aplectrum hyemale (Muhl.) Torr.   Orchid Family
Perennial; 10–16 in. Large single leaf with *distinct pleats* (folds) or
often white lines; leaf lasts through winter, shrivels before plant
flowers. Flowers yellowish to greenish white; *lips purple, crinkle-
edged;* May–June. **Where found:** Rich woods. Que., Vt. to Ga.; west
to Ark., e. Kans., s. Minn. Leave it be! Too rare to harvest.
Uses: American Indians poulticed roots on boils. Root tea formerly
used for bronchial troubles.

SPOTTED CORALROOT   Root
Corallorhiza maculata Raf.   **C. Pl. 17**   Orchid Family
Brownish — *no chlorophyll.* 8–20 in. Stalk *sheathed,* leafless. Flowers grayish yellow to dull purple, with purple-red spots; July–Aug.
Where found: On leaf mold, in woods. Nfld. to N.C.; Ohio, S.D., and
westward. Five species (apparently used interchangeably) occur in
our area.
Uses: Folk remedy for colds, "breaking fevers"; induces profuse
sweating, which reduces temperature. Root tea also used for bronchial irritation, coughs. American Indians used root tea as a blood
"strengthener."

LARGE YELLOW LADY'S-SLIPPER,
AMERICAN VALERIAN   Root
Cypripedium calceolus var. *pubescens* Correll   Orchid Family
[*Cypripedium pubescens* Willd.]
Variable, mostly hairy perennial; 8–36 in. Leaves broadly lance-
shaped; *alternate* on stem. Flowers yellow, often purple-streaked;
May–July. **Where found:** Rich woods, bogs. Nfld. to Ga.; Mo., Kans.
to Minn. Too rare to harvest. Yellow Lady's-slippers were probably
once more common, but heavy harvesting for medicinal use in the
last century decreased populations.
Uses: Lady's-slippers, called "American Valerian," were widely used
in 19th-century America as a sedative for nervous headaches, hysteria, insomnia, nervous irritability, mental depression from sexual
abuse, and menstrual irregularities accompanied by despondency
(PMS?). Active compounds not water-soluble. **Warning:** All lady's-
slippers may cause dermatitis.
Related species: (1) *Cypripedium calceolus* var. *parviflora* (not
shown) is a smaller plant (to 8 in.) with a more northerly range. The
petals are usually more twisted and burgundy-purple to light brown.
It is only slightly hairy compared to its larger relative. (2) The **Pink
Lady's-slipper** (*C. acaule,* p. 138) was considered a substitute for the
more commonly used Yellow Lady's-slippers; its properties were
considered analogous.

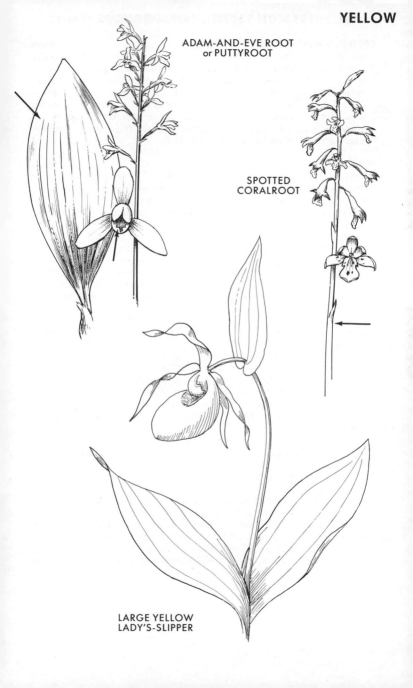

**ADAM-AND-EVE ROOT
or PUTTYROOT**

**SPOTTED
CORALROOT**

**LARGE YELLOW
LADY'S-SLIPPER**

FLOWERS WITH 5 PETALS; LOW-GROWING PLANTS

CREEPING WOOD-SORREL   **Leaves**
Oxalis corniculata L.   Wood-sorrel Family
Creeping perennial; 6–10 in. Leaves cloverlike, with large, brownish stipules. Flowers yellow; April to frost. Seedpods *deflexed*. **Where found:** Waste places. Throughout. Alien.

⚠️ **Uses:** Sour, acidic leaves were once chewed for nausea, mouth sores, sore throats. Fresh leaves were poulticed on cancers, old sores, ulcers. Leaf tea used for fevers, urinary infections, and scurvy. **Warning:** Large doses may cause oxalate poisoning.

PURSLANE   **Leaves**
Portulaca oleracea L.   **C. Pl. 21**   Purslane Family
Prostrate, *smooth*, fleshy annual; to 1 ft. Stems often reddish and forking. Leaves spatula-shaped, *fleshy*. Flowers tiny, yellowish; in leaf rosettes; June–Nov. **Where found:** Waste ground. Throughout our area. Alien.
Uses: American Indians adopted the plant as a poultice for burns, juice for earaches, tea for headaches, stomachaches. Plant juice said to alleviate caterpillar stings; used in Europe for inflammation, sores, painful urination (strangury). Reportedly hypotensive and diuretic. Leaves best known as a wild edible; very nutritious. Recently cited as a vegetarian source of omega-3 fatty acids, though rapeseed and walnuts are magnitudes richer.

DWARF CINQUEFOIL   **Whole plant**
Potentilla canadensis L.   Rose Family
Prostrate perennial, on cylindrical rhizomes; 2–10 in. Leaves palmate; leaflets rounded, *sharply toothed above middle*, strongly wedge-shaped at base. Flowers yellow; March–June. Petals 5, rounded. **Where found:** Fields, woods. N.S. to S.C.; Mo. to Minn.
Uses: American Indians used tea of pounded roots to treat diarrhea; considered astringent. Other cinquefoils are considered astringent as well.

INDIAN STRAWBERRY   **Whole plant, flowers**
Duchesnea indica L.   Rose Family
Small, creeping perennial; to 6 in. Leaves *strawberry-like*. Flowers *yellow*; 3-toothed bracts *longer than petals and sepals*. Flowers April–July. *Strawberry-like* fruit insipid. **Where found:** Yards, waste places. Most of our area. Asian alien.
Uses: In Asia, whole plant poultice or wash (astringent) used for abscesses, boils, burns, insect stings, eczema, ringworm, rheumatism, traumatic injuries. Whole-plant tea used for laryngitis, coughs, lung ailments. Flower tea traditionally used to stimulate blood circulation.

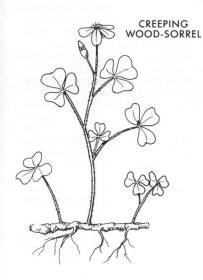

**CREEPING
WOOD-SORREL**

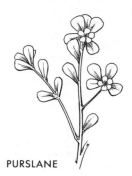

PURSLANE

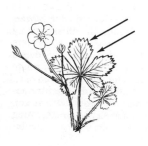

**DWARF
CINQUEFOIL**

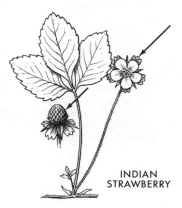

**INDIAN
STRAWBERRY**

FLOWERS IN AXILS, WITH 5 PETALS OR PARTS; LEAVES ALTERNATE

VELVET LEAF   **Leaves, roots, seeds**
Abutilon theophrasti Medic.   Mallow Family
Annual; 3–6 ft. *Entire plant velvety.* Leaves heart-shaped, *large* (4–10 in. long), irregularly toothed. *Single* yellow flowers, each 1–1½ in. across, in leaf axils; June–Nov. Fruit sections beaked. **Where found:** Waste places. Throughout our area. Alien (India).
Uses: Chinese use 1 ounce dried leaf in tea for dysentery, fevers; poultice for ulcers. Dried root used in tea for dysentery and urinary incontinence. Seed powder diuretic; eaten for dysentery, stomachaches. CNS-depressant in mice experiments.

FROSTWEED   **Whole plant, root**
Helianthemum canadense (L.) Michx.   Rockrose Family
Perennial; 6–20 in. Leaves alternate, lance-shaped, *toothless*, green on upper surface; basal leaves absent. First flower *solitary*, yellow, 5-petaled, stamens many; later flowers without petals, few stamens. Flowers May–June. **Where found:** Dry sandy soil, rocky woods. Que., s. Me. to N.C.; Tenn. to Ill., Minn.
Uses: American Indians used leaf tea for kidney ailments, sore throats; "strengthening" medicine. Patients were covered by a blanket "tent" to hold steam; feet soaked in hot tea for arthritis, muscular swellings, and rheumatism. Historically, physicians once used a strong tea for scrofula (tuberculous swelling of lymph nodes), for which it was reported to produce astonishing cures; also diarrhea, dysentery, and syphilis. Externally, used as a wash for skin diseases such as prurigo, and eye infections; gargled for throat infections. Leaves poulticed on "scrofulous tumors and ulcers."

CLAMMY GROUND-CHERRY   **Leaves, root, seeds**
Physalis heterophylla Nees.   Nightshade Family
Perennial; 1–3 ft. Stem sticky-hairy; upper part of stem with slender, soft, wide-spreading hairs. Leaves oval, coarsely toothed; *base rounded*, with *few teeth*. Flower greenish yellow, bell-like; center brownish; June–Sept. Fruit enclosed in a papery bladder. **Where found:** Dry clearings. N.S. to Fla.; Texas to Minn. The most abundant of about 12 highly variable species in our range.
Uses: American Indians used tea of leaves and roots for headaches; wash for burns, scalds; in herbal compounds to induce vomiting for bad stomachaches; root and leaves poulticed for wounds. Seed of this and other *Physalis* species are considered useful for difficult urination, fevers, inflammation, various urinary disorders. Plant compounds are being researched for antitumor activity. **Warning:** Potentially **toxic.**

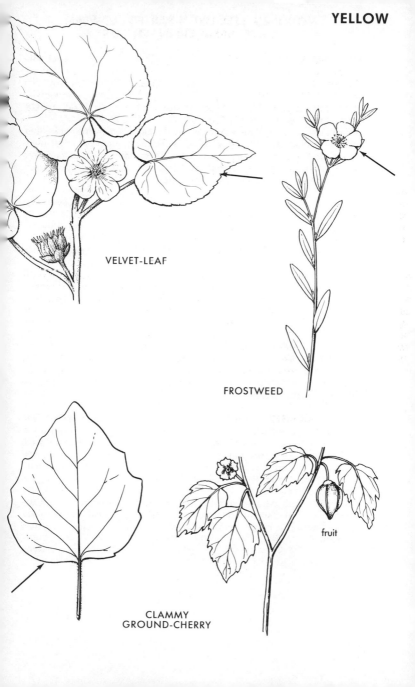

VELVET-LEAF

FROSTWEED

CLAMMY
GROUND-CHERRY

fruit

NODDING, BELL-LIKE, 6-PARTED FLOWERS; LEAVES BASAL OR IN WHORLS

CLINTONIA, BLUEBEARD LILY   Leaf, root
Clintonia borealis (Ait.) Raf.   Lily Family
Perennial; 4–12 in. Leaves basal; leathery, shiny, entire (not
toothed). Flowers bell-like, on a leafless stalk; yellow (or greenish);
May–July. Berries blue. **Where found:** Cool woods. Nfld. to Ga.
mountains; west to Wisc., Minn.
Uses: American Indians poulticed fresh leaves on burns, old sores,
bruises, infections, rabid-dog bites; drank tea of plant for heart medicine, diabetes; root used to aid labor in childbirth. Root contains
anti-inflammatory and estrogenic diosgenin, from which progesterone is made. Science should investigate.

TROUT-LILY   Leaves, root
Erythronium americanum L.   **C. Pl. 11**   Lily Family
Perennial; to 1 ft., with 1–2 *mottled*, lance-shaped leaves. Flowers
lily-like, yellow; March–May. *Petals strongly curved back.* **Where
found:** Moist woods, often in colonies. N.S. to Ga.; Ark., Okla. to
Minn.
Uses: American Indians used root tea for fevers, leaf poultice for
hard-to-heal ulcers and scrofula. Iroquois women ate raw leaves to
prevent conception. Root poultice was used to draw out splinters,
reduce swelling. Fresh and recently dried leaves and roots were considered emetic, expectorant. Water extracts are active against gram-
positive and gram-negative bacteria.
Related species: In **White Trout-lily** (*E. albidum*, not shown), flowers
are white, leaves seldom mottled; it is found from Ont. to Ga.; Ky.,
Ark., Okla. to Minn. Components of *E. grandiflorum* (not shown), a
plant that grows in western N. America, have been shown to be
slightly antimutagenic.

INDIAN CUCUMBER   Root, leaves, fruit
Medeola virginiana L.   Lily Family
Perennial; 1–3 ft. Leaves oval; 6–10, in *1 or 2 whorls* (plants with
only 1 whorl usually do not flower). Flowers yellow, *drooping*; stamens red to purplish, petals and sepals curved back. Flowers April–
June. **Where found:** Rich, moist wooded slopes. N.S. to Fla.; Ala., La.
north to Minn.
Uses: Cucumber-flavored root is crisp, edible; American Indians
chewed root and spit it on hook to make fish bite. Leaf and berry tea
administered to babies with convulsions. Root tea once used as a
diuretic for dropsy.

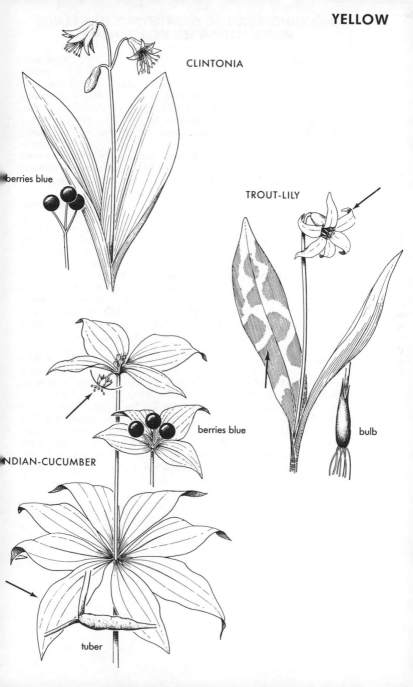

YELLOW

CLINTONIA

berries blue

TROUT-LILY

INDIAN-CUCUMBER

berries blue

bulb

tuber

NODDING, BELL-LIKE, 6-PARTED FLOWERS; LEAVES PERFOLIATE OR SESSILE; BELLWORTS

LARGE BELLWORT   Root, plant
Uvularia grandiflora J.E. Sm.   Lily Family
Perennial; 6–20 in. Solitary or growing in small stands. Leaves oval to lance-shaped, *not glaucous;* clasping or perfoliate; *white-downy beneath.* Leaves have a wilted appearance. Flower a yellow-orange, drooping bell; petals *smooth* within, twisted. Flowers April–June.
Where found: Rich woods. S. Que. to Ga. mountains; Ark. to e. Kans., e. N.D.
Uses: American Indians used the root tea as a wash for rheumatic pains; in fat as an ointment for sore muscles and tendons, rheumatism, backaches. Plant poulticed to relieve toothaches and swellings. Root tea once used for stomach and lung ailments.

PERFOLIATE BELLWORT   Root
Uvularia perfoliata L.   Lily Family
Perennial, forming colonies; 6–18 in. Leaves long-oval; *smooth beneath. Stem* perfoliate — *appears to pass through leaf.* Flowers yellow-orange bells; petals *rough-granular* on inner surface. Flowers April–June. **Where found:** Thin woods. S. Vt. to Fla.; La. to Ont.
Uses: American Indians used root tea as a cough medicine and for sore mouth, sore throat, inflamed gums, and snakebites. Formerly used as a substitute for Large Yellow Lady's-slipper (see p. 94); in tea or ointment for herpes, sore ears, mouth sores, mild cases of erysipelas (acute local skin inflammation and swelling).

WILD OATS   Roots
Uvularia sessilifolia L.   Lily Family
Perennial; 6–12 in. Leaves sessile, *not surrounding stems* as in above species; glaucous beneath. Stem *forked* about ⅔ of way up from the ground. Flowers pale, straw-colored bells; May–June. **Where found:** Alluvial woods, thickets. N.B. to Ga.; Ala. to Ark., north to N.D.
Uses: American Indians used the root tea to treat diarrhea and as a "blood purifier"; taken internally to aid in healing broken bones. Poulticed for boils and broken bones. Root a folk medicine for sore throats and mouth sores; said to be mucilaginous (slimy) and somewhat acrid-tasting when fresh.

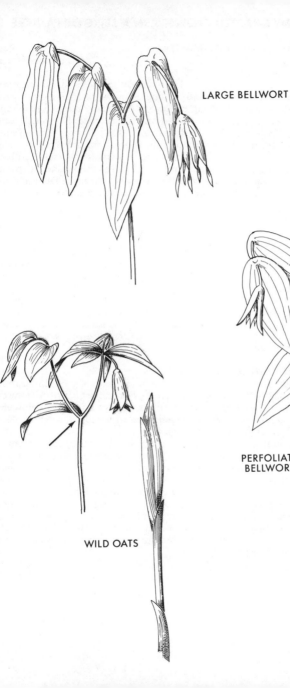

LARGE BELLWORT

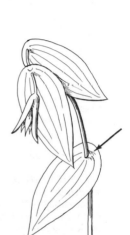

PERFOLIATE
BELLWORT

WILD OATS

FALSE ALOE, RATTLESNAKE-MASTER   Root
Manfreda virginica (L.) Salisb.   Amaryllis Family
[*Agave virginica* L.]   **C. Pl. 37**
Leaves *radiating from root;* lance-shaped, smooth, *fleshy* (mottled purple in form *tigrina*); to 16 in. long. Flowers greenish white to yellow, tubular; fragrant at night. Flowers 6-parted; scattered in a *loose spike on a 3- to 6-ft. stalk;* June–July. **Where found:** Dry soils. Ohio, N.C., W. Va. to Fla.; west to Texas; north to s. Ill.
Uses: American Indians used diuretic root tea for dropsy. Wash used for snakebites. Root nibbled for severe diarrhea, worms; laxative. Like species of *Agave,* this plant might be used as a source for steroid synthesis. **Warning:** May produce a strongly irritating latex. Do not confuse with another plant called Rattlesnake-master (*Eryngium yuccifolium,* p. 18).

DEVIL'S-BIT   Root
Chamaelirium luteum (L.) Gray   Lily Family
Perennial; to 3 ft. (in flower). Leaves smooth, oblong, in basal rosettes. *Male and female flowers on separate plants.* Flowers yellowish, *in crowded spikes* (usually drooping at tip); May–July. **Where found:** Rich woods. W. Mass., N.Y. to Fla.; Ark. to Ill., Mich.
Uses: Small doses of powdered root used for colic, stomach ailments, appetite stimulant, indigestion, and to expel worms. Root tea said to be a uterine tonic. Used for a wide variety of ailments associated with male and female reproductive organs. **Warning:** Avoid during pregnancy.

AMERICAN WHITE or FALSE HELLEBORE   Root
Veratrum viride Ait.   Lily Family
Perennial; 2–8 ft. Leaves large, broadly oval; *strongly ribbed.* Flowers yellowish, turning dull green; small, *star-shaped,* in a many-flowered panicle; April–July. **Where found:** Wet wood edges, swamps. New England to Ga. mountains; Tenn. to Wisc.
Uses: Historically valued as an analgesic for pain, epilepsy, convulsions, pneumonia, heart sedative; weak tea used for sore throat, tonsillitis. Used in pharmaceutical drugs to slow heart rate, lower blood pressure; also for arteriosclerosis and forms of nephritis. Components of the plant (alkaloids) are known to slow heart rate, reduce systolic and diastolic pressure, and stimulate peripheral blood flow to the kidneys, liver, and extremities. Powdered root used in insecticides. **Warning: All parts, especially the root, are highly or fatally toxic.** Leaves have been mistaken, then eaten, for Pokeweed (see p. 56) or Marsh-marigold (p. 88).

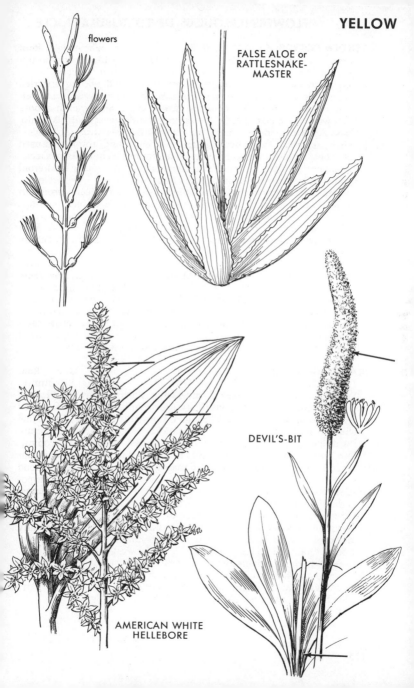

YELLOW

flowers

FALSE ALOE or
RATTLESNAKE-
MASTER

DEVIL'S-BIT

AMERICAN WHITE
HELLEBORE

FLOWERS IRREGULAR, LIPPED, TUBULAR

GOLDEN CORYDALIS **Whole plant, root**
Corydalis aurea (Muhl.) Willd. **C. Pl. 11** Bleeding-heart Family
Perennial; 6–16 in. Leaves finely dissected. Flowers yellow, ½ in. long, with a *blunt spur* at back; upper petal toothed, *without a wing*. Other yellow *Corydalis* species in our area have a projecting wing on the top petal. Flowers March–May. **Where found:** Sandy, rocky soils, open woods. Canada to N.Y., W. Va. mountains; west to Ill., Mo.
Uses: American Indians used tea for painful menstruation, backaches, diarrhea, bronchitis, heart diseases, sore throats, stomachaches; inhaled fumes of burning roots for headaches. Historically, physicians used tea for menstrual irregularities, dysentery, diarrhea, recent syphilitic nodes, and related afflictions.
Related species: Roots of several Chinese *Corydalis* species are used for menstrual irregularities, pain, and hemorrhage. Chinese studies show that alkaloids from the genus are muscle relaxants, painkillers, and inhibit gastric secretions, suggesting usefulness against ulcers. **Warning:** *Corydalis* species are potentially **toxic** in moderate doses.

YELLOW JEWELWEED, PALE TOUCH-ME-NOT **Leaves, stem juice**
Impatiens pallida Nutt. Touch-me-not Family
Annual; 3–5 ft. Similar to Spotted Touch-me-not (*I. capensis*, p. 136) but flowers *yellow*, spurs shorter. Seedpods explode when touched. **Where found:** Wet, shady, limey soils. Nfld. to Ga. mountains; Ark. to Kans.
Uses: Crushed leaves are poulticed on recent poison-ivy rash.

BUTTER-AND-EGGS **Whole plant**
Linaria vulgaris Mill. **C. Pl. 23** Figwort Family
Perennial; 1–3 ft. Leaves many; lance-shaped. Flowers yellow, *orange-marked*; *snapdragon-like, with drooping spurs*; June–Oct. **Where found:** Waste places. Throughout our area. Alien.
Uses: In folk medicine, leaf tea used as a laxative, strong diuretic; for dropsy, jaundice, enteritis with drowsiness, skin diseases, piles. Ointment made from flowers used for piles, skin eruptions. A "tea" made in milk has been used as an insecticide.

LOUSEWORT, WOOD BETONY **Root, leaves**
Pedicularis canadensis L. **C. Pl. 12** Figwort Family
Perennial; 5–10 in. Leaves mostly basal; lance-shaped, deeply incised. Flowers *hooded*, like miniature snapdragons; yellow, reddish (or both), in tight terminal clusters; April–June. **Where found:** Open woods. Que., Me. to Fla.; Texas to Man. and westward.
Uses: American Indians used root tea for stomachaches, diarrhea, anemia, and heart trouble; also in cough medicines; poulticed for swellings, tumors, sore muscles. Finely grated roots were secretly added to food as an alleged aphrodisiac. Not currently studied.

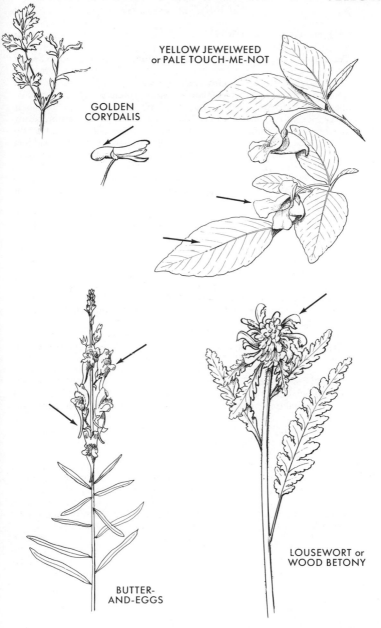

GOLDEN
CORYDALIS

YELLOW JEWELWEED
or PALE TOUCH-ME-NOT

BUTTER-
AND-EGGS

LOUSEWORT or
WOOD BETONY

5 OR MORE PETALS; LEAVES COMPOUND OR STRONGLY DIVIDED

SMALL-FLOWERED AGRIMONY   **Whole plant**
Agrimonia parviflora Ait.   Rose Family
Perennial; 3–6 ft. Stem hairy. Leaves divided; main stem leaves with
11–19 unequal leaflets. Leaflets smooth above, hairy below; strongly
serrated, 1–3 in. long. Tiny yellow flowers, *in slender branched
wands;* July–Sept. **Where found:** Damp thickets, in clumps. W.
Conn., N.Y. to Fla.; e. Texas north to Neb., s. Ont.
Uses: Herbal tea (made from whole plant) astringent, stops bleeding;
used for wounds, diarrhea, inflammation of gall bladder, urinary incontinence, jaundice, and gout. Thought to "strengthen" blood and
aid food assimilation. Gargled for mouth ulcers, throat inflammation.
Related species: *Agrimonia eupatoria* (European alien) is used similarly; in France it is drunk as much for its flavor as for its medicinal
virtues. Tea of the European species is believed to be helpful in diarrhea, blood disorders, fevers, gout, hepatitis, pimples, sore throats,
and even worms. In studies with mice, the European species *A. pi-
losa* has shown antitumor activity.

GOAT'S BEARD   **Root**
Aruncus dioicus (Walter) Fern.   Rose Family
Shrublike; 4–6 ft. Leaves mainly basal; divided into large, serrated,
oval leaflets. Tiny, yellowish white flowers, *crowded in spikes on a
pyramidal plume;* March–May. **Where found:** Rich woods, stream
banks. Ky. to Ga.; west to Okla.; north to Iowa.
Uses: Cherokees poulticed pounded root on bee stings. Root tea
used to allay bleeding after childbirth and to reduce profuse urination. Tea also used externally, to bathe swollen feet.

COMMON or TALL BUTTERCUP   **Root, leaves**
Ranunculus acris L.   Buttercup Family
Erect annual or perennial; 2–3 ft. Leaves palmately divided into *5–7
stalkless, lance-shaped, toothed segments.* Flowers shiny; golden
yellow within, lighter outside; May–Sept. Fruits flat, *smooth, with
distinct margins.* **Where found:** Fields. Throughout our area, but
mostly absent from prairies. Alien (Europe).

Uses: Fresh leaves historically used as external rubefacient in rheumatism, arthritis, neuralgia. American Indians poulticed root for
boils, abscesses. Action based on irritating affected part. **Warning:**
Extremely acrid, causing intense pain and burning of mouth, mucous
membranes; blisters skin. **Avoid use.** Similar warning applies to
other buttercups, and many other plants in the buttercup family.

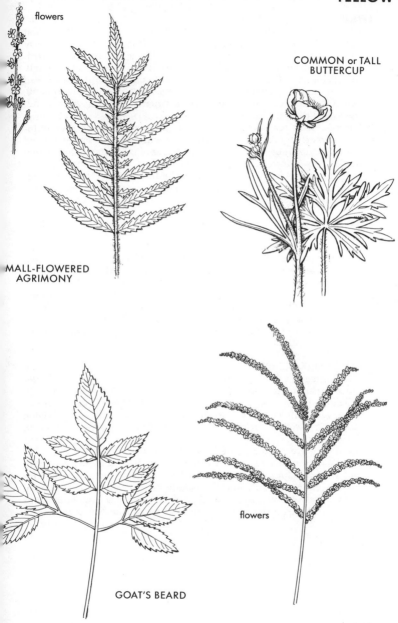

YELLOW

flowers

COMMON or TALL
BUTTERCUP

MALL-FLOWERED
AGRIMONY

GOAT'S BEARD

flowers

FLOWERS IN UMBRELLA-LIKE CLUSTERS (UMBELS)

FENNEL   **Seeds**
Foeniculum vulgare Mill.   **C. Pl. 26**   Parsley Family
Smooth herb; 4–7 ft. *Strongly anise- or licorice-scented.* Leaves
threadlike. Yellowish flowers in flat umbels; June–Sept. **Where
found:** Roadsides. Conn. to Fla.; Neb. to Mich. Very common weed
in California. Alien (Europe). Several different types of Fennel, including annual, biennial and perennial varieties, varying in form and
leaf color are grown in gardens for ornamental, food, flavoring, and
medicinal use.
Uses: Seeds or tea taken to relieve gas, infant colic, stimulate milk
flow. Reportedly diuretic, expectorant, carminative, laxative, soothing to stomach; used to improve the flavor of other medicines. Powdered seeds poulticed in China for snakebites. Experimentally, seed
oil relieves spasms of smooth muscles, kills bacteria, removes hookworms. **Warning:** Fennel or its seed oil may cause contact dermatitis.
Ingestion of oil may cause vomiting, seizures, and pulmonary edema.

WILD PARSNIP   **Root**
Pastinaca sativa L.   Parsley Family
Biennial; 2–5 ft. Stalk *deeply grooved* (ribbed). Leaves in stout rosette in first year, divided into 5–15 stalkless, toothed, oval leaflets.
Tiny golden flowers with 5 petals, in umbels; May–Oct. **Where
found:** Roadsides, waste places. Much of our area. Alien.
Uses: American Indians used roots to treat sharp pains, tea in small
amounts for "female" disorders; poulticed roots on inflammations,
sores. **Warning:** May cause photodermatitis due to xanthotoxin,
which is used to treat psoriasis and vitiligo. Avoid contact and ex-
posure to sunlight.

GOLDEN ALEXANDERS   **Root**
Zizia aurea (L.) W. D. J. Koch   Parsley Family
Smooth perennial; 1–3 ft. Leaves thin; all *twice-compound* with 3–
5 leaflets or divisions, divided again; leaflets *finely sharp-toothed.*
Tiny, yellow flowers in an umbel with 6–20 rays; April–June. **Where
found:** Dry woods, rocky outcrops. New England to Ga.; Texas to
Sask.
Uses: American Indians used root tea for fevers. Historically, the
plant has been referred to as a vulnerary (agent used to heal wounds)
and a sleep inducer; it was also used for syphilis. **Warning:** Possibly
toxic — eating a whole root has caused violent vomiting, which itself was believed to mitigate further adverse reaction. Amateurs fool-
ing with plants in the parsley family are playing herbal roulette.

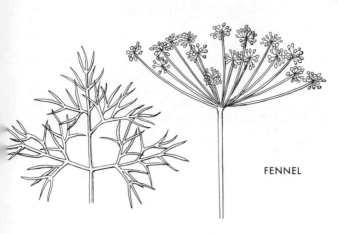

FENNEL

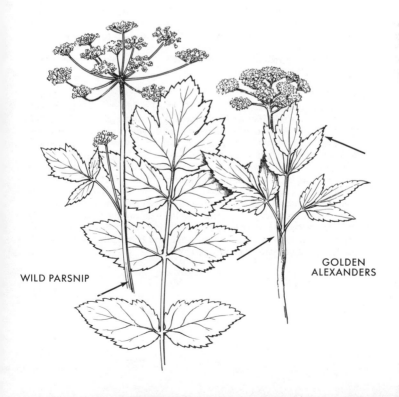

WILD PARSNIP

GOLDEN
ALEXANDERS

YELLOW GIANT HYSSOP
Leaves

Agastache nepetoides (L.) O. Ktze.
Mint Family

Perennial; 3–5 ft. Stems *square*, mostly smooth; branching above. Leaves opposite; narrowly ovate to lance-shaped, sawtoothed. Flowers yellow to whitish, in dense, usually continuous spikes; July–Sept. **Where found:** Rocky wooded hillsides, wood edges. S. Que. to Va.; ne. Texas, e. Okla. to S.D., Minn.

Uses: American Indians used the leaves in a compound mixture to apply to poison-ivy rash.

Remarks: The name *nepetoides* refers to the plant's resemblance to *Nepeta* (Catnip).

STONEROOT, HORSE-BALM
Roots, leaves

Collinsonia canadensis L.
Mint Family

Branching, square-stemmed perennial herb; 2–4 ft. Leaves large, oval, coarsely toothed. Root hard, broader than long. Flowers greenish yellow, *lower lip fringed, stamen strongly protruding*; lemon-like scent; July–Sept. **Where found:** Rich woods. Ont., Vt. to Fla.; Mo. to Wisc.

Uses: Folk uses include leaf poultice for burns, bruises, wounds, sores, sprains; root tea for piles, laryngitis, indigestion, diarrhea, dysentery, dropsy, kidney and bladder ailments. Contains alkaloids; strongly diuretic, useful in cystitis. Roots contain more than 13,000 parts per million of rosmarinic acid, the same anti-oxidant (preservative) found in Rosemary. **Warning:** Minute doses of fresh leaves may cause vomiting.

HORSEMINT
Leaves

Monarda punctata L.　　　**C. Pl. 41**　　　Mint Family

Strongly aromatic biennial or short-lived perennial; 1–4 ft. Leaves lance-shaped. Flowers like gaping mouths; yellowish, purple-dotted; in tiered whorls, *with yellowish to lilac bracts beneath*; July–Oct. **Where found:** Dry soils. L.I. to Fla.; La., Texas, Ark., Kans.

Uses: American Indians used leaf tea for colds, fevers, flu, stomach cramps, coughs, catarrhs, bowel ailments. Historically, doctors used this mint as a carminative, stimulant, digestive, and diuretic, and to regulate menses. Oil high in thymol; antiseptic, expels worms. Thymol, now manufactured synthetically, was once commercially derived from thyme (*Thymus* species). During World War I, commercial thyme fields were destroyed in Europe and Horsemint was grown in the U.S. as a substitute source of thymol.

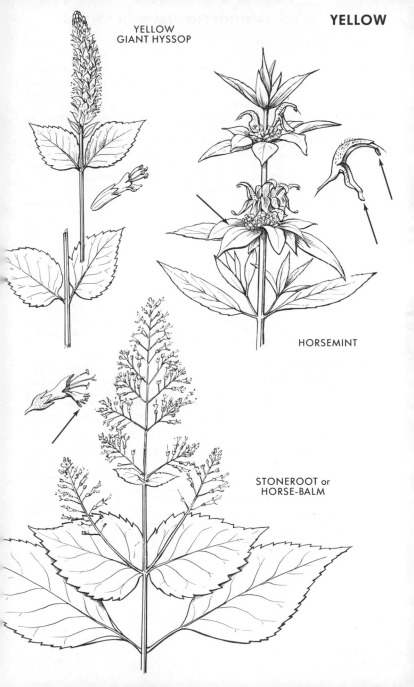

YELLOW
GIANT HYSSOP

HORSEMINT

STONEROOT or
HORSE-BALM

MISCELLANEOUS FLOWERS WITH 5 PETALS

COMMON ST. JOHNSWORT
Leaves, flowers

Hypericum perforatum L.   **C. Pl. 36**   St. Johnswort Family
Perennial; 1–3 ft. Leaves oblong, dotted with translucent glands.
Flowers yellow; stamens in a bushy cluster; petals 5, with *black dots
on margins*. Flowers June–Sept. **Where found:** Fields, roadsides.
Throughout. Alien (Europe).

⚠️ **Uses:** Fresh flowers in tea, tincture, or olive oil, once a popular domestic medicine for treatment of external ulcers, wounds (especially
those with severed nerve tissue), sores, cuts, bruises, etc. Tea a folk
remedy for bladder ailments, depression, dysentery, diarrhea, worms.
Experimentally, sedative, anti-inflammatory, antibacterial. Contains the biologically active compounds choline, pectin, rutin, sitosterol, hypericin, and pseudohypericin. Recent studies (1988) have
found that hypericin and pseudohypericin have potent anti-retroviral
activity, without serious side effects. Being researched for AIDS
treatment. **Warning:** Taken internally or externally, hypericin may
cause photodermatitis (skin burns) on sensitive persons exposed to
light.

WHORLED LOOSESTRIFE
Leaves, root

Lysimachia quadrifolia L.   Primrose Family
Delicate perennial; 1–3 ft. Leaves in *whorls of 4* (3–6). Flowers *yel-
low; red-dotted or streaked*; from leaf axils; May–Aug. **Where found:**
Calcareous bogs, moist thickets. Me to Va., Ga.; Ill. to Wisc.
Uses: American Indians used plant tea for "female ailments," kid-
ney trouble, bowel complaints; root tea emetic.

COMMON MULLEIN
Leaves, flowering tops

Verbascum thapsus L.   **C. Pl. 39**   Figwort Family
Biennial; 1–8 ft. in flower. Leaves, large, broadly oval, *very hairy
(flannel-like)*; hairs branching. Flowers yellow, in tight, long spikes;
July–Sept. **Where found:** Poor soils. Common throughout our area.
Alien (Europe).

⚠️ **Uses:** Traditionally, leaf and flower tea expectorant, demulcent, antispasmodic, diuretic, for chest colds, asthma, bronchitis, coughs,
kidney infections; leaves poulticed for ulcers, tumors, piles; flowers
soaked in olive or mineral oil used as earache drops. Leaves high in
mucilage, soothing to inflamed mucous membranes; experimentally, strongly anti-inflammatory. Asian Indians used the stalk for
cramps, fevers, and migraine. The seed is a narcotic fish poison.
Warning: The leaves contain rotenone and coumarin, neither viewed
with great favor by the FDA. Hairs may irritate skin.

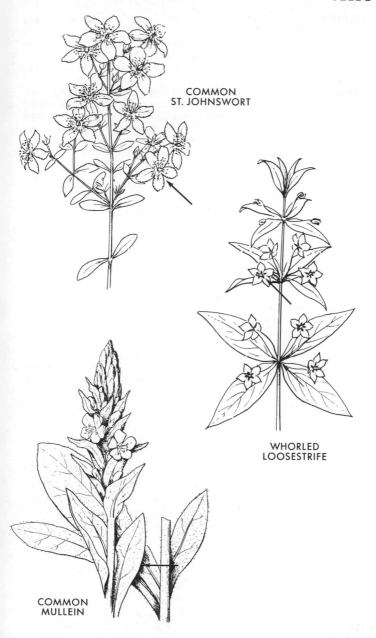

COMMON
ST. JOHNSWORT

WHORLED
LOOSESTRIFE

COMMON
MULLEIN

PEA-LIKE FLOWERS; 3 LEAFLETS

CREAM WILD INDIGO
Baptisia leucophaea Nutt. **C. Pl. 36**

Seeds, roots, leaves

Pea Family

Hairy, bushy perennial; 10–30 in. Leaves with 3 spatula-shaped leaflets. Flowers *cream-yellow*, on showy lateral, drooping racemes, *with large, leaflike bracts beneath*; April–June. **Where found:** Dry soils. Ark., Texas, Neb. to Minn.

Uses: Ointment of seed powder mixed in buffalo fat applied to stomach for colic (by Pawnees). Root tea formerly used for typhoid and scarlet fever; leaf tea in "mercurial salivation"; used externally on cuts and wounds (astringent). Recent research suggests immune-system stimulant activity. **Warning:** Potentially **toxic.**

WILD INDIGO
Baptisia tinctoria (L.) R. Br.

Root

Pea Family

Smooth, blue-glaucous perennial; 1–3 ft. Leaves narrowly cloverlike, nearly stalkless. Flowers yellow, few, on numerous racemes on upper branchlets; May–Sept. **Where found:** Dry open woods, clearings. Va. to Fla.; less common from s. Me. to Ind., se. Minn.

Uses: American Indians used the root tea as an emetic and purgative; cold tea to stop vomiting. A poultice of the root was used for toothaches, to allay inflammation; wash used for cuts, wounds, bruises, and sprains. Historically, fresh root tea considered laxative, astringent, antiseptic. Used for typhus and scarlet fever; gargled for sore throats. Tea used as a wash for leg, arm, and stomach cramps, wounds. Said to stimulate bile secretion. Root poultice for gangrenous ulcers. German studies have shown the extract stimulates the immune system. **Warning:** Large or frequent doses are potentially harmful.

YELLOW SWEET-CLOVER
Melilotus officinalis (L.) Lam. **C. Pl. 22**

Flowering plant

Pea Family

Straggly biennial; 2–6 ft. Leaves in cloverlike arrangement; leaflets narrow, elongate, slightly toothed. Flowers small, yellow, pea-like, in long, tapering spikes; *fragrant when crushed*; April–Oct. **Where found:** Roadsides. Throughout our area. Alien (Europe).

Uses: Dried flowering plant traditionally used in tea for neuralgic headaches, painful urination, nervous stomach, colic, diarrhea with flatulence, painful menstruation with lameness and cold sensation, aching muscles; poulticed for inflammation, ulcers, wounds, rheumatism; smoked for asthma. **Warning:** Moldy hay causes uncontrollable bleeding in cattle due to coumarins. Science has developed compounds like warfarin from such coumarins to prevent blood clotting in rodents.

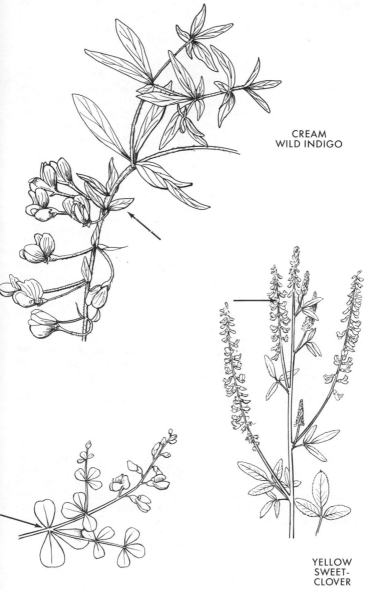

CREAM
WILD INDIGO

YELLOW
SWEET-
CLOVER

WILD INDIGO

LEGUMES (PEA FAMILY); MANY LEAFLETS

WILD SENNA
Leaves, seedpods

Cassia marilandica L.   **C. Pl. 34**   Pea Family

Erect perennial; 3–6 ft. Leaves compound, with 4–8 pairs of elliptical leaflets. Note *rounded gland at base of leaf stalk.* Yellow flowers in loose clusters at leaf axils; July–Aug. Seedpods with joints twice as wide as they are long. **Where found:** Dry thickets. Pa. to Fla.; Kans. to Iowa.

Uses: Powdered leaves or tea given as a strong laxative, also for fevers. One teaspoon of ground Coriander seeds was added to leaf tea to prevent griping (cramps), tea of pods milder, slower-acting. Laxatives made from **Alexandrian Senna** (*C. senna*, Africa) and **Indian Senna** (*C. angustifolia*, India) are found in every pharmacy.

WILD SENSITIVE-PLANT
Roots

Cassia nictitans L.   Pea Family

Perennial; 6–15 in. Leaves *fold when touched.* Leaflets in 6–15 pairs. Flowers yellow, small (¼ in. long), with 5 stamens; July–Sept. **Where found:** Sandy soil. Mass., N.Y. to Fla.; Texas, Kans., Mo. to Ohio.

Uses: Cherokees used root tea with other plants, to relieve fatigue.

Related species: *C. fasciculata* (not shown) has been used similarly.

SICKLEPOD
Leaves, seeds

Cassia obtusifolia L.   **C. Pl. 27**   Pea Family

Annual; to 3 ft. Leaflets in 3 pairs; obovate; tip rounded, often with an abrupt point. Note cylindrical gland between 2 lowermost leaflets. Flowers July–Sept. Pods to 9 in. long; curved. **Where found:** Waste places. Pa., Ky., Mo. and southward.

Uses: Seed tea of *C. obtusifolia* was once used for headaches, fatigue, and stomachaches. In Africa, leaves are used to make a fermented protein paste. Seeds of *C. tora* (see below) are roasted as a coffee substitute, eaten during famine. Chinese use seeds of *C. tora* for boils (internal and external), eye diseases. Fruit tea used for headaches, hepatitis, herpes, and arthritis.

Related species: *C. obtusifolia* is considered distinct from *and* synonymous with *C. tora.* Taxonomy confused. *C. tora* has foul-smelling leaves that are used for leprosy, psoriasis, and ringworm.

GOAT'S RUE
Root, leaves

Tephrosia virginiana (L.) Pers.   Pea Family

Silky-hairy perennial; 1–2 ft. Leaves pinnate; 17–29 leaflets. Flowers *bi-colored* — yellow base, pink wings; May–Aug. Legume (seedpod) hairy. **Where found:** Prairies, sandy soil. N.H. to Fla.; Texas to Man.

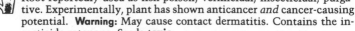

Uses: American Indians used root tea to make children muscular and strong; cold tea used for male potency, and to treat tuberculosis, coughs, bladder problems; leaves put in shoes to treat rheumatism. Root reportedly used as fish poison; vermicidal, insecticidal, purgative. Experimentally, plant has shown anticancer *and* cancer-causing potential. **Warning:** May cause contact dermatitis. Contains the insecticide rotenone. Seeds **toxic.**

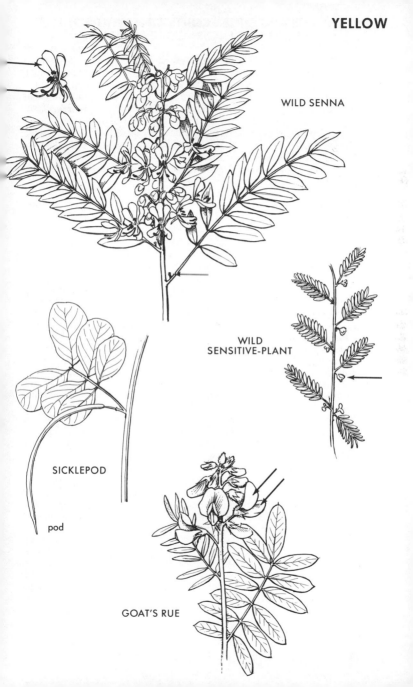

YELLOW

WILD SENNA

WILD
SENSITIVE-PLANT

SICKLEPOD

pod

GOAT'S RUE

THISTLES AND OTHER COMPOSITES WITH FERNLIKE LEAVES OR LACERATED UPPER LEAVES

SPANISH NEEDLES, SOAPBUSH NEEDLES   Leaves
Bidens bipinnata L.   Composite Family
Square-stemmed annual; 1–3 ft. Leaves *strongly dissected,* fernlike.
Flowers yellow, rays absent; Aug.–Oct. Elongate seeds ("needles") in
spreading clusters; each seed topped with 2–4 barbs. **Where found:**
Waste places, sandy soil. Mass., N.Y. to Fla.; Texas to Kans.
Uses: Cherokees used leaf tea as a worm expellent. Leaves were
chewed for sore throats. Plant juice once used for eardrops and as a
styptic. **Warning:** May be an irritant.
Related species: A related species has CNS-depressant and blood-
sugar lowering activity.

BLESSED THISTLE   Whole plant
Cnicus benedictus L.   **C. Pl. 26**   Composite Family
Hairy annual herb; 10–30 in. Both leaves and stems hairy. Stems 5-
sided. Leaves *broadest at base;* lacerated, spiny-toothed. Flowers yellow, *with a large leafy bract beneath;* April–Sept. Reddish, spinelike
projections surround yellow tufts of flowers. **Where found:** Roadsides, waste places. Local. Alien.

 Uses: Weak tea (2 teaspoons to 1 cup of water) of dried flowering
plant traditionally used in Europe to stimulate sweating, appetite,
milk production; diuretic. Folk reputation as remedy for boils, indigestion, colds, deafness, gout, headaches, migraines, suppressed
menses, chilblains, jaundice, and ringworm. Experimentally, it increases gastric and bile secretions; antibacterial. Seeds have served
as emergency oil seeds. **Warning:** Large doses may cause irritation,
vomiting.

GOLDEN RAGWORT, SQUAW-WEED   Leaves, roots
Senecio aureus L.   **C. Pl. 3**   Composite Family
Perennial; 2–4 ft. Has 2 leaf types, unlike other *Senecio* species in
our range — basal leaves *heart-shaped, rounded;* upper leaves lance-
shaped, incised. Highly variable. Flowers yellow, in flat-topped clusters; late March–July. **Where found:** Stream banks, moist soil,
swamps. Most of our area.

Uses: Root and leaf tea traditionally used by American Indians, settlers, and herbalists to treat delayed and irregular menses, leukorrhea, and childbirth complications; also used for lung ailments, dysentery, difficult urination. **Warning:** Many ragworts (*Senecio* species)
contain **highly toxic** pyrrolizidine alkaloids.

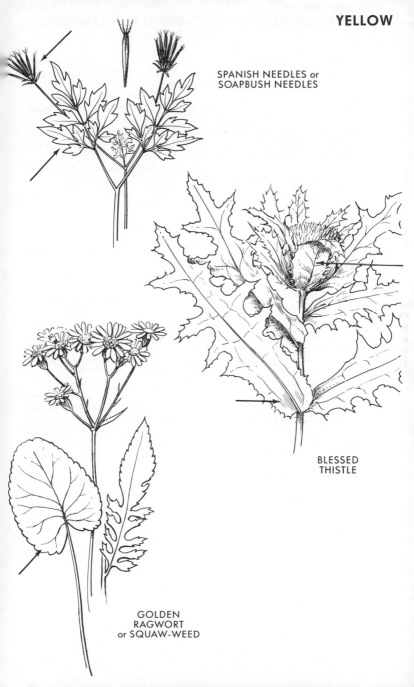

YELLOW

SPANISH NEEDLES or
SOAPBUSH NEEDLES

BLESSED
THISTLE

GOLDEN
RAGWORT
or SQUAW-WEED

COMPOSITES WITH PROMINENT OVERLAPPING BRACTS

GUMWEED, ROSINWEED   Leaves, flowers
Grindelia squarrosa (Pursh) Dunal   Composite Family
Highly variable; 1–3 ft. Leaves *strongly aromatic*, mostly serrate,
linear-oblong; mostly clasping. Flowers yellow, with *very gummy
bracts*; bract tips recurved; July–Sept. **Where found:** Prairies, roadsides. Prairie states; spreading locally eastward.
Uses: Plant tea traditionally used for asthma, coughs, kidney ailments, bronchitis. Tea of flowering tops used for colic, stomachaches. Externally, a leaf poultice or wash was used for sores, skin
eruptions, wounds. This and other *Grindelia* species have been used
in folk remedies for cancers of the spleen and stomach, burns, colds,
fever, gonorrhea, pneumonia, rashes, rheumatism, smallpox, and tuberculosis. Said to be sedative and spasmolytic. Should be investigated for asthma.
Related species: *G. lanceolata* (see C. Pl. 36) differs in that the individual bracts surrounding the flowerhead are spreading rather than
strongly curved back, among other technical details. Its general
range is more eastern than that of *G. squarrosa*. For all practical historical medicinal purposes, both plants were used interchangeably.

ELECAMPANE   Roots, leaves, flowers
Inula helenium L.   **C. Pl. 35**   Composite Family
Perennial; 4–8 ft. Leaves large, burdock-like, but narrower and
woolly beneath; upper ones reduced. Flowers yellow, *large — to 4 in.
across; rays slender*; July–Sept. Broad bracts beneath flowerhead.
Where found: Fields, roadsides. Locally established. Alien.
Uses: Root tea (½ ounce to 1 pint water) a folk remedy for pneumonia, whooping cough, asthma, bronchitis, upset stomach, diarrhea, worms; used in China for certain cancers. Wash used for facial
neuralgia, sciatica. Experimentally, tea strongly sedative to mice; antispasmodic, expectorant, worm expellent, anti-inflammatory, antibacterial, and fungicidal. In studies of mice, the root infusion (tea)
had pronounced sedative effects. Contains alantolactone, which is a
better wormer than santonin and less toxic. In small doses, it lowers
blood-sugar levels, but in larger doses, it raises blood sugar, at least
in experimental animals.

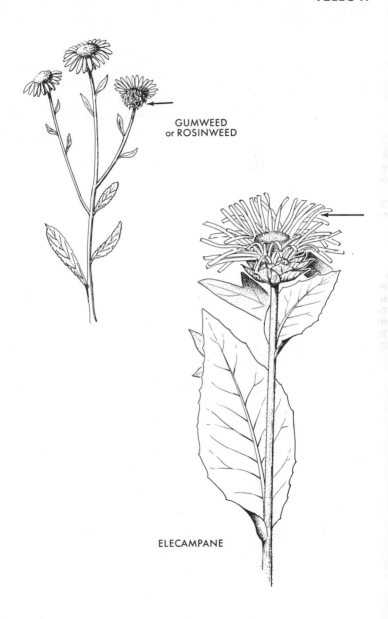

GUMWEED
or ROSINWEED

ELECAMPANE

PINEAPPLE-WEED
Leaves, flowers

Matricaria matricarioides
(Lessing) Porter   **C. Pl. 21**   Composite Family
Pineapple-scented annual; 4–16 in. Leaves *finely dissected; segments linear.* Flowers tiny, *without rays;* May–Oct. **Where found:** Waste places, roadsides. Throughout our area. Alien.
Uses: Traditionally, plant tea used for stomachaches, flatulence, colds, menstrual cramps; wash used externally, for sores, itching. **Warning:** Some individuals may be allergic to this plant.

CANADA GOLDENROD
Roots, flowers

Solidago canadensis L.   Composite Family
Our most common goldenrod. 1–5 ft. Stem smooth at base, hairy below lower flower branches. Leaves many; lance-shaped, 3-veined, sharp-toothed. Flowers in a broad, triangular panicle; July–Sept. **Where found:** Fields, roadsides. Most of our area.
Uses: American Indians used root for burns; flower tea for fevers, snakebites; crushed flowers chewed for sore throats. Contains quercetin, a compound reportedly useful in treating hemorrhagic nephritis. Seeds eaten as survival food. **Warning:** Causes allergies, though most allergies attributed to goldenrods are due to Ragweed pollen.

SWEET GOLDENROD
Leaves

Solidago odora Ait.   **C. Pl. 41**   Composite Family
Anise-scented perennial; 2–5 ft. Leaves lance-shaped, not toothed (but tiny prickles catch skin when rubbed backward along edge of leaf). Flowers on 1 side of branch; July–Oct. **Where found:** Dry open woods. S. N.H. to Fla.; Texas to Okla., Mo.
Uses: Leaf tea pleasant-tasting. Formerly used as a digestive stimulant, diaphoretic, diuretic, mild astringent; for colic, to regulate menses, stomach cramps, colds, coughs, fevers, dysentery, diarrhea, measles; externally, a wash for rheumatism, neuralgia, headaches. **Warning:** May cause allergic reactions.

COMMON TANSY
Whole plant

Tanacetum vulgare L.   **C. Pl. 35**   Composite Family
Strong-scented perennial; 1–4 ft. Leaves *fernlike.* Flowers to ½ in., in flat terminal clusters. June–Sept. **Where found:** Roadsides, fields. Scattered throughout our area. Alien (Europe).
Uses: Traditionally, weak, cold leaf tea was used for dyspepsia, flatulence, jaundice, worms, suppressed menses, weak kidneys; externally, as a wash for swelling, tumors, inflammations; spray or inhalant of tea for sore throats. Experiments have confirmed that Tansy is antispasmodic and antiseptic. Leaves insecticidal. **Warning:** Oil is **lethal** — ½ ounce can kill in 2–4 hours. It is illegal to sell this herb as food or medicine. May cause dermatitis.

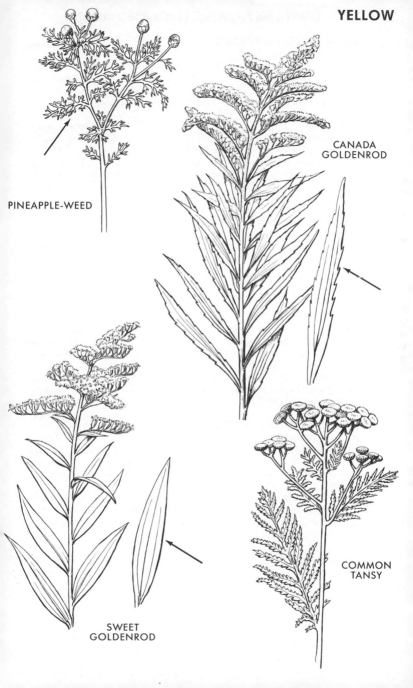

YELLOW

PINEAPPLE-WEED

CANADA
GOLDENROD

SWEET
GOLDENROD

COMMON
TANSY

DAISY-LIKE FLOWERS, BLACK-EYED SUSANS

GARDEN COREOPSIS, TICKSEED   **Whole plant**
Coreopsis tinctoria Nutt.   Composite Family
Smooth-stemmed annual; 2–4 ft. Leaves divided into slender seg-
ments. Flowers yellow; *base of rays brown*; June–Sept. **Where found:**
Moist fields. Minn. to Texas. Garden escape westward.
Uses: American Indians used root tea for diarrhea and as an emetic.

SNEEZEWEED   **Disk florets, leaves**
Helenium autumnale L.   Composite Family
Perennial; 2–5 ft. Winged, angled stems. Leaves lance-shaped to
ovate-oblong, coarsely toothed. Flowers yellow; *disk globular; rays
wedge-shaped, 3-toothed*; July–Nov. **Where found:** Rich thickets,
wet fields. Que. to Fla. and westward.

Uses: American Indians used powdered dried disk florets as a snuff
for head colds and catarrh, or drank tea for "catarrh of stomach."
Powdered leaves induce sneezing. Flower tea used to treat intestinal
worms. Folk remedy for fevers. Helenalin, a lactone found in this and
other species of *Helenium*, has shown significant antitumor activity
in the cancer-screening program of the National Cancer Institute.
Warning: Poisonous to cattle. May cause contact dermatitis. Helenalin is poisonous to fishes and worms as well as to insects.

BLACK-EYED SUSAN   **Root**
Rudbeckia hirta L.   **C. Pl. 34**   Composite Family
Biennial or short-lived perennial; 1–3 ft. Leaves lance-shaped to oblong, *bristly-hairy*. Flowers yellow, daisy-like, with 8–21 rays around
a deep brown center; June–Oct. **Where found:** Fields, roadsides, waste
places. Most of our area.
Uses: American Indians used root tea for worms, colds; external
wash for sores, snakebites, swelling; root juice for earaches. **Warning:**
Contact sensitivity to the plant has been reported.

GREEN-HEADED CONEFLOWER   **Root, flowers, leaves**
Rudbeckia lacinata L.   Composite Family
Large, branched perennial; 3–12 ft. Leaves deeply divided into 3–5
sharp-toothed lobes. Flowers yellow; rays drooping, disk *greenish
yellow*; June–Sept. **Where found:** Moist, rich thickets. Throughout
our area and beyond.
Uses: American Indians used root tea (with Blue Cohosh, p. 206) for
indigestion. Flower poultice (with Blue Giant or Anise-Hyssop, p.
190, and a Goldenrod species) applied to burns. Cooked spring greens
were eaten for "good health."

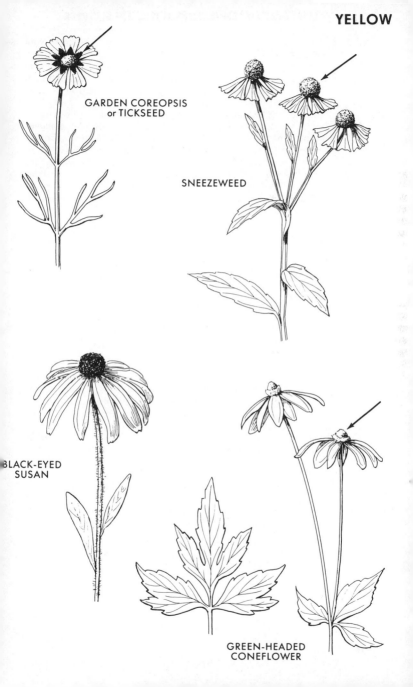

YELLOW

GARDEN COREOPSIS
or TICKSEED

SNEEZEWEED

BLACK-EYED
SUSAN

GREEN-HEADED
CONEFLOWER

TALL PLANTS WITH DANDELION-LIKE FLOWERS

WILD LETTUCE
Lactuca canadensis L.

Leaves, sap
Composite Family

Biennial; usually over 30 in. tall. Stem smooth, branched, with whitish film. Highly variable. Leaves lance-shaped, wavy-margined to deeply lobed. Flowers in panicles of yellow, dandelion-like heads; July–Sept. **Where found:** Thickets. Most of our area.

Uses: American Indians used plant tea as a nerve tonic, sedative, pain reliever. Milky latex from stem used for warts, pimples, poison-ivy rash, and other skin irritations. Used similarly by settlers. The milky juices of this and other lettuces, wild and "tame," have been used to make the so-called lettuce opium ("head lettuce"), which has been openly sold as a sedative here in the U.S. We suspect it might make a better substitute for rubber than for opium or chicle. **Warning:** This species and other Lactucas may cause dermatitis or internal poisoning.

PRICKLY LETTUCE
Lactuca scariola L.

Leaves, sap
Composite Family

Annual or biennial; 2–7 ft. Leaves oblong to lance-shaped or dandelion-like but *prickly*; margins with weak spines. Flowers yellow, dandelion-like. July–Oct. **Where found:** Waste places. Much of our area. Alien. (Europe).
Uses: American Indians used leaf tea to stimulate milk flow; diuretic. Also used like other Wild Lettuces. **Warning:** May cause dermatitis or internal poisoning.

FIELD SOW-THISTLE
Sonchus arvensis L.

Root, sap, leaves
Composite Family

Perennial; 1½–4 ft. Leaves divided, dandelion-like; base *heart-shaped, clasping; weak-spined.* Flowers dandelion-like; July–Oct. Bracts often glandular-hairy. **Where found:** Fields, waste places. Nfld. to Del.; Mo. to N.D., Alaska. Alien (Europe).
Uses: American Indians used leaf tea to calm nerves; wash for caked breasts. Asian Indians use the root in tea for asthma, bronchitis, cough, and whooping cough; leaves (poultice or wash) for swellings; latex (juice) for severe eye inflammations. In Europe, leaves are poulticed as an anti-inflammatory. Folk tumor remedy. Young shoots are eaten as a salad or potherb.

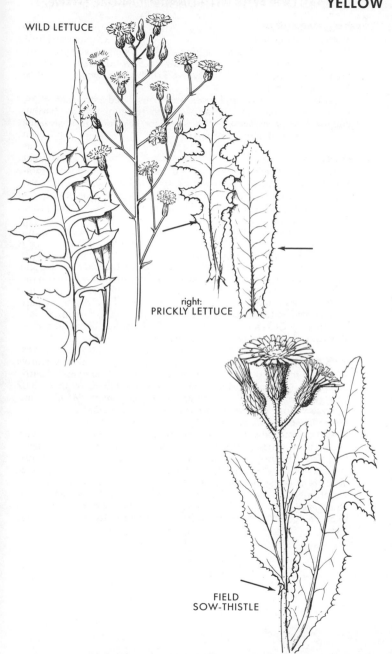

WILD LETTUCE

right:
PRICKLY LETTUCE

FIELD
SOW-THISTLE

SMALLER PLANTS WITH DANDELION-LIKE FLOWERS

RATTLESNAKE-WEED   Leaves, root
Hieracium venosum L.   Composite Family
Perennial; 1–2 ft. Leaves oblong to lance-shaped at base; veins *strongly purple-red*. Flowers small, yellow, dandelion-like; on branching stalks; May–Oct. **Where found:** Open woods, clearings. Much of our area.
Uses: Powdered leaves and roots were considered astringent, expectorant. Tea used for hemorrhages, spitting-up blood, diarrhea, coughs. One of numerous snakebite remedies. Juice in fresh leaves used as folk medicine (external) for warts.

DANDELION   Roots, leaves
Taraxacum officinale Weber   **C. Pl. 21**   Composite Family
Familiar weed; 2–18 in. Flowering stalk hollow, with milky juice. Leaves jagged-cut. Flowers yellow; March–Sept. (sporadically all year). Bracts reflexed. **Where found:** Lawns, fields, waste places. Throughout our area.
Uses: Fresh root tea traditionally used for liver, gall bladder, kidney, and bladder ailments; diuretic (not indicated when inflammation is present). Also used as a tonic for weak or impaired digestion, constipation. Dried root thought to be weaker, often roasted as coffee substitute. Dried leaf tea a folk laxative. Experimentally, root is hypoglycemic, weak antibiotic against yeast infections (*Candida albicans*), stimulates flow of bile and weight loss. All plant parts have served as food. Leaves and flowers are rich in vitamins A and C. **Warning:** Contact dermatitis reported from handling plant, probably caused by latex in stems and leaves.

COLT'S FOOT   Leaves, flowers
Tussilago farfara L.   **C. Pl. 23**   Composite Family
Perennial; 4–8 in. Leaves rounded, slightly lobed, toothed; base strongly heart-shaped. Flowers *appear before leaves*; March–April. Flowers yellow, *with many slender rays*, on a *reddish-scaled* stalk. **Where found:** Fields. N.S. to N.J.; Ohio to Minn. Alien.
Uses: Leaf and flower tea traditionally used as a demulcent and expectorant for sore throats, coughs, asthma, bronchitis, lung congestion. One of Europe's mostly popular cough remedies; dried leaves smoked for coughs and asthma. Smoke believed to impede impulse of fibers of parasympathetic nerves, and act as an antihistamine. Research suggests leaf mucilage soothes inflamed mucous membranes, and leaves have spasmolytic activity. **Warning:** Contains traces of liver-affecting pyrrolizidine alkaloids; potentially **toxic** in large doses.

YELLOW

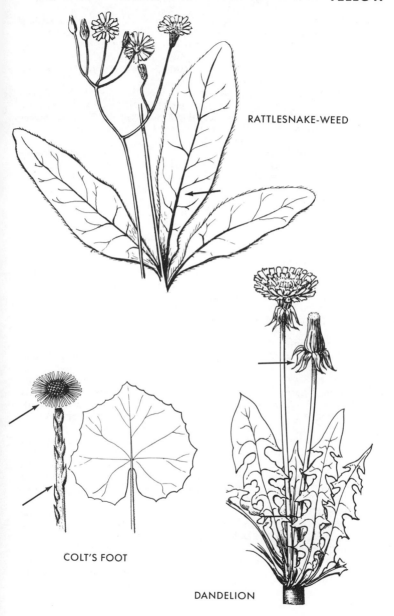

RATTLESNAKE-WEED

COLT'S FOOT

DANDELION

PLANTS WITH SUNFLOWERLIKE FLOWERS

SUNFLOWER   **Whole plant**
Helianthus annuus L.   **C. Pl. 35**   Composite Family
Annual; 6–10 ft. Leaves *mostly alternate, rough-hairy, broadly heart- or spade-shaped.* Flowers orange-yellow; disk flat; July–Oct. **Where found:** Prairies, roadsides. Minn. to Texas; escaped elsewhere. Wild parent of our domesticated sunflower.
Uses: American Indians used flower tea for lung ailments, malaria. Leaf tea taken for high fevers; astringent; poultice on snakebites and spider bites. Seeds and leaves said to be diuretic, expectorant. **Warning:** Pollen or plant extracts may cause allergic reactions.

JERUSALEM ARTICHOKE   **Tubers, stalks, flowers**
Helianthus tuberosus L.   **C. Pl. 35**   Composite Family
Hairy, tuber-bearing perennial; 5–10 ft. Leaves oval, thick, hard; sandpapery above, 3-nerved; leafstalk winged. Yellow flowers; Aug.– Oct. **Where found:** Thickets, fields. Throughout our area.
Uses: American Indians drank leaf and stalk tea or ate flowers to treat rheumatism. Folk use has suggested that the edible tubers, which contain inulin, may aid in treating diabetes.

COMPASS-PLANT   **Root, leaves, resin**
Silphium laciniatum L.   Composite Family
Perennial; 3–10 ft. Leaves large, *deeply divided, rough-hairy; aromatic.* Flowers yellow, with few rays; July–Sept. **Where found:** Prairies, glades. Mich. to Ark., Texas; Okla. to N.D.
Uses: American Indians used root tea as a general tonic for debility; worm expellent. Leaf tea emetic, once used for coughs, lung ailments, asthma. Resin said to be diuretic. Root tea used for coughs, asthma, gonorrhea. **Warning:** Of unknown toxicity.

CUP-PLANT   **Root**
Silphium perfoliatum L.   Composite Family
Square-stemmed perennial; 3–8 ft. Upper leaves united at base, *forming a cup.* Flowers like small sunflowers; July–Sept. **Where found:** Rich, moist thickets. Ont. to Ga.; Okla. to S.D.
Uses: American Indians used root tea for lung bleeding, back or chest pain, profuse menstruation, and to induce vomiting; inhaled smoke for head colds, neuralgia, and rheumatism. Historically, root tea used for enlarged spleen, fevers, internal bruises, debility, liver ailments, and ulcers. **Warning:** Of unknown toxicity.

PRAIRIE-DOCK   **Root**
Silphium terebinthinaceum Jacq.   Composite Family
Perennial; 2–9 ft. Leaves *huge,* heart-shaped; *odor of turpentine when crushed.* Flowers like small sunflowers; Aug.–Oct. **Where found:** Prairies, glades. Ont. to Tenn.; Mo. to Ohio, Ind.
Uses: Same as for *S. laciniatum* (above). **Warning:** Potentially **toxic.**

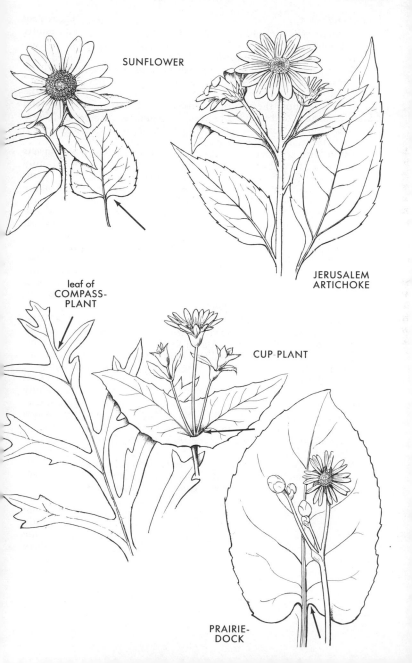

SUNFLOWER

JERUSALEM ARTICHOKE

leaf of COMPASS-PLANT

CUP-PLANT

PRAIRIE-DOCK

ORANGE LILIES

DAYLILY   **Root, flower buds**
Hemerocallis fulva L.   **C. Pl. 25**   Lily Family
Perennial; 3–6 ft. Leaves in clumps, *swordlike.* Flowers *face upward or outward, not downward;* striped in middle, petals curved back. Large, showy flowers; May–July. **Where found:** Escaped from gardens. Grows near abandoned homesites and gardens throughout. Alien (Asia).

 Uses: In China, the root tea is used as a diuretic in turbid urine, edema, poor or difficult urination; for jaundice, nosebleeds, leukorrhea, uterine bleeding; poultice for mastitis. A folk cancer remedy for breast cancer. Experimentally, Chinese studies indicate that root extracts are antibacterial, useful against blood flukes (parasites), and diuretic. The edible flower buds are used for diuretic and astringent properties in jaundice and to "relieve oppression and heat in the chest"; poulticed for piles. **Warning:** The roots and young leaf shoots are considered potentially **toxic.** Chinese reports indicate that the toxin accumulates in the system and can adversely affect the eyes, even causing blindness in some cases. Chinese studies hint that the roots may also contain the carcinogen and teratogen colchicine, which, though poisonous, has long been used in the treatment of acute gout crises. Foragers beware.

CANADA LILY   **Root**
Lilium canadense L.   **C. Pl. 6**   Lily Family
Perennial; 2–5 ft. Leaves lance-shaped, usually in whorls. *Nodding* yellow, orange, or reddish flowers; spotted, bell-shaped; July–Aug. **Where found:** Moist meadows, openings. Se. Canada. to e. Md., Va. mountains, N.C., Ga., Fla.; Ala. to Ky.
Uses: American Indians used root tea for stomach ailments, irregular menses, dysentery, rheumatism; root poultice used externally, for snakebites.

WOOD LILY   **Root, flowers**
Lilium philadelphicum L.   **C. Pl. 20**   Lily Family
Perennial; 1–3 ft. Leaves in whorls. Flowers bright orange, *upturned, spotted;* June–July. **Where found:** Acid woods, openings, clearings. Me. to W. Va., Ga. mountains; north to Ky., Ont.
Uses: American Indians used root tea for stomach disorders, coughs, consumption, fevers; to expel placenta; externally, for swelling, bruises, wounds, sores. Flowers poulticed for spider bites.

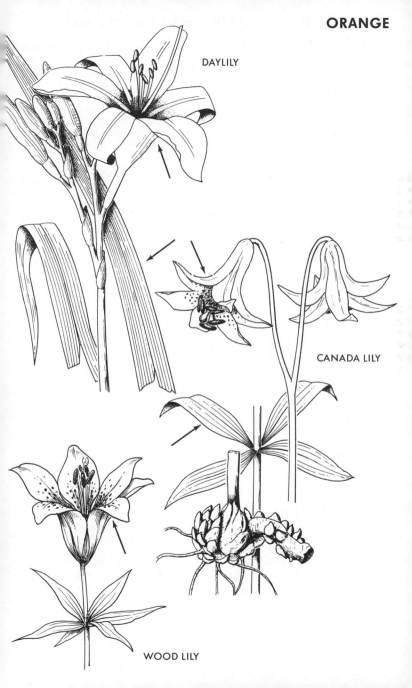

DAYLILY

CANADA LILY

WOOD LILY

MISCELLANEOUS ORANGE-RED FLOWERS

COLUMBINE   **Roots, seeds, whole plant**
Aquilegia canadensis L.   **C. Pl. 12**   Buttercup Family
Perennial; 1–2 ft. Leaves divided in *3's*. Flowers drooping, bell-like, with *5 spurlike appendages at top*; April–July. **Where found:** Moist, rich woods. S. Canada southward. Throughout our area.

⚠ **Uses:** Astringent, diuretic, anodyne. American Indians used minute amounts of crushed seeds for headaches, "love charm" (uses related?), fevers. Seeds rubbed into hair to control lice. Root chewed or weak tea for diarrhea, stomach troubles, diuretic. Root tea for uterine bleeding. **Warning:** Potentially **poisonous.**

BUTTERFLYWEED, PLEURISY-ROOT   **Root**
Asclepias tuberosa L.   **C. Pl. 41**   Milkweed Family
Perennial; 1–3 ft. Stem *without milky juice*. Leaves *lance-shaped*. Flowers showy orange (rarely yellow); May–Sept. **Where found:** Dry roadsides, prairies. S. N.H. to Fla.; Texas, Kans., Minn.

⚠ **Uses:** Tea or tincture of large, tuberous root once widely used for lung inflammations (pleurisy), asthma, and bronchitis; anodyne, laxative, diuretic, expectorant. Root poultice used for bruises, swellings, rheumatism, and lameness. **Warning:** Potentially **toxic** in large quantities.

JEWELWEED, SPOTTED TOUCH-ME-NOT   **Leaves, juice**
Impatiens capensis Meerb.   **C. Pl. 3**   Touch-me-not Family
Smooth annual; 3–5 ft. Leaves oval, toothed; lower ones opposite, upper ones alternate. Flowers pendantlike, *with red spots*; June–Sept. **Where found:** Wet, shady soil. Most of our area.
Uses: Crushed leaves are poulticed on recent poison-ivy rash — a well-known folk remedy. Mucilaginous stem juice (harvested before flowering) also applied to rash. A 1957 study by a physician found it effective (in 2–3 days) in treating 108 of 115 patients. Some people swear by the leaf tea as a poison-ivy rash preventative; others rub on frozen tea (in the form of ice cubes) as a remedy. Poultice a folk remedy for bruises, burns, cuts, eczema, insect bites, sores, sprains, warts, ringworm.

HOARY PUCCOON   **Whole flowering plant**
Lithospermum canescens   **C. Pl. 38**   Forget-me-not Family
(Michx.) L.
Perennial, with *very fine, soft white hairs*; 4–18 in. Leaves alternate, lance-shaped. Flowers orange to yellow; April–June. Flowers 5-petaled, in curled or flat clusters; stamens concealed in tube. **Where found:** Dry soils, prairies. S. Ont. to Ga., Miss.; Texas to Sask.
Uses: American Indians used leaf tea (as a wash) for fevers accompanied by spasms. Wash rubbed on persons thought to be near convulsions.

ORANGE

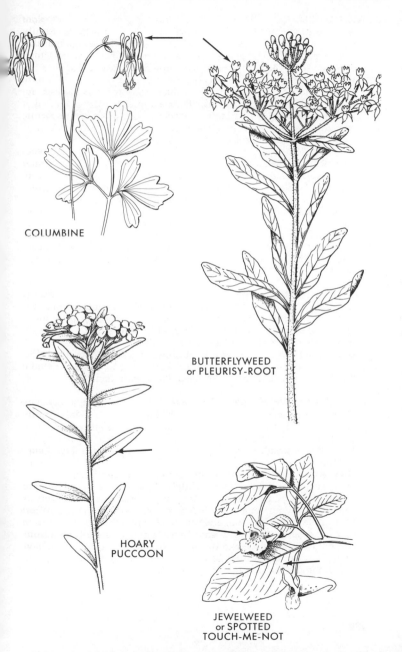

COLUMBINE

BUTTERFLYWEED
or PLEURISY-ROOT

HOARY
PUCCOON

JEWELWEED
or SPOTTED
TOUCH-ME-NOT

PLANTS WITH 3 "PARTS"

WILD GINGER   Root
Asarum canadense L.   **C. Pl. 11**   Birthwort Family
Creeping perennial. Leaves *strongly heart-shaped*. Flowers maroon,
urn-shaped, with 3 "petals" (actually sepals); between crotch of
leaves; April–May. Root strongly aromatic. **Where found:** Rich
woods. Canada to S.C., Ala.; Okla. north to N.D.
Uses: American Indians highly valued root tea for indigestion,
coughs, colds, heart conditions, "female ailments," throat ailments,
nervous conditions, and cramps. Relieves gas, promotes sweating,
expectorant; used for fevers, colds, sore throats. Contains the antitumor compound aristolochic acid. Ginger substitute.

PINK LADY'S-SLIPPER   Root
Cypripedium acaule Ait.   **C. Pl. 19**   Orchid Family
Perennial orchid; 6–15 in. Leaves 2; *basal.* Flower pink (rarely
white), strongly veined; pouch with a deep furrow; May–June. **Where
found:** Acid woods. Nfld. to Ga.; Ala., Tenn. to Minn. Too rare to
harvest.

Uses: Called "American Valerian." Widely used in 19th century as
sedative for nervous headaches, hysteria, insomnia, and "female"
diseases. See Yellow Lady's-slipper (p. 94). **Warning:** May cause dermatitis.

INDIAN PAINTBRUSH, PAINTED CUP   Flower
Castilleja coccinea (L.) K. Spreng.   **C. Pl. 38**   Snapdragon Family
Annual; to 2 ft. Leaves in basal rosettes. Flowers with *3-lobed, scar-
let-tipped bracts* (rarely yellow); April–July. **Where found:** Meadows,
prairies. S. N.H. to Fla.; Texas, Okla. to s. Man.
Uses: American Indians used weak flower tea for rheumatism, "female" diseases; also as a secret love charm in food, and as a poison,
"to destroy your enemies." **Warning:** Potentially **toxic.**

RED TRILLIUM, WAKEROBIN, BETHROOT   Root, whole plant
Trillium erectum L.   **C. Pl. 11**   Lily Family
Perennial; 6–16 in. Leaves triangular-oval; *3, in a single whorl.* Flowers dull red (to white), with 3 triangular petals and sepals; April–
June. **Where found:** Rich woods. N.S. to Ga. mountains, Fla.; Tenn.
to Mich., Ont.
Uses: American Indians used root tea (made from "birth root") for
menstrual disorders, to induce childbirth, aid in labor; for "change
of life" (menopause); uterine astringent, aphrodisiac (root contains
steroids). Used for coughs and bowel troubles. Whole plant poulticed
for tumors, inflammation, and ulcers. Historically, physicians used
root tea as above, and for hemorrhages, asthma, difficult breathing,
chronic lung disorders; externally, for snakebites, stings, skin irritations. A tea of equal parts of Bugleweed (*Lycopus virginicus*, p. 70)
and Bethroot was once used for diabetes.

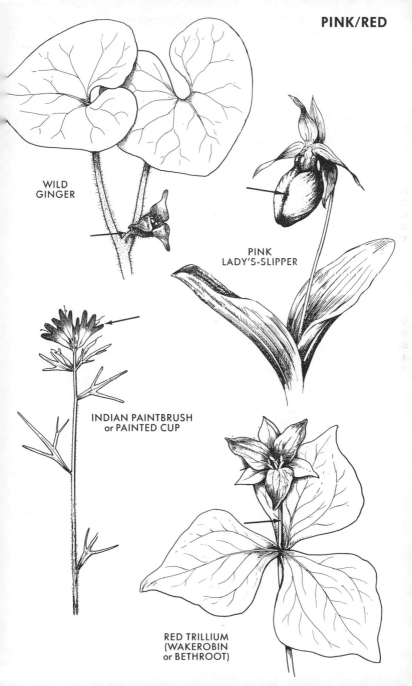

WILD
GINGER

PINK
LADY'S-SLIPPER

INDIAN PAINTBRUSH
or PAINTED CUP

RED TRILLIUM
(WAKEROBIN
or BETHROOT)

MISCELLANEOUS PLANTS WITH PINK OR RED FLOWERS

NODDING WILD ONION   Bulb, whole plant
Allium cernuum Roth   Lily Family
Perennial; 1–2 ft. Leaves soft, flat. Stem *arching* at top. Flowers pink-white; July–Aug. **Where found:** Open woods, rocky soil. N.Y. to Ga.; west to Texas; west from Mich., Minn. to B.C.
Uses: Cherokees used slender bulbs for colds, colic, croup, and fevers. After a dose of Horsemint (*Monarda punctata*) tea, the juice of this wild onion was taken for "gravel" (kidney stones) and dropsy. Poultice of plant applied to chest for respiratory ailments. Effects probably similar to, but weaker than those of Garlic (see p. 30).

FEVERWORT, COFFEE PLANT   Root, leaves
Triosteum perfoliatum L.   Honeysuckle Family
Perennial; 2–4½ ft. Leaves opposite; *connected around stem* (perfoliate). Flowers greenish to dull purple, in leaf axils; *5 prominent sepals;* May–July. Fruit bright red-orange. **Where found:** Moist woods. Mass. to Ga.; Ala., Okla. to Minn.
Uses: American Indians used the root tea for irregular to profuse menses, constipation, urinary disorders; cold tea for bad colds and sore throats. Root poulticed for snakebites, sores, and felons. Leaf tea taken to induce sweating. Historically, root was used by physicians for headaches, colic, vomiting, diarrhea, and indigestion. Diuretic for chronic rheumatism. In large doses it is cathartic and emetic. Seeds used as coffee substitute.

VALERIAN   Root
Valeriana officinalis L.   **C. Pl. 25**   Valerian Family
Perennial; 4–5 ft. Leaves strongly divided, *pinnate;* lower ones toothed. Tiny, pale pink to whitish flowers, in tight clusters; June–July. **Where found:** Escaped, along roadsides, especially in ne. U.S. Que., Me. to N.J., Pa.; Ohio to Minn. Alien (from Europe).
Uses: A well-known herbal calmative, antispasmodic, nerve tonic, used for hypochondria, nervous headaches, irritability, mild spasmodic affections, depression, despondency, insomnia. Active components are called valepotriates. Research has confirmed that teas, tinctures, and/or extracts of this plant are CNS-depressant, antispasmodic, and sedative when agitation is present, but also a stimulant in fatigue; antibacterial, antidiuretic, liver-protective. Valerian is a leading over-the-counter tranquilizer in Europe. Cats are said to be attracted to the scent of the root as they are to Catnip. Folklore says the root repels rats.
Related species: *Valeriana sitchensis* (not shown), native to the western U.S., is thought to have higher levels of valepotriates, thus stronger medicinal activity.

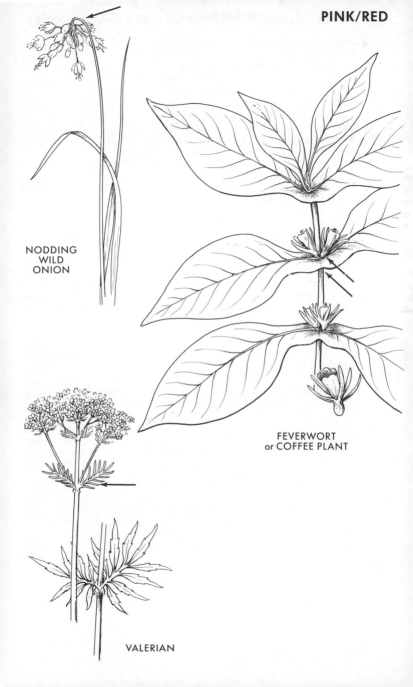

PINK/RED

NODDING
WILD
ONION

FEVERWORT
or COFFEE PLANT

VALERIAN

MISCELLANEOUS PLANTS OF BOGS AND SWAMPS

WATER or PURPLE AVENS   **Root**
  Geum rivale L.   **C. Pl. 17**   Rose Family
  Perennial; 1–2 ft. Basal leaves much divided; leaflets toothed, *outermost one largest*; stem leaves divided into *3 parts*. Nodding, dull reddish (rarely yellow) globular flowers, mostly in 3's; May–Aug. Fruits hooked. **Where found:** Bogs, moist ground. Lab. to W. Va.; Minn. west to B.C.
  Uses: Powdered root was once used as astringent for hemorrhage, fevers, diarrhea, dysentery, indigestion, leukorrhea.
  Related species: In China and Japan, a tea of the whole plant of *Geum japonicum* is used as a diuretic and as an astringent for treating coughs and spitting up of blood. The root and leaves of *G. japonicum* are used as a poultice or wash for skin diseases and boils. Other Geums are used similarly.

SWAMP PINK
  Helonias bullata L.   Lily Family
  Perennial; 1–3 ft. Leaves spatula- or lance-shaped, in an evergreen rosette. Flowers vibrant pink, in a tight, egg-shaped cluster, borne on a tall, hollow stem; April–July. **Where found:** Swamps, bogs. Coastal plain from N.Y., N.J. to Va.; n. Ga. to Pa. mountains. Rare — should not be harvested at all.
  Uses: Confused in the literature with Devil's-bit (*Chamaelirium luteum*, p. 104).

PITCHER-PLANT   **Leaves, root**
  Sarracenia purpurea L.   **C. Pl. 4**   Pitcher-plant Family
  Unique perennial; 8–24 in. Leaves red-veined, *pitcherlike*, often partially filled with water; downcurved hairs within. Flowers dull red, nodding, with a *large flat pistil*; May–July. **Where found:** Peat or sphagnum bogs, savannas, and wet meadows. Nfld. to Fla.; Ohio to Minn.; scattered elsewhere. May be a threatened species; best left undisturbed in the wild.
  Uses: American Indians used root to treat smallpox, lung and liver ailments, spitting up of blood; childbirth aid; diuretic. Dried leaf tea used for fevers, chills, and shakiness. Historically, physicians considered the herb to be a stimulating tonic, diuretic, and laxative. The plant was thought to be a preventive for smallpox. It was used in an effort to modify the disease and shorten its duration, though it was believed to be ineffective by those who tried it. European physicians researched the plant as a possible smallpox cure in the 19th century, but without success. Medicinal merit not proved, or disproved.

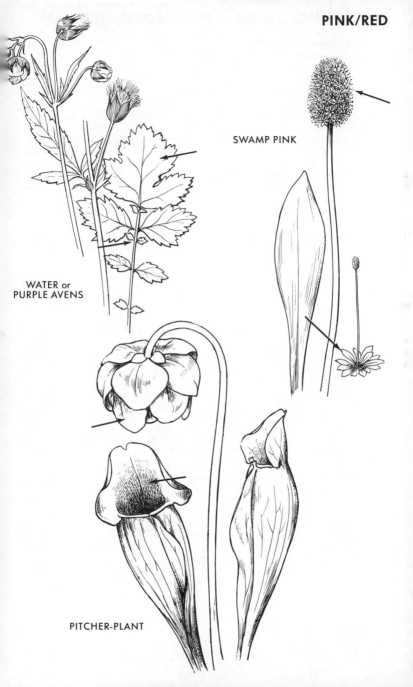

PINK/RED

SWAMP PINK

WATER or
PURPLE AVENS

PITCHER-PLANT

MISCELLANEOUS SHOWY FLOWERS; WET SOILS

QUEEN-OF-THE-PRAIRIE   **Root**
Filipendula rubra (Hill) Robinson   Rose Family
Smooth perennial; 2–8 ft. Leaves deeply divided; *segments interrupted.* Flowers pink-red, *in spreading terminal clusters;* June–Aug.
Where found: Moist meadows, bogs. Pa. to Ga.; west to Iowa; north to Mich. Rare in southern extensions of range.
Uses: Fox Indians (Wisc.) used root for heart trouble and in "love potions." Due to high tannin content, the root was valued as a folk medicine for its astringent properties in diarrhea, dysentery, and to stop bleeding. Like the European **Queen-of-the-Meadow** or **Meadowsweet,** *Spiraea (Filipendula) ulmaria,* this plant probably contains chemical forerunners of aspirin. Salicin, the popular analgesic derived from poplars and willows, probably decomposes in the digestive tract to salicylic acid, a compound first isolated from Meadowsweet flower buds in 1839. The semisynthetic acetyl-salicylic acid (aspirin) is said to have fewer side effects than the natural compound from which it is derived. Still, nonsteroidal anti-inflammatory drugs, including aspirin, account for 10,000–20,000 deaths per year. Probably all medicines, natural and synthetic, have side effects.

SWAMP ROSE-MALLOW   **Leaves, root**
Hibiscus moscheutos L.   Mallow Family
Musky-scented perennial; 5–7 ft. Lower leaves often 3-lobed; median leaves lance-shaped. Flowers to 8 in. across; white, with a *purple-red center;* June–Sept. **Where found:** Marshes. Md. to Fla.; Ala. to Ind.
Uses: Abounds in mucilage. Leaves and roots of this plant, like those of related species and genera, used as demulcent and emollient in dysentery and lung and urinary ailments.

CARDINAL FLOWER   **Root, leaves**
Lobelia cardinalis L.   **C. Pl. 2**   Bluebell Family
Perennial; 2–3 ft. One of our most showy wildflowers. Leaves oval to lance-shaped, toothed. Flowers vibrant scarlet (rarely white), in brilliant spikes. July–Sept. **Where found:** Moist soil, stream banks. N.B. to Fla.; Texas to Minn.
 Uses: American Indians used root tea for stomachaches, syphilis, typhoid, worms; ingredient of "love potions." Leaf tea used for colds, croup, nosebleeds, fevers, headaches, rheumatism. It was once thought to help cramps, expel worms, and act as a nerve "tonic." Historically, this plant was considered a substitute for Lobelia or Indian-tobacco (*L. inflata,* p. 184), but with weaker effects; it was seldom if ever used. **Warning:** Potentially **toxic;** degree of toxicity unknown.

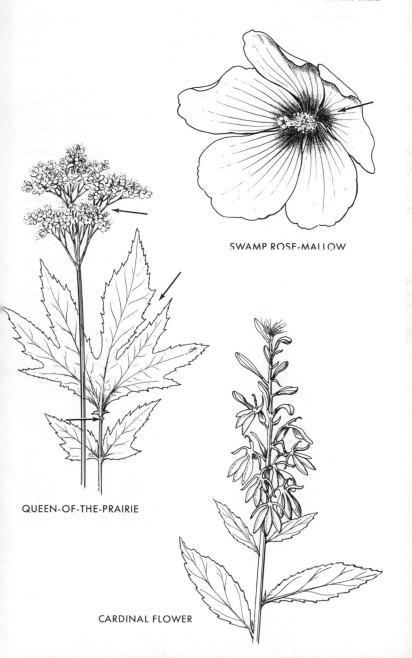

PINK/RED

SWAMP ROSE-MALLOW

QUEEN-OF-THE-PRAIRIE

CARDINAL FLOWER

4–5 PETALS; FRUITS UPTURNED; "STORK'S BILLS"

FIREWEED   **Leaves, root**
Epilobium angustifolium L.   **C. Pl. 6**   Evening-primrose Family
Perennial; 1–7 ft. Leaves lance-shaped. Flowers rose-pink; July–Sept.
Petals 4, rounded; buds drooping. **Where found:** Clearings; invasive
after fires. Subarctic to Ga. mountains; Ind. to Iowa.
Uses: American Indians poulticed peeled root for burns, skin sores,
swelling, boils, carbuncles. Leaf and root tea a folk remedy for dysentery, abdominal cramps, "summer bowel troubles." Leaf poultice
used for mouth ulcers. Leaves used in U.S.S.R. as "kaporie" tea (10
percent tannin). Leaf extract shown to reduce inflammation.

STORK'S BILL, ALFILERIA   **Leaves**
Erodium cicutarium (L.) L'Her.   Geranium Family
Winter annual or biennial; 3–12 in. Leaves fernlike, twice-pinnate,
often in a basal rosette. Flowers pinkish, 5-petaled; less than ½ in.
long; April–Oct.; almost all year round, at least in the South. Seeds
smooth, elongate, sharp — like a stork's bill. **Where found:** Waste
places. Much of our area. Alien.
Uses: Leaf tea a folk medicine used to induce sweating, allay uterine
hemorrhage; diuretic. Seed poultice used for gouty tophus. Source of
vitamin K. Leaves soaked in bath water for rheumatic patients.

WILD or SPOTTED GERANIUM   **Root**
Geranium maculatum L.   **C. Pl. 13**   Geranium Family
Perennial; 1–2 ft. Leaves broad, *deeply 5-parted;* segments toothed.
Flowers pink to lavender (rarely white), 5-petaled; April–June. Distinct "crane's bill" in center of flower enlarges into seedpod. **Where
found:** Woods. Me. to Ga.; Ark., Kans. to Man.
Uses: Tannin-rich (10–20 percent) root highly astringent, styptic;
once used to stop bleeding, diarrhea, dysentery, relieve piles, gum
diseases, kidney and stomach ailments; diuretic. Powdered root applied to canker sores. Externally, used as a folk cancer remedy.

HERB ROBERT   **Leaves**
Geranium robertianum L.   Geranium Family
Perennial; 6–18 in. Stems often reddish; scent bitter-aromatic.
Leaves pinnate, with 3–5 toothed segments; end segment *long-stalked.* Flowers pinkish, usually in pairs; *petals not notched;* May–
Oct. **Where found:** Rocky woods. Nfld. to Md.; Ohio, Ill. to Man.
Uses: Leaf tea formerly used for malaria, tuberculosis, stomach and
intestinal ailments, jaundice, kidney infections; to stop bleeding;
gargled for sore throats. Externally, wash or poultice used to relieve
pain of swollen breasts; folk cancer remedy, applied externally to
fistulas, tumors, and ulcers.

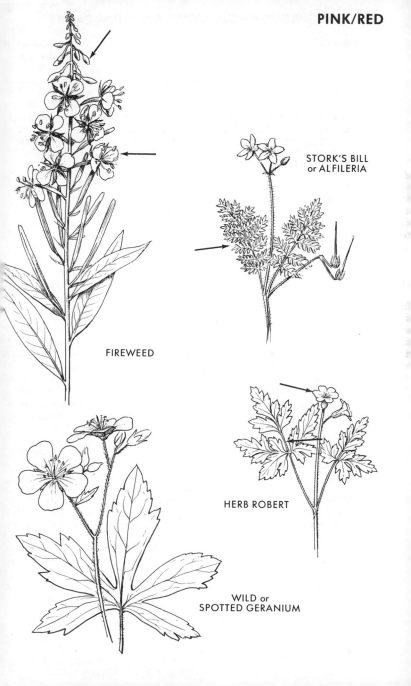

STORK'S BILL
or ALFILERIA

FIREWEED

HERB ROBERT

WILD or
SPOTTED GERANIUM

5-PARTED FLOWERS WITH A TUBULAR CALYX

CORN-COCKLE
Agrostemma githago L.

Seeds
Pink Family

Silky annual or biennial; 1–3 ft. Leaves lance-shaped. Petals deep pink, veined. Calyx inflated; *strongly 10-ribbed*. Hairy, linear sepals extend beyond petals. Flowers June–Sept. **Where found:** Noxious weed of grain fields, waste places. Throughout our area. Alien.

 Uses: Minute amounts of powdered seeds once taken in honey as a diuretic, expectorant, vermifuge (dewormer); used for jaundice, dropsy, gastritis. European folk use for cancers, warts, hard swellings in uterus. **Warning:** Seeds **toxic,** especially when broken; dangerous saponins are concentrated in seed embryo.

BOUNCING BET, SOAPWORT
Saponaria officinalis L.

Whole plant
Pink Family

Stem *thick-jointed;* smoothish perennial; 1–2 ft. Leaves opposite, oval to lance-shaped. Flowers white or rose, 1 in. across; July–Sept. Petals *reflexed, notched.* **Where found:** Throughout our area. Alien.

⚠ **Uses:** Crushed leaves and roots make lather when mixed with water. American Indians poulticed leaves for spleen pain, boils. In European tradition, plant tea is used as a diuretic, laxative, expectorant; poulticed on acne, boils, eczema, psoriasis, poison-ivy rash. Root tea used as above; also for lung disease, asthma, gall disease, and jaundice. **Warning:** Contains saponins. Large doses may cause **poisoning.**

FIRE PINK
Silene virginica L.

Root
Pink Family

Perennial; 8–20 in. Leaves *opposite,* in 2–6 pairs on stems. Flowers brilliant scarlet; 5 petals, *notched at tips;* April–June. **Where found:** Rocky woods. S. Ont. to Ga.; Ark., Okla. to Minn.

⚠ **Uses:** Unconfirmed historical reports speak of worm-expellent properties (may result from same confusion cited below). **Warning:** Reports state American Indians considered the plant **poisonous.** It may have been confused with *Spigelia* (see below).

PINK-ROOT
Spigelia marilandica L.   **C. Pl. 15**

Root
Logania Family

Perennial; 12–24 in. Leaves opposite, united by stipules; ovate to lance-shaped. Flowers *scarlet,* 5-lobed flaring trumpets, with a *cream yellow interior;* May–June. **Where found:** Rich woods, openings. Md. to Fla.; Texas, e. Okla. to Mo., Ind.

 Uses: American Indians used root tea as a worm expellent. This plant was also once used by physicians for worms, especially in children. **Warning:** Side effects include increased heart action, vertigo, convulsions, and possibly death.

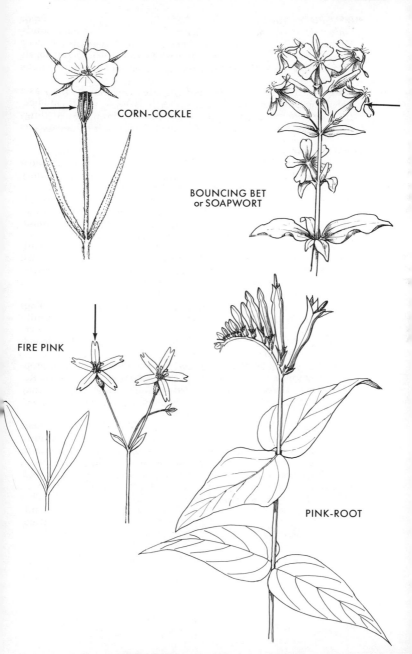

CORN-COCKLE

BOUNCING BET
or SOAPWORT

FIRE PINK

PINK-ROOT

FLOWERS WITH 5 SHOWY PETALS; MALLOWS

PURPLE POPPY-MALLOW   **Root**
Callirhoe involucrata (T. & G.) Gray   Mallow Family
Creeping herb. Leaves palmate; divided into 5–7 parts with pointed, toothed lobes (especially lower leaves). Flowers *poppy-like*, reddish purple; May–Aug. **Where found:** Prairies. S. Mo. to Texas; N.D. west to Utah, Wyo.
Uses: The Teton Dakotas crushed the dried root, burned it, and inhaled the smoke to treat head colds. Aching limbs were exposed to the smoke to reduce pain. Root boiled, then tea drunk for pains. One Dakota name for the plant means "smoke-treatment medicine."

COMMON MALLOW, CHEESES   **Leaves, root**
Malva neglecta Wallr.   Mallow Family
Deep-rooted herb; to 1 ft. Stems trailing. Leaves rounded, toothed; *slightly 5- to 7-lobed.* Flowers pale rose-lavender to whitish, in axils; April–Oct. Petals *notched* (heart-shaped) on ends; *pistils smoothish, not veined.* The common name "Cheeses" is derived from the similarity of the shape of the flat, rounded fruits to a "round" of cheese. **Where found:** Yards. Throughout our area. Alien.
Uses: Leaves edible, highly nutritious. Used as a soup base in China. As with Okra, also of the mallow family, the mucilaginous properties tend to thicken soup. Leaf or root tea of this mallow soothing to irritated membranes, especially of digestive system. Tea also used for angina, coughs, bronchitis, stomachaches; anti-inflammatory, mildly astringent. Poulticed on wounds and tumors. Root extracts show activity against tuberculosis.

HIGH MALLOW   **Leaves, flowers, root**
Malva sylvestris L.   **C. Pl. 27**   Mallow Family
Erect, hairy biennial; 8–36 in. Leaves long-stalked; rounded, with 5–7 *distinct lobes.* Flowers rose-purple, with darker veins; *pistils wrinkle-veined.* Flowers May–July. **Where found:** Waste places. Frequently cultivated, then escaped, but not considered naturalized. Scattered over much of our area. Alien.
Uses: Leaves edible. Leaf or root tea soothing to irritated membranes, especially of digestive system; also used for coughs, bronchitis, stomachaches; anti-inflammatory, mildly astringent. In China the leaves and flowers have been used as an expectorant, a gargle for sore throats, and a mouthwash. Diuretic properties are also attributed to the plant and it is said to be good for the stomach and spleen. Other *Malva* species are used similarly.

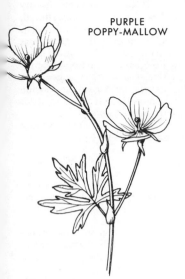

PURPLE
POPPY-MALLOW

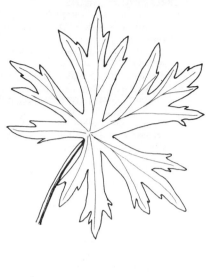

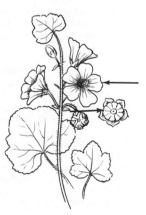

COMMON MALLOW
or CHEESES

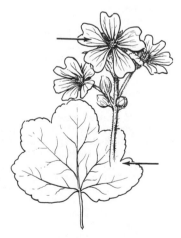

HIGH MALLOW

5-PARTED, BELL-SHAPED FLOWERS

SPREADING DOGBANE   **Root**
Apocynum androsaemifolium L.   **C. Pl. 43**   Dogbane Family
Shrublike; 1–4 ft. *Milky latex within.* Leaves oval, opposite; smooth above. Flowers drooping pink bells, *rose-striped within;* in leaf axils *and* terminal; June–July. **Where found:** Scattered throughout our area. Fields, roadsides. Absent from Kans., south of N.C. highlands. **Uses:** American Indians used root of this plant for many ailments. Induces sweating and vomiting; laxative. Used in headaches with sluggish bowels, liver disease, indigestion, rheumatism, and syphilis. **Warning: Poisonous.** Cymarin, a cardioactive glycoside, poisons cattle. Nonetheless, the plant has shown antitumor activity.
Related species: Indian Hemp (*A. cannabinum*), a close relative, is also used medicinally but is also considered **poisonous.**

TWINFLOWER   **Whole plant**
Linnaea borealis L.   Honeysuckle Family
Delicate creeper; 3–5 in. Leaves *paired.* Flowers fragrant, *nodding bells, in pairs* on a slender stalk; June–July. **Where found:** Cold, moist woods. Canada to L.I.; W. Va. mountains, Ohio to n. Ind. Locally too rare for harvest.
Uses: Algonquins used plant tea as a tonic for pregnancy and in difficult or painful menstruation; also for children's cramps, fevers. Historical use only.

HEART-LEAVED FOUR O'CLOCK   **Root, leaves**
Mirabilis nyctaginea (Michx.) MacM.   Four O'Clock Family
Perennial; 1–5 ft. Leaves opposite, heart-shaped. Pink to purple flowers *atop a 5-lobed, green, veiny cup or bracts;* June–Oct. **Where found:** Prairies, rich soil. Wisc. to Ala.; Texas to Mont.; escaped and weedy eastward.
Uses: American Indians used root tea for burns, fevers, and to expel worms; externally, root poulticed for sprains, burns, sores, and swellings. Leaf (or root) tea used for bladder ailments. **Warning:** Considered **poisonous.**

TOBACCO   **Leaves**
Nicotiana tabacum L.   Nightshade Family
Acrid, rank, clammy-hairy, large annual; 3–9 ft. Leaves lance-shaped to oval. Funnel-shaped flowers, to 3 in. long; greenish to pink, 5-parted; Aug.–Sept. **Where found:** Escaped from recent cultivation. Alien (from tropical America).
Uses: Well-known addictive narcotic. American Indians employed it in rituals; leaf tea diuretic, emetic, strongly laxative, worm expellent, anodyne; used for cramps, sharp pains, toothaches, dizziness, dropsy, colic. Poulticed for boils, snakebites, insect stings. **Warning:** Hazards of Tobacco use are well known. Still, the toxic insecticidal alkaloid, nicotine, is offered in pills or perhaps even in skin patches to help curb the nicotine habit.

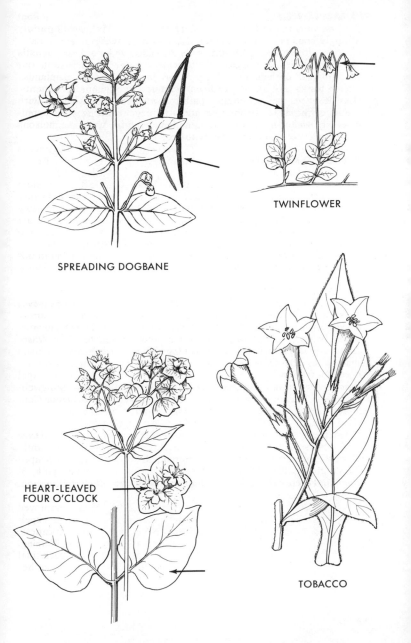

TWINFLOWER

SPREADING DOGBANE

HEART-LEAVED
FOUR O'CLOCK

TOBACCO

FLOWERS IN DOMED CLUSTERS; MILKWEEDS

SWAMP MILKWEED   Root
Asclepias incarnata L.   **C. Pl. 1**   Milkweed Family
Strongly branched, smooth perennial; 2–4 ft. Leaves numerous, *opposite; narrowly lance-shaped* or oblanceolate (wider at base); veins ascending; soft-hairy, especially beneath. Flowers reddish to deep rose, in small umbels; June–Sept. **Where found:** Wet areas, marshes, stream banks, and moist meadows. Scattered throughout our area.

 Uses: Root tea used in "tonic" bath for weak patients. Root tea diuretic, carminative, strongly laxative; induces vomiting. American colonists used it for asthma, rheumatism, syphilis, worms, and as a heart tonic. **Warning:** Potentially **toxic.**

FOUR-LEAVED MILKWEED   Root
Asclepias quadrifolia Jacq.   Milkweed Family
Perennial; stems solitary, 1–2½ ft. Leaves ovate-elliptical; upper and lowermost ones paired. Largest middle pair of leaves appears to be in a *whorl of 4.* Flowers pale pink to lavender, whitish, or greenish; in sparse umbels. May–July. **Where found:** Open deciduous woods and forest margins. N.H. to S.C., Ala.; Ark., Kans. to Minn.

Uses: Cherokees used root tea as laxative, diuretic for "gravel" (kidney stones), dropsy. Leaves have been rubbed on warts to remove them. **Warning:** Potentially **toxic.**

COMMON MILKWEED   Root, latex
Asclepias syriaca L.   **C. Pl. 34**   Milkweed Family
Milky-juiced, *downy* perennial; 2–4 ft. Stems usually solitary. Leaves opposite, large, widely elliptical; to 8 in. long. Flowers pink-purple (variable), in globe-shaped (often drooping) clusters from leaf axils; June–Aug. Pods *warty.* **Where found:** Fields, roadsides. S. Canada to Ga., Ala.; Okla., Kans. to N.D. The most common milkweed in the Northeast.

Uses: American Indians used root tea as a laxative, and as a diuretic for "gravel" (kidney stones) and dropsy; applied milky latex to warts, moles, ringworm. Root tea expectorant, diuretic; induces sweating. Used by early American physicians for asthma, rheumatism. Latex chewed as gum, a dangerous practice — see warning below. Silky seed tassels used in pillows, feather beds. Folk cancer remedy. One Mohawk antifertility concoction contained Milkweed and Jack-in-the-Pulpit (p. 202), both considered dangerous and contraceptive. **Warning:** Potentially **toxic** — contains cardioactive compounds.

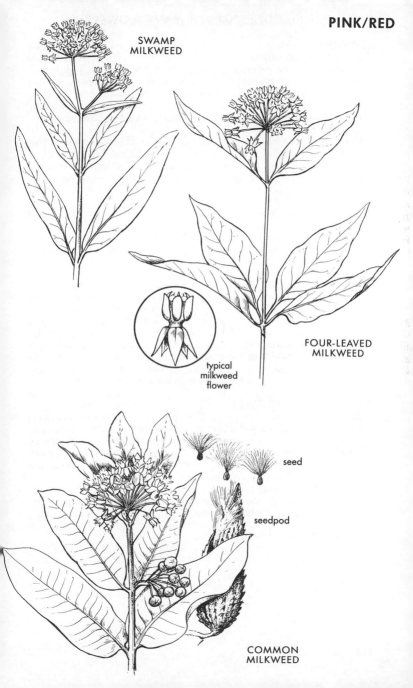

PINK/RED

SWAMP
MILKWEED

FOUR-LEAVED
MILKWEED

typical
milkweed
flower

seed

seedpod

COMMON
MILKWEED

SLENDER SPIKES OF MANY FLOWERS

LOPSEED   Roots
Phryma leptostachya L.   Lopseed Family
Slender-branched perennial; 1–3 ft. Stems swollen for a short dis-
tance (1 in. or less) above each pair of leaves. Leaves opposite, oval,
toothed. Leaf stalks on middle leaf pairs longer than those on upper
or lower leaves. Flowers small, purplish, snapdragon-like; in terminal spikes; July–Sept. **Where found:** Woods, thickets. Throughout our
area.
Uses: American Indians gargled root tea (or chewed root) for sore
throats; drank root tea for rheumatism. Also found in e. Asia, where
it is used for fevers, ulcers, ringworm, scabies, and insect bites. Root
poulticed for boils, carbuncles, sores, and cancers. Also considered
insecticidal.

EUROPEAN VERVAIN   Root, leaves
Verbena officinalis L.   Verbena Family
Mostly smooth, loosely branched annual; 1–3 ft. Leaves paired, with
deeply cut lobes and sharp teeth. Flowers tiny, purple to pinkish; in
slender spikes; June–Oct. **Where found:** Waste places. Escaped from
gardens; locally established. Alien.
Uses: In Europe, plant tea used for obstructions of liver and spleen,
headaches, and nervous disorders. Leaves considered diuretic, milk-
inducing; extracts analgesic. Used experimentally in China to control malaria symptoms, kill blood flukes (parasites) and germs, stop
pain and inflammation. Chinese studies suggest that herbage of this
plant is synergistic with a prostaglandin (E_2). Russian studies show
adaptogenic activity of the alcoholic extract or tincture. Said to be
milder than Blue Vervain (*Verbena hastata*, p. 172) and other species. **Warning:** Plant suspected of poisoning cattle in Australia.

PURPLE or SPIKE LOOSESTRIFE   Flowering plant
Lythrum salicaria L.   **C. Pl. 5**   Loosestrife Family
Downy perennial; 2–4 ft. Leaves whorled or opposite; *rounded or
heart-shaped at base.* Purple-pink, *6-petaled* flowers, in spikes;
June–Sept. **Where found:** Invasive in swampy meadows, often forming large stands and blanketing moist meadows in a sea of color. New
England to N.C.; Mo. to Minn. Alien.
Uses: Tea made from whole flowering plant, fresh or dried, is a European folk remedy (demulcent, astringent) for diarrhea, dysentery;
used as a gargle for sore throats, a douche for leukorrhea, and a
cleansing wash for wounds. Experimentally, plant extracts stop
bleeding, kill some bacteria.

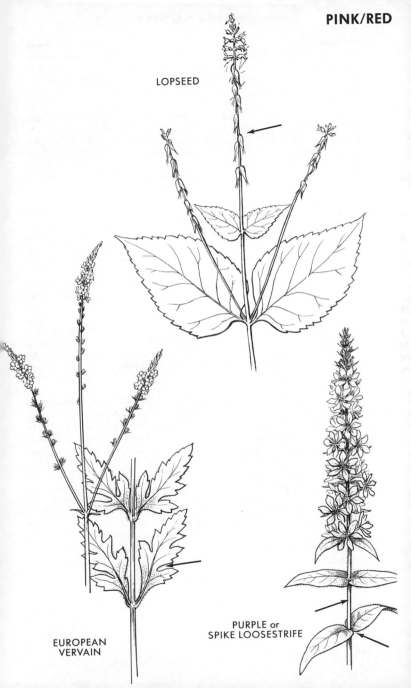

PINK/RED

LOPSEED

EUROPEAN
VERVAIN

PURPLE or
SPIKE LOOSESTRIFE

PEA-LIKE FLOWERS

GROUNDNUT   **Root**
Apios americana Medic.   Pea Family
Twining vine. Leaves with 5–7 oval, sharp-pointed leaflets. *Sweetly fragrant, maroon or purple-brown* flowers, in crowded clusters in leaf axils; July–Sept. **Where found:** Rich, moist thickets. N.B. to Fla.; west to Texas; north to Minn., N.D.
Uses: Delicious tubers used as food by Pilgrims during first bleak winters. Favorite Indian food. With 3 times the protein of potatoes, each Groundnut plant, under cultivation, may produce 5 pounds of tubers. The plant has been suggested as a nitrogen-fixing edible ornamental for permaculturists. John Josselyn (1672) suggested a poultice of Groundnut root be used for cancerous conditions known as "proud flesh."

NAKED-FLOWERED TICK-TREFOIL   **Root**
Desmodium nudiflorum (L.) DC.   Pea Family
Perennial; 18–36 in. Leaves in whorls; 3 oval leaflets, middle one on a longer stalk. *Leaf stalk separate from flower stalk.* Pinkish red flowers on a *leafless stalk;* July–Aug. Pods jointed; "beggar's ticks" adhere to clothes. **Where found:** Woods. Me. to Fla.; Texas to Minn.
Uses: Cherokees chewed the root for inflammation of mouth, sore bleeding gums, periodontal diseases with pus discharge. Root tea was used as a wash for cramps.

RED CLOVER   **Flowering tops**
Trifolium pratense L.   **C. Pl. 22**   Pea Family
Familiar biennial or short-lived perennial; to 18 in. Leaves divided into 3 oval leaflets; leaflets fine-toothed, with *prominent "V" marks.* Flowers pink to red, in rounded heads; May–Sept. **Where found:** Weed. Fields, roadsides. Throughout our area.

 Uses: Historically, flower tea has been used as an antispasmodic, expectorant, mild sedative, "blood purifier"; for asthma, bronchitis, spasmodic coughs; externally, a wash has been used as a folk cancer remedy, including the famous Hoxsey treatment, and for athlete's foot, sores, burns, and ulcers. Flowers formerly smoked in anti-asthma cigarettes. Science has not confirmed traditional uses, though the plant contains many biologically active compounds, including estrogens. **Warning:** Fall or late-cut hay in large doses can cause frothing, diarrhea, dermatitis, and decreased milk production in cattle. Diseased clover, externally showing no symptoms, may contain the indolizidine alkaloid slaframine, which is much more poisonous than castanospermine, now being studied for anti-AIDS and antidiabetic activity.

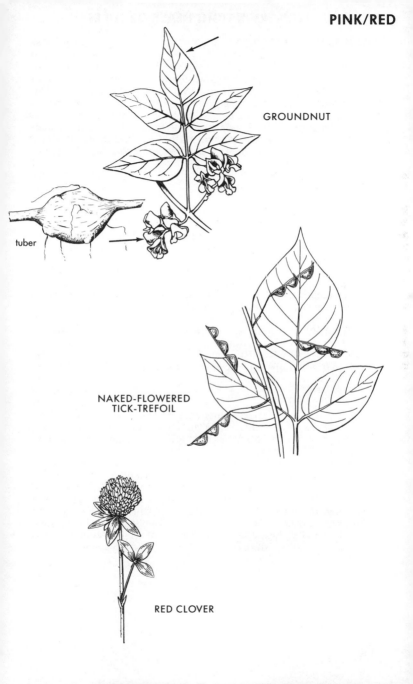

PINK/RED

GROUNDNUT

tuber

NAKED-FLOWERED
TICK-TREFOIL

RED CLOVER

FLOWERS IN TIGHT HEADS OR SPIKES

PENNSYLVANIA SMARTWEED
Polygonum pensylvanicum L.

Leaves, tops
Buckwheat Family

Erect or sprawling annual; 1–5 ft. Leaves lance-shaped; sheaths *not fringed* (see Lady's Thumb, below). Flowers rose-pink (or white); in crowded, elongate clusters; July–Nov. Flower stalks often have *minute glandular hairs* near top. Highly variable. **Where found:** Waste ground. Throughout our area.

Uses: American Indians used tea made from whole plant for diarrhea; poulticed leaves for piles. Bitter leaf tea used to stop bleeding from mouth. Tops were used in tea for epilepsy. **Warning:** Fresh juice acrid; may cause irritation.

LADY'S THUMB, HEART'S EASE
Polygonum persicaria L.

Leaves
Buckwheat Family

Reddish-stemmed, sprawling perennial; 6–24 in. Leaves lance-shaped, often with a purplish triangular blotch in the middle of leaf; papery sheath at leaf nodes has *fringes*. Pinkish flowers in elongate clusters; June–Oct. **Where found:** Waste places. Throughout our area. Alien (Europe).

Uses: American Indians adopted the leaf tea for heart troubles, stomachaches, and as a diuretic for "gravel" (kidney stones). The whole herb was poulticed for pain, rubbed on poison-ivy rash, and on horses' backs to keep flies away. Leaf tea used as a foot soak for rheumatic pains of the legs and feet. In European tradition, leaf tea was used for inflammation, stomachaches, and sore throats. **Warning:** Fresh juice may cause irritation.

Related species: Other *Polygonum* species in our range, many naturalized from Europe, have been used similarly.

SALAD BURNET
Sanguisorba officinalis L.

Leaves, root
Rose Family

Perennial; 1–5 ft. Leaves compound; leaflets 7–15, *toothed.* Tiny, purplish red flowers, in oval or thickly rounded heads; May–Oct. **Where found:** Me. to Minn. Escaped elsewhere. Alien. Mostly cultivated in herb gardens.

Uses: In Europe leaf tea was used for fevers, and as a styptic. American soldiers drank tea before battles in Revolutionary War to prevent bleeding if wounded. Root tea astringent, allays menstrual bleeding. In China the root tea is used to stop bleeding, "cool" blood; for piles, uterine bleeding, dysentery; externally for sores, swelling, burns. Experimentally, the plant is antibacterial (in China); stops bleeding and vomiting. Powdered root used clinically for 2nd- and 3rd-degree burns. **Warning:** Contains tannins, contraindicated for burns in Western medicine.

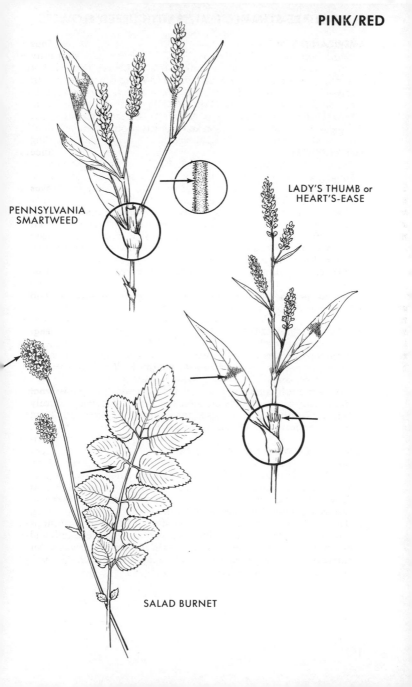

PENNSYLVANIA
SMARTWEED

LADY'S THUMB or
HEART'S-EASE

SALAD BURNET

SQUARE-STEMMED PLANTS WITH LIPPED FLOWERS

AMERICAN DITTANY   **Leaves**
Cunila origanoides (L.) Britton   Mint Family
Wiry-stemmed, branched perennial; 1–2 ft. Leaves oval, to 1 in.; toothed, *oregano-scented*. Small, violet to white flowers, in clusters; July–Oct. *stamens 2; throat hairy*. **Where found:** Dry woods, thickets. Se. N.Y. to Fla.; Texas, Okla., Mo., Ill.
Uses: Leaf tea a folk remedy for colds, fevers, headaches, snakebites; thought to induce perspiration and menstruation.

MOTHERWORT   **Leaves**
Leonurus cardiaca L.   **C. Pl. 29**   Mint Family
Square-stemmed perennial; 3–5 ft. Leaves 3-lobed; lobes toothed. Pinkish flowers in whorls in axils; May–Aug. *Upper lip furry*. **Where found:** Weed. Much of our area. Alien.
Uses: Traditionally, leaf tea is used to promote menstruation, regulate menses, aid in childbirth (hence the common name); also used for asthma and heart palpitations. Said to be sedative; used for insomnia, neuralgia, sciatica, spasms, fevers, and stomachaches. Scientists have found extracts to be antispasmodic, hypotensive, and sedative. Experimentally, leonurine, a leaf constituent, is a uterine tonic.
Related species: Chinese species, well documented with laboratory and clinical reports, have been used similarly.

BEE-BALM, OSWEGO TEA   **Leaves**
Monarda didyma L.   **C. Pl. 24**   Mint Family
Perennial; 2–5 ft. Leaves paired. Flowers red, tubular, in crowded heads; June–Sept. Bracts often red or purplish. **Where found:** Thickets, stream banks. N.Y. to Ga.; Tenn. to Mich.
Uses: American Indians used leaf tea for colic, gas, colds, fevers, stomachaches, nosebleeds, insomnia, heart trouble, measles, and to induce sweating. Poultice used for headaches. Historically, physicians used leaf to expel worms and gas.

GERMANDER, WOOD SAGE, WILD BASIL   **Leaves**
Teucrium canadense L.   Mint Family
Variable perennial; 1–3 ft. Leaves oval to lance-shaped, toothed, white-hairy beneath. Flowers purple, pink, or whitish; June–Sept. Calyx felty; *stamens protude from cleft of upper lip*. **Where found:** Woods, thickets. Throughout our area.
Uses: Leaf tea traditionally used to induce menstruation, urination, and sweating. Used like the bugleweeds or water-horehounds (*Lycopus*, p. 70) for lung ailments, worms, piles; externally, as a gargle and antiseptic dressing. A widespread adulterant to commercial supplies of Skullcap (*Scutellaria lateriflora*, p. 186).

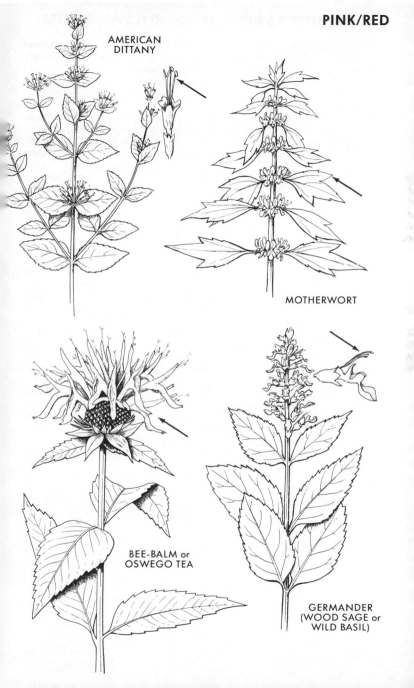

AMERICAN
DITTANY

MOTHERWORT

BEE-BALM or
OSWEGO TEA

GERMANDER
(WOOD SAGE or
WILD BASIL)

COMPOSITES WITH FLAT-TOPPED FLOWER CLUSTERS

DAISY FLEABANE
Whole plant
Erigeron philadelphicus L.   Composite Family
Slender, hairy perennial; 1–3 ft. Basal leaves oblong; stem leaves smaller, *clasping at base.* Flowers less than 1 in. across; pinkish to magenta, with *numerous slender rays* and a yellow disk. April–July.
Where found: Thickets. Most of our area.
Uses: Plant tea diuretic, astringent; a folk remedy for diarrhea, "gravel" (kidney stones), diabetes, painful urination; also used to stop hemorrhages of stomach, bowels, bladder, kidneys, and nose. Once used for fevers, bronchitis, tumors, piles, and coughs. **Warning:** May cause contact dermatitis.

SPOTTED JOE-PYE-WEED
Leaves, root
Eupatorium maculatum L.   Composite Family
Perennial; 2–6 ft. Stem *purple or purple-spotted.* Leaves lance-shaped, in *whorls* of 4–5. Purple flowers in flat-topped clusters; July–Sept.
Where found: Wet meadows. N.S. to mountains of N.C.; Neb. to B.C.
Uses: American Indians used tea of whole herb as a diuretic for dropsy, painful urination, gout, kidney infections, rheumatism. Root tea once used for fevers, colds, chills, sore womb after childbirth, diarrhea, liver and kidney ailments; a wash for rheumatism. Name derived from "Joe Pye," a 19th-century Caucasian "Indian theme promoter" who used the root to induce sweating in typhus fever.

SWEET JOE-PYE-WEED, GRAVEL ROOT
Leaves, root
Eupatorium purpureum L.   Composite Family
Similar to *E. maculatum* (above). Perennial, to 12 ft. tall; stems green, purple at leaf nodes. Pale pink-purple flowers, in a somewhat rounded cluster; July–Sept. **Where found:** Thickets. N.H. to Fla.; Ark., Okla., w. Neb. to Minn.
Uses: Leaf and root tea traditionally used to eliminate stones in urinary tract, and treat urinary incontinence in children, and dropsy; also for gout, rheumatism, impotence, uterine prolapse, asthma, chronic coughs. Homeopathically used for gall bladder and urinary ailments.
Remarks: Also known as Queen-of-the-Meadow, a name that is shared with a European species (*Spiraea ulmaria* — see p. 144).
Related species: German researchers report immunologically active polysaccharides from other *Eupatorium* species, both American and European.

DAISY
FLEABANE

SPOTTED
JOE-PYE-WEED

SWEET
JOE-PYE-WEED
or GRAVEL ROOT

THISTLE-LIKE, BRISTLY FLOWERS;
BURDOCKS AND THISTLES

GREAT BURDOCK   **Leaves, root, seeds**
Arctium lappa L.   Composite Family
Biennial; 2–9 ft. Lower leaves *large, rhubarb-like*. Stalk solid, celery-like — *grooved* above. Reddish purple, thistle-like flowers, 1–1½ in. across; *long-stalked*, in flat-topped clusters; July–Oct. Seedpods (familiar "burs") stick to clothing. **Where found:** Waste places. Canada south to Pa., N.C.; west to Ill., Mich. Local elsewhere. Alien. A widespread Eurasian weed used in traditional medicine in China, Japan, Europe, and N. America.

Uses: Traditionally, root tea (2 ounces dried root in 1 quart of water) used as a "blood purifier"; diuretic, stimulates bile secretion, sweating; also used for gout, liver and kidney ailments, rheumatism, gonorrhea. In China, a tea of leafy branches was used for vertigo, rheumatism, and (in tea mixed with brown sugar) for measles. Externally, used as a wash for hives, eczema, and other skin eruptions. Seeds diuretic; thought to be antiseptic. Seeds used for abscesses, sore throats, insect and snake bites, flu, constipation; once used to treat scarlet fever, smallpox, and scrofula. Crushed seeds poulticed on bruises. Leaves poulticed on burns, ulcers, sores. Japanese studies suggest roots contains compounds that may curb mutations (and hence cancer?). **Warning:** Leaf hairs may irritate skin. Do not confuse leaves with the toxic leaves of Rhubarb.

COMMON BURDOCK   **Root, seeds, leaves**
Arctium minus (Hill) Bernh.   Composite Family
Smaller than *A. lappa* (see above); 2–5 ft. Leaf stems *hollow, not furrowed*. Flowers smaller — to ¾ in. across; *without stalks or short-stalked*; July–Oct. **Where found:** Waste places. Most of our area. Alien.
Uses: Same as for *A. lappa*. Used extensively by American Indians.

CANADA THISTLE   **Leaves, root**
Cirsium arvense (L.) Robson   Composite Family
Perennial; 1–5 ft., with vigorous taproots; usually forms colonies. Stems smooth; leafy near top. Leaves oblong to lance-shaped; *margins very prickly*. Flowers small, pink to violet (rarely white); to 3–4 in. across; July–Sept. *Bracts strongly appressed.* **Where found:** Fields, pastures, roadsides. Throughout our area. Serious alien weed from Europe.
Uses: Leaf tea "tonic" and diuretic. Once used for tuberculosis; externally, for skin eruptions, skin ulcers, and poison-ivy rash. Root tea used for dysentery, diarrhea. American Indians used root tea as a bowel tonic and dewormer.

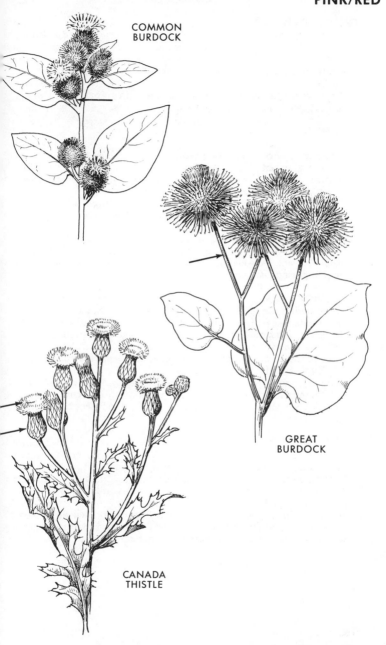

PINK/RED

COMMON
BURDOCK

GREAT
BURDOCK

CANADA
THISTLE

PETALS IN 3'S

CRESTED DWARF IRIS   **Root**
Iris cristata Ait.   **C. Pl. 15**   Iris Family
Spreading perennial; 4–8 in. Leaves *short*, lance-shaped; *sheathed* on stem. Blue (rarely white) flowers with yellow crests on downcurved sepals; April–May. **Where found:** Wet woods. Md. to N.C.; Miss., Ark., e. Okla. to Ind.
Uses: American Indians used root ointment (in animal fats or waxes) on cancerous ulcers. Root tea used for hepatitis.

BLUE FLAG   **Root**
Iris versicolor L.   Iris Family
Perennial; 1–2 ft. Leaves swordlike, similar to those of garden irises. Flowers violet-blue, sepals violet at outer edge; veins prominent; *sheaths papery.* Flowers May–July. **Where found:** Wet meadows, moist soil. Lab. to Va.; Ohio, Wisc. to Minn., Man.
Uses: American Indians poulticed root on swellings, sores, bruises, rheumatism; analgesic agent; internally root tea used as strong laxative, emetic, and to stimulate bile flow. Physicians formerly used root of this plant in small, frequent doses to "cleanse" blood and stimulate the bowels, kidney, and liver. Homeopathically used for migraines and as a cathartic, diuretic, and emetic. **Warning:** Considered **poisonous.**

SPIDERWORT   **Leaves, root, whole plant**
Tradescantia virginiana L.   **C. Pl. 42**   Spiderwort Family
Perennial; 1–3 ft. Leaves grass- or iris-like, sheathing stem. Purple flowers in a terminal cluster; April–June. Petals 3; stamens many, with *prominent, large-celled hairs.* (Individual stamen hair cells are so large they may be seen with naked eye.) **Where found:** Me. to W. Va., Ky., Ga., Miss.; Ark. to Minn.
Uses: Root tea of this and other spiderwort species used by American Indians for "female," kidney, and stomach ailments, and as a laxative. Smashed plant (leaf poultice) applied to insect bites, stings, and cancers.

ASIATIC DAYFLOWER   **Leaves**
Commelina communis L.   **C. Pl. 6**   Spiderwort Family
Sprawling perennial; 1–3 ft. Leaves oval, clasping stem. Flowers with 2 prominent, earlike blue petals and a *smaller whitish petal beneath*; May–Oct. **Where found:** Waste places throughout our area. Troublesome weed. Alien (Asia).
Uses: In China, leaf tea gargled for sore throats; used for cooling, detoxifying, and diuretic properties in flu, acute tonsillitis, urinary infections, dysentery, and acute intestinal enteritis.

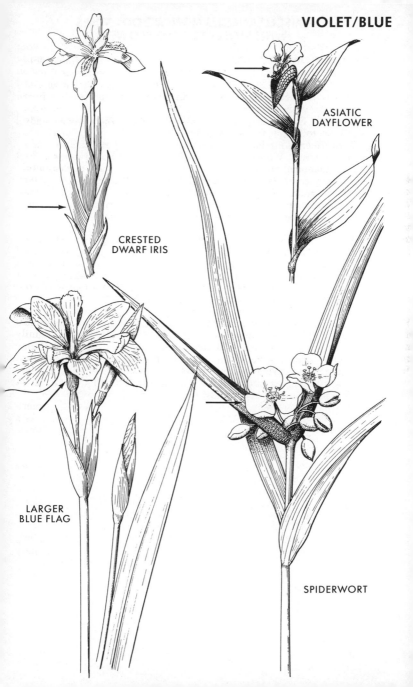

VIOLET/BLUE

ASIATIC
DAYFLOWER

CRESTED
DWARF IRIS

LARGER
BLUE FLAG

SPIDERWORT

MISCELLANEOUS NON-WOODY VINES
WITH VIOLET TO BLUE FLOWERS

PASSION-FLOWER, MAYPOP   **Whole plant**
Passiflora incarnata L.   **C. Pl. 32**   Passion-flower Family
Climbing vine; to 30 ft. Tendrils *springlike*. Leaves *cleft* with 2–3
slightly toothed lobes. Flowers large, showy, unique — whitish to
purplish, with *numerous threads* radiating from center. Flowers
July–Oct. Fruits fleshy, egg-shaped; Aug.–Nov. **Where found:** Sandy
soil. Pa. to Fla.; e. Texas to s. Mo.

⚠ **Uses:** American Indians poulticed root for boils, cuts, earaches, and
inflammation. Whole plant has traditionally been used in tea as an
antispasmodic, and a sedative for neuralgia, epilepsy, restlessness,
painful menses, insomnia, tension headaches. Research shows plant
extracts are mildly sedative, slightly reduce blood pressure, increase
respiratory rate, and decrease motor activity. Fruits edible, delicious. **Warning:** Potentially harmful in large amounts.

KUDZU   **Root, flowers, seeds, stems, root starch**
Pueraria lobata (Willd.) Ohwi   **C. Pl. 32**   Pea Family
Noxious, robust, trailing, or climbing vine. Leaves *palmate, 3-
parted*; leaflets entire or palmately lobed. Flowers reddish purple,
grape-scented; in a loose raceme; July–Sept. **Where found:** Waste
ground. Pa. to Fla.; Texas to Kans. Asian alien.
Uses: In China, root tea used for headaches, diarrhea, dysentery,
acute intestinal obstruction, gastroenteritis, deafness; to promote
measle eruptions, induce sweating. Experimentally, plant extracts
lower blood sugar and blood pressure. Flower tea used for stomach
acidity; "awakens the spleen," "expels drunkenness." Seeds used for
dysentery, and to expel drunkenness. Stem poulticed for sores, swellings, mastitis; tea gargled for sore throats. Root starch (used to stimulate production of body fluids) eaten as food.

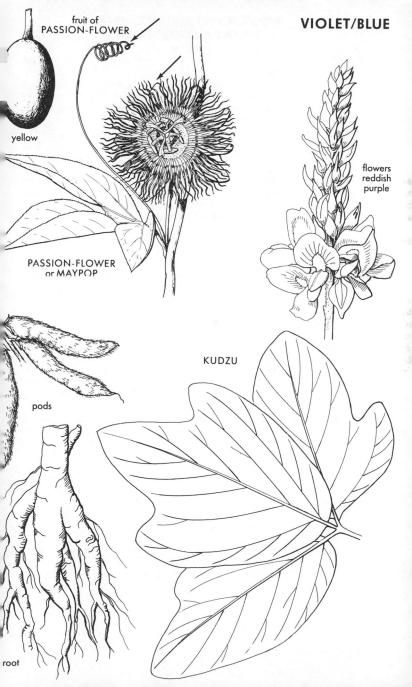

VIOLET/BLUE

fruit of
PASSION-FLOWER

yellow

PASSION-FLOWER
or MAYPOP

flowers
reddish
purple

pods

KUDZU

root

MISCELLANEOUS PLANTS WITH
SHOWY FLOWER SPIKES

TALL BELLFLOWER   **Leaves**
Campanula americana L.   Bellflower Family
Annual; to 6 ft. Leaves lance-shaped to oblong-ovate (3–6 in.). Blue
flowers in terminal spikes; July–Sept. Star-shaped petals are fused
together. Note *long, curved style.* **Where found:** Moist woods, stream
banks. Ont. to Fla.; Texas to Minn.
Uses: American Indians used leaf tea for coughs and tuberculosis.
Crushed root was used for whooping cough.

FOXGLOVE   **Leaves**
Digitalis purpurea L.   **C. Pl. 28**   Figwort Family
Biennial; 3–6 ft. Leaves in a basal rosette; ovate to lance-shaped, soft-
hairy, toothed; to 1 ft. long. Flowers purple to white *spotted thimbles*, 1¼ in. long, on spikes; *in summer of second year.* **Where found:**
Garden escape. New England. Alien.
Uses: Dried leaves a source of heart-tonic glycosides. Used in modern medicine to increase force of systolic contractions in congestive
heart failure; lowers venous pressure in hypertensive heart ailments;
elevates blood pressure in weak heart; diuretic, reduces edema. **Warning: Lethally toxic.** First-year's leaf growth (rosette) has been mistaken for leaves of Comfrey (*Symphytum* — see p. 180), with fatal
results. Therapeutic dose of *Digitalis* is dangerously close to lethal
dose. **For use by physicians only.**

BLUE VERVAIN   **Leaves, root**
Verbena hastata L.   **C. Pl. 34**   Verbena Family
Perennial; 2–4 ft. Stem 4-angled, grooved. Leaves mostly lance-
shaped, sharp-toothed; base sometimes lobed. Flowers blue-violet;
tops branched in *pencil-like* spikes; July–Sept. **Where found:** Fields,
thickets. Most of our area.
Uses: American Indians used leaf tea as a "female tonic"; also for
colds, coughs, fevers, bowel complaints, dysentery, stomach cramps;
emetic in large doses. Root considered more active than leaves. Used
similarly by 19th-century physicians.

PURPLE or SPIKE LOOSESTRIFE   **Flowering plant**
Lythrum salicaria L.   **C. Pl. 5**   Loosestrife Family
Downy perennial; 2–4 ft. Leaves whorled or opposite; *rounded or
heart-shaped at base.* Flowers purple-pink, *6-petaled;* in spikes;
June–Sept. **Where found:** Invasive in swampy meadows. New England to N.C.; Mo. to Minn. Alien.
Uses: Tea made from whole flowering plant (fresh or dried) a European folk remedy (demulcent, astringent) for diarrhea, dysentery;
gargle for sore throats; douche for leukorrhea, cleansing wash for
wounds. Experimentally, stops bleeding, antibacterial.

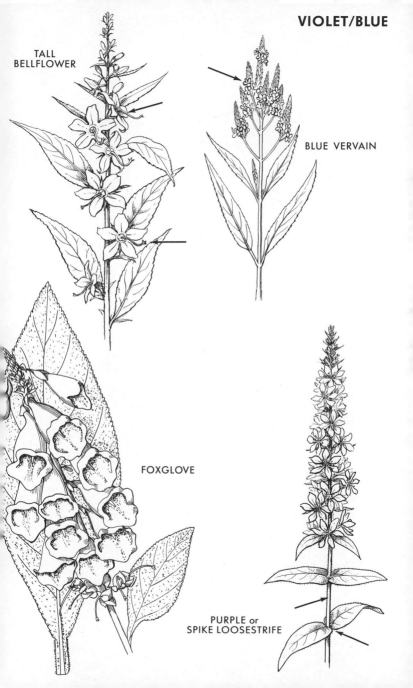

VIOLET/BLUE

TALL
BELLFLOWER

BLUE VERVAIN

FOXGLOVE

PURPLE or
SPIKE LOOSESTRIFE

PLATES

Symbols: = **Poisonous.** Dangerous or deadly to ingest, or perhaps even to touch.

 = **Caution.** See warning in text.

 = Known to cause **allergic reactions** in some individuals.

 = Known to cause **dermatitis** in some individuals.

 = Used in **modern medicine** in the U.S.

An Important Note to Our Readers: This book is intended to be a field guide to medicinal plants, and as such, it focuses on plant identification — recognition, not recommended treatments or prescriptions. Only your doctor or another health-care professional who is licensed to do so can prescribe medication — herbal or synthetic — for you. Moreover, any medicine can be toxic in overdoses. Never eat or taste any part of a wild plant, or use it in any medicinal preparation, unless you have consulted an expert on its identification and a licensed medical professional on correct dosage and usage.

PLATE 1

AQUATIC PLANTS;
IN OR NEAR WATER

Ponds, lakes, streams, and other waterways provide specialized habitats for many aquatic species, including several medicinal plants.

FRAGRANT WATER-LILY
Nymphaea odorata   **p. 14**

 Aquatic perennial with large, round, floating leaves, notched at base. Flowers white, to 5 in. across; sweetly fragrant. **Flowers June–Sept.** Grows in ponds, slow waters. Nfld. to Fla. and Texas to Neb. The large, spongy, fleshy roots were used by American Indians and as a folk medicine for various conditions, especially lung ailments, but the plant may be **toxic.**

SWAMP MILKWEED
Asclepias incarnata   **p. 154**

Found throughout much of our range in swamps, wet thickets, and along pond edges, this showy, highly variable milkweed usually has many lance-shaped, opposite leaves; small amounts of milky juice; and flower clusters in branched, flat-topped groupings (umbels). **Flowers June–Aug.** The root has been used in folk medicine, but is potentially **toxic.**

WATERCRESS
Nasturtium officinale   **p. 34**

Watercress, well known for its edible, mustard-like leaves, forms large colonies in cool running water. **Flowers March–June.** The leaves, high in vitamins A and C, are harvested before flowers appear. Traditionally used as a diuretic and "blood purifier." **Caution:** Harvest leaves from unpolluted waters. Poisonings have resulted from eating leaves from plants growing in polluted waters, from which the plant has absorbed heavy metals and toxins.

ARROWHEADS
Sagittaria species   **p. 16**

 The 15 or so species occurring in ponds or lakes throughout our range are separated based on technical details. They have been used interchangeably. **Flowers June–Sept.** The edible tubers have been used in tea for indigestion and externally, in a poultice for wounds and sores. The leaves have also been used medicinally, but may cause dermatitis.

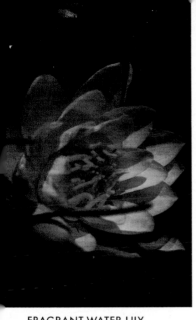

FRAGRANT WATER-LILY

SWAMP MILKWEED

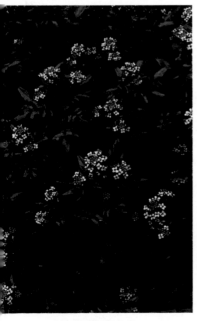

WATERCRESS

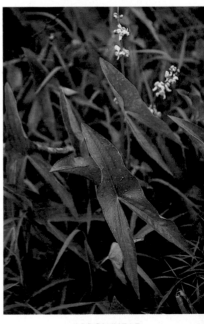

ARROWHEAD

PLATE 2
NEAR RUNNING WATER (1)

Banks of slow- or fast-flowing streams and edges of springs or ponds provide habitats for many medicinal plants. See also Pl. 3.

TURTLEHEAD
Chelone glabra   p. 12

This 2- to 3-ft.-high perennial grows in moist areas in much of our range, though it is largely absent from the South. The white to pink-tinged flowers have a swollen, strongly arching upper lip, resembling a turtle's head in form. **Flowers July–Oct.** The leaf tea or ointment was once used as a folk remedy.

CARDINAL FLOWER
Lobelia cardinalis   p. 144

Many consider this one of our most showy wildflowers. The vibrant scarlet flower spikes flag its presence along stream or pond edges in mid- to late summer. **Flowers July–Sept.** The root was used to expel worms in 19th-century medicine. The leaves were also used in tea as a folk medicine. See warning in text.

SCOURING RUSH, GREATER HORSETAIL
Equisetum hyemale   p. 304

This evergreen, hollow-stemmed, primitive perennial is often found in moist sandy soils, along stream banks and pond edges and in moist depressions throughout our range and beyond. The jointed, apparently leafless, rough, finely ribbed, nonbranching stems make this plant easy to distinguish from other species of horsetail. It has been widely used throughout the Northern Hemisphere as a diuretic for kidney and bladder ailments. See warning in text.

GREAT LOBELIA
Lobelia siphilitica   p. 184

Often found growing on wet ground with Cardinal Flower, this is a common fall wildflower along southern streams. It occurs as far north as Maine, where it is rare, and Minnesota. **Flowers Aug.–Oct.** Early medical writers observed that American Indians used the root to treat syphilis, hence the species name *siphilitica*. Potentially **toxic.**

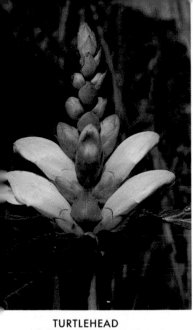

TURTLEHEAD

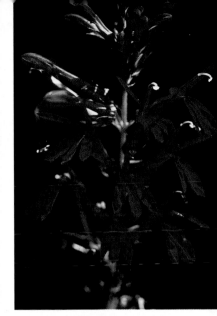

CARDINAL FLOWER

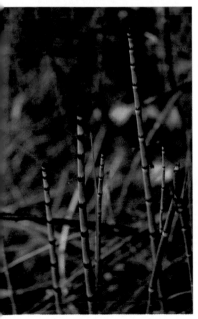

SCOURING RUSH

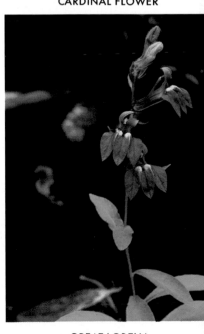

GREAT LOBELIA

PLATE 3

NEAR RUNNING WATER (2)

Pond outlets and inlets, spring seepage, and streams, brooks, or creeks provide dozens of wild medicinal curios for the forager to observe.

BONESET
Eupatorium perfoliatum **p. 78**

Clumps of this 3- to 4-ft.-tall, white-flowered perennial in the composite family are common along waterways, especially in the North, though it occurs throughout our range. It is easily distinguished by its opposite pairs of perfoliate leaves, which are joined and appear to be pierced at the base by the stem. The leaves resemble a stretched diamond (if you stretch your imagination). **Flowers July–Oct.** The leaves were once used to treat "break-bone fever," (perhaps a flu epidemic), hence the common name "Boneset." Widely acclaimed as useful during flu epidemics in 19th-century America, Boneset shows potential in recent research as an immune-system stimulant. These findings, coupled with the historical uses, suggest the plant should be investigated further.

GOLDEN RAGWORT, SQUAW-WEED
Senecio aureus **p. 120**

This early spring wildflower, often growing in clumps among exposed rocks in streams, is easily distinguished from other ragworts (*Senecio* species) by the heart-shaped leaves at the base of the plant. **Flowers late March–July.** Traditionally, the leaves and roots have been used for a variety of "female" diseases, so the plant acquired an alternate common name, "Squaw-weed." **Caution:** Many ragworts contain high levels of **toxic** pyrrolizidine alkaloids.

JEWELWEED
Impatiens capensis **p. 136**

Common along stream and river banks, or around seepage in woods throughout our range. The fresh crushed leaves, rubbed on the skin, have gained a wide reputation as a preventative or treatment for poison-ivy rash. **Flowers June–Sept.**

GIANT CANE
Arundinaria gigantea **p. 312**

One of our largest native grasses, this distinctly bamboo-like perennial forms large thickets along rivers and creeks and in moist soils south of Delaware. The root was once used as a diuretic. **Caution:** Ergot, a poisonous fungus, occasionally forms on the seeds of this plant. Do not collect from areas with diseased plants.

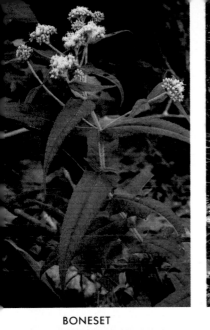

BONESET

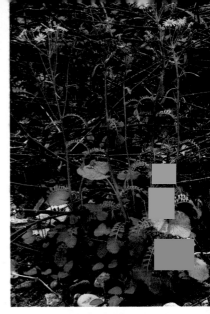

GOLDEN RAGWORT

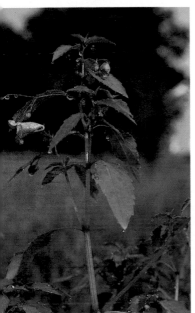

JEWELWEED

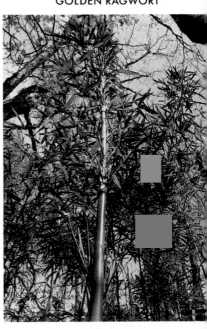

GIANT CANE

PLATE 4
SPHAGNUM BOGS

Highly acidic bogs composed of mats of Sphagnum Moss, often several feet thick, are best known as the source of peat moss. These habitats harbor fascinating medicinal plants. **Habitat:** The "cottony" seedheads are those of Cotton Grass or Bog Cotton (*Eriophorus* species), a common sedge in sphagnum bogs, and a good habitat indicator.

PITCHER-PLANT
Sarracenia purpurea **p. 142**
The tubular, pitcher-shaped leaves, which often contain water, have evolved to capture and digest insects. The "pitchers" have smooth surfaces and downward-pointing hairs, making it difficult for insects to crawl out. Once the insect drowns, the leaves secrete enzymes that digest the insect's soft body parts, which allows the plant to obtain nutrients that would otherwise be unavailable in its habitat. The leaves were once used as an unsuccessful treatment for smallpox. The flowers *(center left)*, usually reddish and with a large flat pistil, are distinctive. **Flowers May–July.**

ROUND-LEAVED SUNDEW
Drosera rotundifolia **p. 28**
Another insectivorous (insect-eating) bog plant. This sundew's unusual leaves are barely 2 inches tall, and are covered with reddish hairs exuding a sticky, dewlike secretion that traps unwary insects. The leaves fold over the captured insect and digest it. The leaves have traditionally been used for lung ailments, perhaps reflecting the "doctrine of signatures" (see p. 6). Research has confirmed the antibacterial activity of a chemical component in the plant. **Flowers June–Aug.**

LABRADOR TEA
Ledum groenlandicum **p. 230**
This 3-ft.-tall shrub can be recognized by its leathery leaves with edges rolled under and white or rusty woolly hairs beneath. **Flowers May–July.** The leaves were used in tea as a remedy for colds, asthma, stomachaches, and other ailments. *Photo by Phillip E. Keenan.*

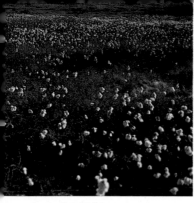

Bog Habitat

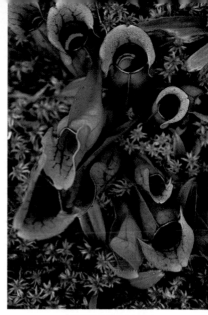

PITCHER-PLANT

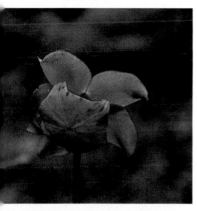

Flower of PITCHER-PLANT

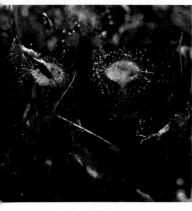

SUNDEW

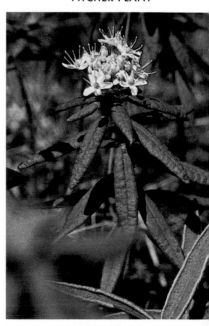

LABRADOR TEA

PLATE 5
MOIST MEADOWS, POND EDGES (1)

Moist meadows and pond edges are rich habitats for medicinal plants. See also Pl. 6.

PURPLE or SPIKE LOOSESTRIFE
Lythrum salicaria **p. 156**
This European plant has become an invasive, though beautiful, weed of swampy meadows, especially in the Northeast. **Flowers June–Sept.** The whole flowering plant, fresh or dried, is used in European folk medicine, primarily as an astringent to stop bleeding, diarrhea, and dysentery, and as a soothing gargle for sore throats.

SWEETFLAG
Acorus americanus **p. 86**
Often found in large clumps in low spots of pastures or moist meadows and along pond edges or in ditches, this member of the arum family has rigid, grasslike leaves. It produces aromatic fleshy rhizomes that are used in traditional medicine. The fingerlike flowerheads, jutting at an angle about ⅓ of the way up the stem, are usually found on a low percentage of plants in a given population. **Flowers May–Aug.** See warning in text.

AMERICAN BUGLEWEED, CUT-LEAVED WATER-HOREHOUND
Lycopus americanus **p. 70**
The most abundant of about 7 or so species in our range; distinguished by its lance-shaped, strongly cut or toothed leaves. Found on low ground throughout much of our area. **Flowers July–Sept.** The leaves of this and other bugleweeds (*Lycopus* species) are traditionally used as a mild sedative and astringent in heart diseases, lung ailments, and so on. Scientists should investigate this folk remedy further.

AMERICAN WHITE HELLEBORE
Veratrum viride **p. 104**
This **highly toxic** plant, up to 8 ft. tall, produces large panicles of greenish, star-shaped flowers. It occurs along edges of wet woods and in swampy areas. In minute, controlled doses, this poisonous plant has been used for a variety of medicinal purposes.

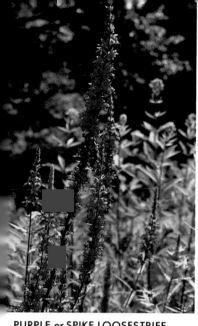

PURPLE or SPIKE LOOSESTRIFE

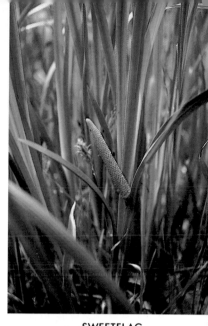

SWEETFLAG

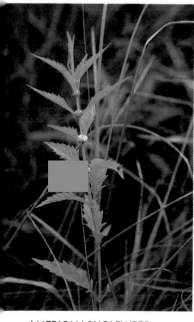

AMERICAN BUGLEWEED

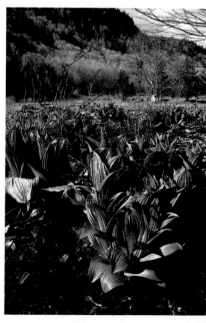

AMERICAN WHITE HELLEBORE

PLATE 6
MOIST MEADOWS (2)

DAYFLOWERS
Commelina species **p. 168**

Each dayflower blooms for only 1 day, hence the common name. One common Asiatic species, *Commelina communis*, is a widespread, troublesome weed in much of our range. The 3-petaled flowers have 2 large, earlike petals and 1 petal, usually much smaller, beneath. **Flowers May–Oct.** In China the leaf tea is gargled for sore throats and is used for its cooling, detoxifying, and diuretic properties in flu, acute tonsillitis, urinary infections, dysentery, and acute enteritis.

ANGELICA
Angelica atropurpurea **p. 60**

Angelica grows in swampy or moist soils. It has large, inflated sheaths at the leaf bases and has a smooth purple or purple-tinged stem, hence the species name *atropurpurea* (which means "dark purple"). **Flowers June–Aug. Caution:** Although all parts of the plant can be used medicinally, it should not be harvested unless it has been positively identified by a trained botanist, because it may be confused with the deadly Poison Hemlock or Water-hemlock (p. 58), which grows in the same habitat.

FIREWEED
Epilobium angustifolium **p. 146**

This common weed is invasive in burned areas and on land that has been cleared recently. Fireweed occurs throughout northern temperate regions and is used as a traditional medicine by native peoples of N. America, Europe, and Asia. **Flowers July–Sept.**

CANADA LILY
Lilium canadense **p. 134**

Note the nodding, yellow to orange flowers of this large native lily. **Flowers July–Aug.** The root is among the multitude of snakebite remedies.

STINGING NETTLE
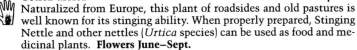
Urtica dioica **p. 212**

Naturalized from Europe, this plant of roadsides and old pastures is well known for its stinging ability. When properly prepared, Stinging Nettle and other nettles (*Urtica* species) can be used as food and medicinal plants. **Flowers June–Sept.**

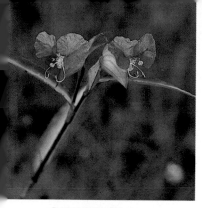

DAYFLOWERS

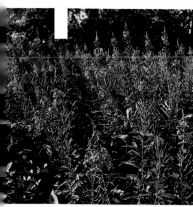

FIREWEED

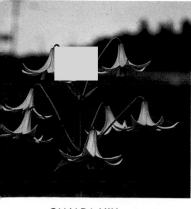

CANADA LILY

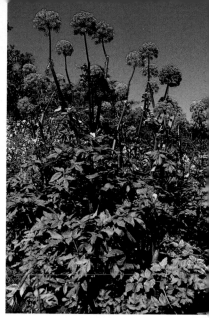

ANGELICA

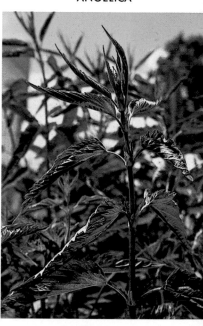

STINGING NETTLE

PLATE 7

MOIST GROUND, OFTEN SHADED; WEEDY PLANTS

The widespread plants depicted here thrive in moist soil, often in shady areas around barnyards, streambanks, or wherever their seeds may land.

FIELD HORSETAIL
Equisetum arvense   **p. 304**

This horsetail occurs in moist sandy soils in much of our range and beyond. Horsetails (*Equisetum* species) have been widely used throughout the Northern Hemisphere as a diuretic for kidney and bladder ailments. See warning in text.

CELANDINE
Chelidonium majus   **p. 92**

When the stem of this plant is broken, it exudes a bright yellow juice (do not touch). The root juice is sometimes bright orange. This member of the poppy family has been used in the folk medicine of N. America, Europe, and China. **Caution:** Celandine is potentially **poisonous. Flowers March–Aug.**

PERILLA
Perilla frutescens   **p. 186**

This Asian alien has become an invasive weed in the South. In the Ozarks it is called "Rattlesnake Weed" because the dried seed cases rattle as one walks by. An important medicinal and culinary herb of e. Asia. See warning in text. **Flowers July–Sept.**

WINTER CRESS
Barbarea vulgaris   **p. 90**

A European weed; widespread in ditches, along roadsides, and in meadows. The large leaves poking through the yellow Winter Cress flowers belong to an unrelated plant, Yellow or Curly Dock *(Rumex crispus)*. **Flowers April–Aug.**

CHICKWEED
Stellaria media   **p. 42**

A common European weed, widespread throughout the U.S. **Flowers March–Sept.** Used as a home remedy to stop itching. Scientists have not yet thoroughly researched the plant.

CLEAVERS
Galium aparine   **p. 36**

A weak-stemmed annual with raspy prickles. This European weed is common in moist shaded areas throughout our area and beyond. Flowers insignificant — the plant depicted here is in full bloom. Used as a diuretic. **Flowers April–Sept.** See warning in text.

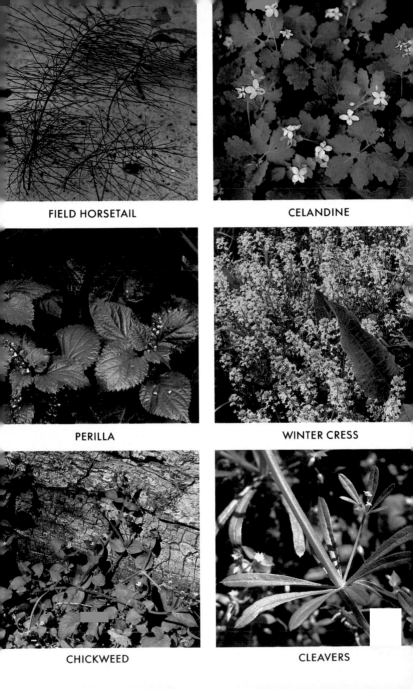

FIELD HORSETAIL

CELANDINE

PERILLA

WINTER CRESS

CHICKWEED

CLEAVERS

PLATE 8
WOODY PLANTS OF STREAM BANKS

SPICEBUSH
Lindera benzoin   **p. 252**

This shrub is common along stream banks and in rich, moist woods from New England south. The scarlet, strongly spice-scented berries, and the pleasant-scented, entire (toothless) leaves distinguish this plant. The berries often persist on branches after leaves drop in autumn. They have been used as an Allspice substitute, as well as in folk medicine. The small yellow flowers *(top right)* appear in early spring, before the leaves unfold. **Flowers March–May.**

SWEETGUM
Liquidambar styraciflua   **p. 280**

To some, the 5–7 finely toothed lobes make the leaves resemble stars. The crushed leaves have a pine-like scent. This is a common deciduous tree, mostly along streams and river banks, and in moist low woods. Common in the South. The "gum" produced in pockets in the bark is used medicinally. The hard, spiny fruits *(below)* make this tree a poor choice for lawn plantings, though the ornamental value of the brilliantly colored autumn leaves offsets negative aspects.

WAHOO
Euonymus atropurpureus   **p. 244**

This shrub or small tree is found in moist woods, often along streams. It can be recognized by the unusual structure of its fruit (shown here) after the leaves drop in autumn. The stem and root bark and seeds have been used in traditional medicine, but are considered **poisonous.**

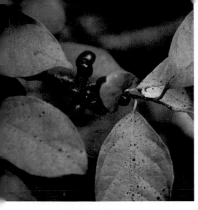

SPICEBUSH

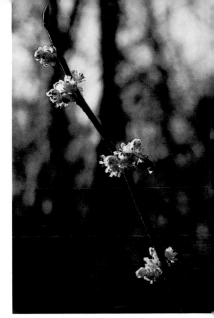

SPICEBUSH flowers

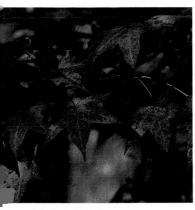

SWEETGUM

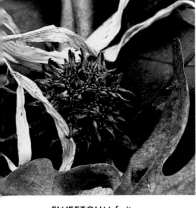

SWEETGUM fruit

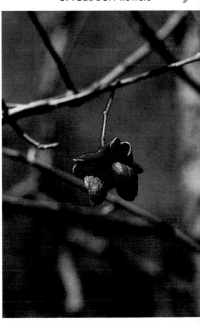

WAHOO

PLATE 9

MOIST UNDERSTORY SHRUBS; ALONG
STREAMS OR WET ROCKY OUTCROPS

BUTTONBUSH

Cephalanthus occidentalis **p. 242**

Common along stream banks and pond edges. The showy, 1–1½ in. wide, globe-shaped flowerheads with strongly protruding stamens make this plant easy to identify when it is in bloom. **Flowers July–Aug.** Historically, the bark has been used medicinally, though it may be **poisonous.**

WILD HYDRANGEA

Hydrangea arborescens **p. 242**

Like familiar cultivated hydrangeas, our native Wild Hydrangea has flowerheads surrounded by sterile, papery, white, flowerlike structures that attract bees and other pollinators to the tiny, inconspicuous fertile blooms. **Flowers June–Aug.** The root has been used by American Indians for centuries, and in herbal medicine as a diuretic, primarily for bladder ailments and kidney stones. The root bark was formerly marketed under the name "Gravel Root," referring to its use for kidney stones. **Caution:** Research has shown that this plant is potentially **toxic;** see text.

NINEBARK

Physocarpus opulifolius **p. 234**

This shrub often escapes from cultivation. The bark on the older branches separates, peeling into several layers, hence the common name "Ninebark." The inner bark is the medicinal part. The species name, *opulifolius*, refers to the resemblance of the leaves to those of Crampbark (*Viburnum opulus*, p. 246). **Flowers May–July. Warning:** Said to be toxic.

WITCH-HAZEL

Hamamelis virginiana **p. 256**

The leaves have scalloped margins (large wavy teeth) and uneven, wedge-shaped bases. End buds are scalpel-shaped. The yellow flowers, each with 4 1-in.-long slender yellow petals, have a spiderlike appearance. The flowers appear after the leaves drop. **Flowers late Sept.–Dec.** Witch-hazel "extract," used externally as a skin toner, is a common item in American medicine cabinets.

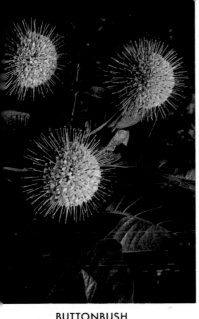

BUTTONBUSH

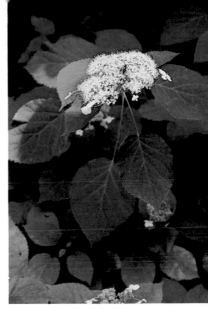

WILD HYDRANGEA

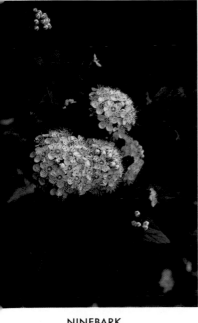

NINEBARK

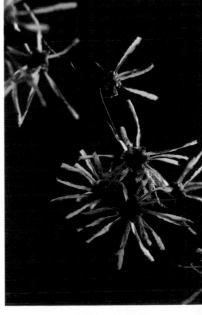

WITCH-HAZEL

PLATE 10
NEAR SEASHORES

Seaside habitats of the Atlantic Coast have long been a favorite foraging ground for wild edibles. A number of medicinal plants occur in the same habitats.

BAYBERRY
Myrica pensylvanica   **p. 254**

Bayberry is a shrub that grows to 12 ft. in infertile soils from the Canadian Atlantic Coast from southern Nfld. south to Va. and N.C., where it is rare. The hard seeds are covered in a white or gray wax, long used in candle-making. The leaves, fruits, and root bark have been used medicinally. **Caution:** The wax can be irritating.

RUGOSA or LARGE-HIP ROSE
Rosa rugosa   **p. 234**

Common; often found in large thickets along coastal beaches and dunes. This Asian introduction has larger fruits (rose hips) than any of our native roses. In Traditional Chinese Medicine the flowers are used to "regulate vital energy," promote circulation, and treat stomachaches. The fruits, high in vitamin C, have been used to treat scurvy (vitamin-C deficiency).

BEARBERRY
Arctostaphylos uva-ursi   **p. 26**

A trailing shrub found in sandy soils and on exposed rock from the Arctic south to the northern tier of the U.S. Shown here is a plant with immature (green) fruits, which turn bright red when ripe. The leaves have been used for their diuretic qualities and as an ingredient in smoking mixtures.

SWEETFERN
Comptonia peregrina   **p. 254**

The distinctively shaped, leathery, aromatic leaves give Sweetfern a fernlike appearance. Though this plant is often found in infertile soils near shores, it is also a common weedy shrub of dry roadsides, gravel banks, and woodland clearings. The species name, *peregrina*, means "foreign." This is a misnomer from an American perspective: although the plant was foreign to the European botanist who first named it, it is native to N. America. The leaves are used medicinally.

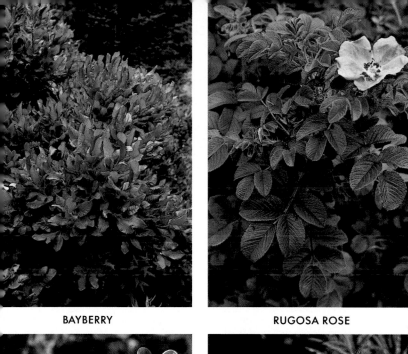

BAYBERRY

RUGOSA ROSE

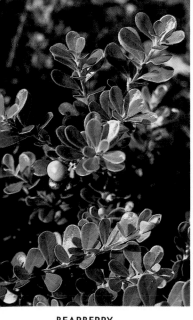

BEARBERRY

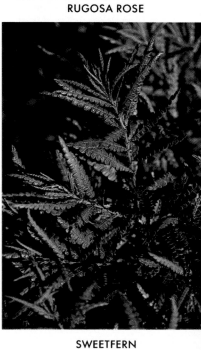

SWEETFERN

PLATE 11

MOIST, RICH WOODS;
SPRING-FLOWERING PLANTS (1)

Many early spring wildflowers in moist woods throughout our range are used medicinally. See also Pls. 12–17.

WILD GINGER
Asarum canadense **p. 138**
This creeping perennial produces urn-shaped maroon flowers, often hidden beneath the leaf litter. The leaves are distinctly heart-shaped. **Flowers April–May.** The root is used medicinally.

SKUNK CABBAGE
Symplocarpus foetidus **p. 202**
In the North, the unusual reddish green blooms of Skunk Cabbage are among the first wildflowers to appear in spring. **Flowers Feb.–May.** Temperature within the flower spathe is often 60° F. higher than the ambient air; the flower may melt snow as it begins to bloom. **Caution:** Although the root is used medicinally, it is considered **toxic.**

TROUT-LILY
Erythronium americanum **p. 100**
A yellow-flowered lily, recognized by its backcurving petals and shiny leaves mottled with white spots. **Flowers March–May.** Both the leaves and roots are used medicinally.

PARTRIDGEBERRY
Mitchella repens **p. 26**
A familiar creeping evergreen perennial of oak forests. The inner lobes of the trumpet-shaped, paired flowers are hairy. **Flowers May–July.** Produces red berries in fall. Also called "Squaw Vine," the plant has historically been used for menstrual difficulties.
Photo by Phillip E. Keenan.

CORYDALIS
Corydalis species **p. 106**
Corydalis flowers have a spur on the back side, so the flower appears to be attached to its stalk toward the middle of the flower. Near the tip, the upper and lower petals have flat vertical lips. There are about 7 species in our range; all have been used interchangeably. **Flowers March–June;** *C. aurea* blooms May–June. **Caution:** Potentially **toxic.**

RED TRILLIUM, WAKEROBIN, BETHROOT
Trillium erectum **p. 138**
Leaves are in a single whorl of 3, below the dull red or white, 3-petaled flowers. The root was traditionally used as an aid in childbirth, hence the name "Bethroot" ("birth root"). **Flowers April–June.**

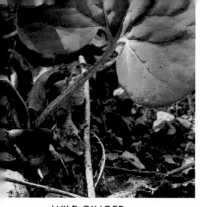

WILD GINGER

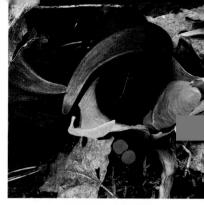

SKUNK CABBAGE

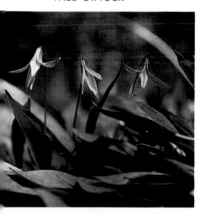

TROUT-LILY

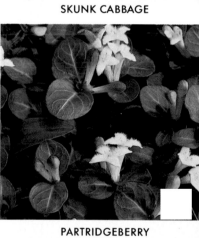

PARTRIDGEBERRY

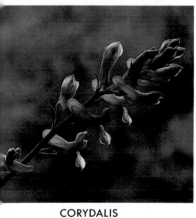

CORYDALIS

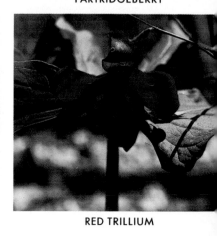

RED TRILLIUM

PLATE 12

MOIST, RICH WOODS;
SPRING-FLOWERING PLANTS (2)

ROUND-LOBED HEPATICA
Hepatica americana   **p. 176**
The flowers appear before the round-lobed, semi-evergreen leaves become lush. **Flowers March–early June.** The genus name *Hepatica* refers to the liverlike shape of the leaves. The leaves were traditionally used for liver ailments.

SHARP-LOBED HEPATICA
Hepatica acutiloba   **p. 176**
The flowers, usually violet-blue, appear in early spring, before the liver-shaped, semi-evergreen leaves with pointed tips become erect. **Flowers Feb.–early June.** The range of this species is more southern than that of *H. americana.*

LOUSEWORT, WOOD BETONY
Pedicularis canadensis   **p. 106**
The flowers, which look like miniature snapdragons, are yellow to reddish. They appear early in the spring in tight spiraling whorls. **Flowers April–June.** The leaves are deeply incised, giving them a fernlike appearance. The root and leaves are traditionally used for stomachaches, diarrhea, anemia, and heart trouble, as well as in cough medicine; they are also used externally, as a poultice for swellings, sore muscles, and other ailments.

COLUMBINE
Aquilegia canadensis   **p. 136**
The drooping, bell-like, reddish orange and yellow flowers have 5 spurlike appendages at the top. This plant occurs in rich, moist woods, often on wet, shaded rocky outcrops. **Flowers April–July.** The roots, seeds, and leaves have been used medicinally. The crushed seeds have been used to control lice, to relieve headaches, and as a "love charm." See warning in text.

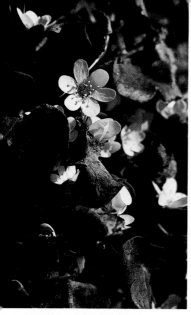

ROUND-LOBED HEPATICA

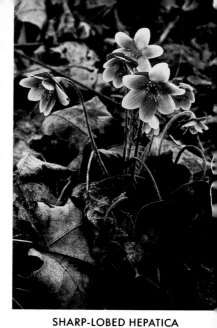

SHARP-LOBED HEPATICA

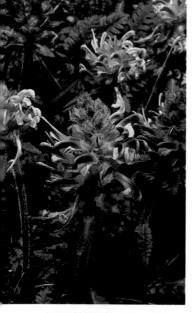

LOUSEWORT

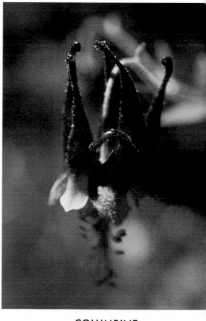

COLUMBINE

PLATE 13

MOIST, RICH WOODS;
SPRING-FLOWERING PLANTS (3)

These plants, often found growing alongside one another, are important sources of roots used in modern herbal medicine or sold in health and natural food stores.

GOLDENSEAL
Hydrastis canadensis **p. 50**

The bright yellow roots of Goldenseal are one of the most widely consumed products sold through health and natural food stores. The plant grows in colonies. Individual plants have 1–2 leaves. The flowers lack petals but have numerous stamens. **Flowers April–May.** The root, high in the alkaloid berberine, is employed as an antibacterial, and as a "tonic" for irritated or inflamed mucous membranes.

BLOODROOT
Sanguinaria canadensis **p. 48**

Both the common name and the genus name refer to the blood-red juice in the roots. This **poisonous** member of the poppy family blooms early in spring, before its leaves appear and usually before the leaves on trees emerge. **Flowers March–June.** Today, components of the root are used in minute amounts in commercial toothpastes and mouthwashes to fight plaque.

WILD GERANIUM
Geranium maculatum **p. 146**

Flowers April–June. The leaves of Wild Geranium are often confused with those of Goldenseal (see above), though Wild Geranium leaves are not wrinkled and have more deeply cut lobes. The roots, high in tannins, have been used to stop bleeding, and to treat diarrhea, dysentery, piles, gum diseases, and other ailments.

MAYAPPLE
Podophyllum peltatum **p. 46**

Mayapple not only occurs in rich, moist woods, but also along wood margins, and in moist fields and other habitats. **Flowers April–June.** The **poisonous** root of this plant contains components that are used today in ointments to treat venereal warts; it is also the source of a semisynthetic compound used in the treatment of testicular cancer and small-cell lung cancer.

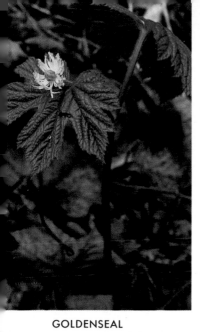

GOLDENSEAL

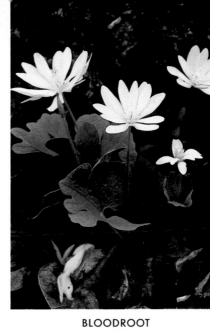

BLOODROOT

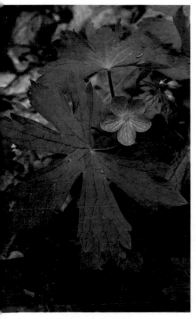

WILD GERANIUM

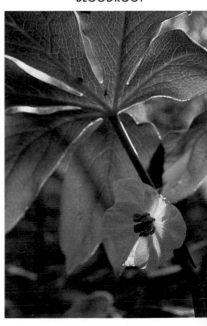

MAYAPPLE

PLATE 14

MOIST, RICH WOODS (4);
ON NORTH SLOPES

North-facing slopes provide deep shade with rich, moist soil that harbors many important medicinal herbs.

AMERICAN GINSENG
Panax quinquefolius   **p. 50**
No medicinal herb is more famous than Ginseng. For over 200 years, wild American Ginseng has been harvested and shipped to the Orient. Today, over 95 percent of the American Ginseng crop (wild-harvested and cultivated) is shipped to e. Asia. Interstate commerce of the root is regulated by the federal government. It is unethical and illegal to harvest the roots before the red berries ripen and set seed in late summer or early autumn. **Flowers June–July.** Considered a "tonic." See warning in text.

MAIDENHAIR FERN
Adiantum pedatum   **p. 308**
This is one of the easiest ferns to recognize, with the arrangement of the wedge-shaped leaflets in a circular or horseshoe-shaped frond, and the ebony-colored stems. American Indians throughout N. America used the leaves as a hair wash to make their hair shiny.

SOLOMON'S-SEAL
Polygonatum species   **p. 32**
The root of Solomon's-seal has been used to treat indigestion, lung ailments, "general debility," and other ailments. The plant often droops under its own weight. Flowers are in pairs hanging below the leaf axils. **Flowers May–June.**

AMERICAN GINSENG
Panax quinquefolius   **p. 50**
The rhizome at the top of the root, often referred to as the "neck," has scars left by each year's leaf stem. The age of the root, which affects its quality and price, is determined by counting the annual leaf scars. Only roots at least 5 years old are desirable. The root shown here is about 14 years old.

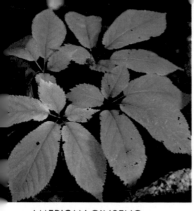

AMERICAN GINSENG

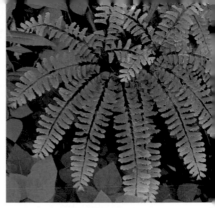

MAIDENHAIR FERN

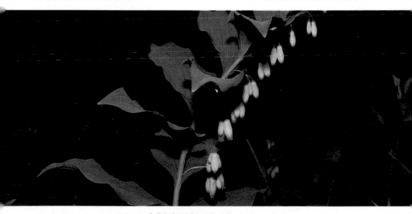

SOLOMON'S-SEAL

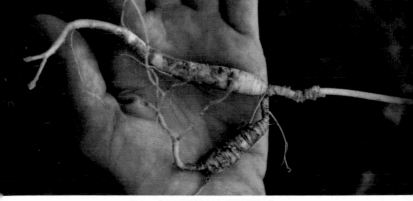

Root of AMERICAN GINSENG

PLATE 15
MOIST, RICH WOODS (5)

PINK-ROOT
Spigelia marilandica **p. 148**

When blooming, Pink-root can be identified by its 5-lobed, trumpet-shaped flowers, which are scarlet on the outside and cream-yellow within. **Flowers May–June.** Found from Md. south, the plant is considered **poisonous.** The root was once used to expel worms.

CRESTED DWARF IRIS
Iris cristata **p. 168**

This diminutive iris of southern woods, growing to 8 in. tall, is named for the yellow crests on the downcurved blue sepals. **Flowers April–May.** In the background of the photo is Scouring Rush *(Equisetum hyemale)*, often found in the same habitat (see also Pl. 2). American Indians used the root of this iris in ointments for cancerous ulcers, and in tea for hepatitis.

SPIKENARD
Aralia racemosa **p. 54**

This large, herbaceous (usually non-woody) member of the ginseng family grows to 5 ft. It has compound leaves with 6–21 toothed, weakly heart-shaped leaflets. The tiny white flowers are in small clusters on a raceme. **Flowers June–Aug.** The root has been used as a "blood purifier" and was once valued as a remedy for lung ailments.

WILD YAM
Dioscorea villosa **p. 204**

The alternate, heart-shaped leaves of this perennial twining vine are often in whorls of 3 or more leaves toward the base of the plant. The flowers are insignificant. Roots of tropical plants in this genus *(Dioscorea)* have been used in recent years to provide chemical starting material for the manufacture of progesterone and other steroid drugs, including contraceptives. See warning in text.

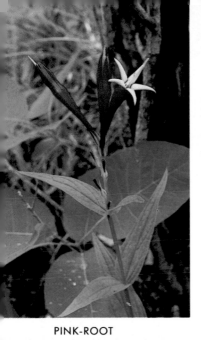

PINK-ROOT

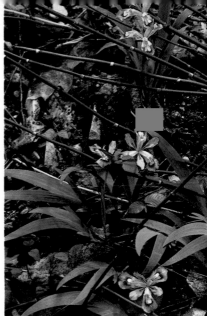

CRESTED DWARF IRIS

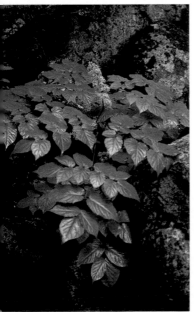

SPIKENARD

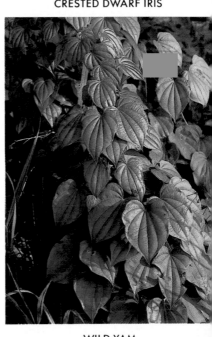

WILD YAM

PLATE 16

MOIST, RICH WOODS (6);
POTENTIALLY POISONOUS PLANTS

Safety/efficacy and risk/benefit ratios are often related to dose, method of preparation, and other variables. These plants are best appreciated for their historical value, and left alone by amateurs.

WHITE BANEBERRY, DOLL'S EYES
Actaea pachypoda   p. 52

The fleshy white berries with a dark dot at the tip earn this plant the common name "Doll's Eyes." The tiny white flowers are in an oblong cluster. **Flowers April–June. Fruits July–Oct.** Though tiny amounts of the root have been used medicinally, the plant is generally considered to be **poisonous.**

RED BANEBERRY
Actaea rubra   p. 50

Closely related to White Baneberry, Red Baneberry has red fruits on less stout stalks, and the flowerheads are in more rounded rather than oblong clusters. The root has been used in small doses to treat menstrual irregularity and colds and coughs. It, too, is generally considered potentially **poisonous.**

DRAGON or GREEN ARUM
Arisaema dracontium   p. 202

Most common in southern woods, this arum has leaflets arranged in a semicircle or curved groupings. The distinctive greenish yellow flower has a long spadix surrounded by a narrow spathe. **Flowers May–July.** The roots, after elaborate processing, are considered edible, and have been used medicinally. The fresh roots have an acrid, burning effect and are considered **poisonous.**

JACK-IN-THE-PULPIT
Arisaema triphyllum   p. 202

The cuplike spathe, with a curved flap overhanging the erect spadix, and the 3 terminal leaflets distinguish this species. The root of this species was used like that of Dragon Arum and the same warnings apply. **Flowers April–early July.**

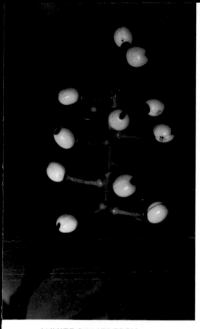

WHITE BANEBERRY

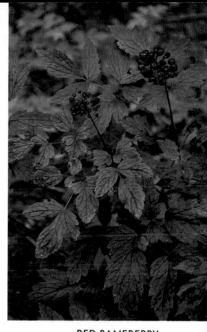

RED BANEBERRY

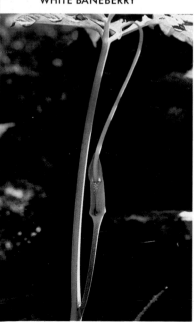

DRAGON or GREEN ARUM

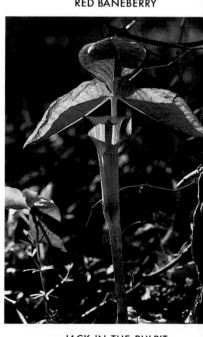

JACK-IN-THE-PULPIT

PLATE 17
MOIST, RICH WOODS (7)

GREEK VALERIAN, JACOB'S LADDER
Polemonium reptans   **p. 178**
A perennial with violet-blue, bell-like flowers in loose clusters. The
stamens of this species are not strongly protruding. **Flowers April–
June.** The name "Jacob's Ladder" refers to the ladderlike arrange-
ment of the leaves. The root was once used in herbal prescriptions.

CORALROOTS
Corallorhiza species   **p. 94**
Coralroots are a brownish, chlorophyll-lacking group of orchids,
found growing on leaf mold in rich woods throughout our area. It
takes a careful eye to find them. **Flowers July–Aug.** The root was a
folk remedy for fevers. Five species occur in our area. All species in
the genus appear to have been used interchangeably, though *C. maculata* is listed in most herbals.

BLUE COHOSH
Caulophyllum thalictroides   **p. 206**
The bluish green leaves are thrice-divided into leaflets with 2–3
lobes. The greenish yellow flowers (not shown) appear before the
leaves unfold. **Flowers April–June.** The root has historically been
used to aid in childbirth and treat menstrual problems. Science confirms the plant's anti-inflammatory and estrogenic activity, and its
ability to check spasms. See warning in text.

WATER or PURPLE AVENS
Geum rivale   **p. 142**
The amateur giving this plant a cursory glance would not associate
it with other plants in the rose family. The dull reddish, nodding
flowers characterize the plant. **Flowers May–Aug.** The root was
once used as an astringent to stop bleeding and for other ailments.
Most *Geum* species were used similarly.

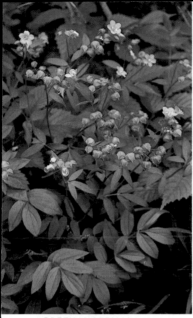

**GREEK VALERIAN
(JACOB'S LADDER)**

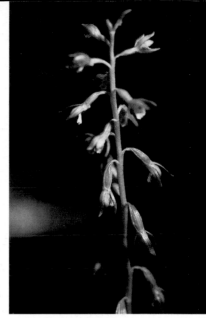

CORALROOT

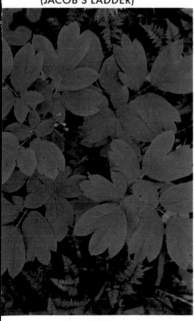

BLUE COHOSH

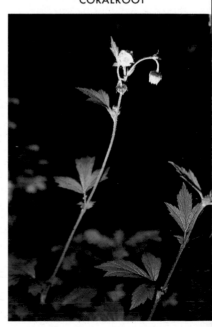

WATER or PURPLE AVENS

PLATE 18

MOIST TO DRY RICH WOODS

The plants depicted here are found in a variety of woodland conditions.

WINDFLOWER, RUE ANEMONE
Anemonella thalictroides **p. 48**

Flowers of this common and widespread woodland wildflower often vary from pink to white in the same population. The 5 showy, petal-like sepals are a common sight in spring. **Flowers March–May.** The tuberous roots were once used for medicinal purposes and have been used experimentally to treat piles. See warning in text.

INDIAN-PIPE
Monotropa uniflora **p. 28**

This chlorophyll-lacking perennial is translucent white, with scale-like leaves that are barely visible. The species name, *uniflora,* refers to the single flower atop each stalk. **Flowers June–Oct.** Old herbals list this plant as "bird's nest root," referring to the shape of the root. The root was once used as a sedative and the juice of the plant was used to treat eye inflammations, but the safety of these medicinal uses is undetermined.

DUTCHMAN'S-BREECHES
Dicentra cucullaria **p. 12**

With finely dissected gray-green leaves and drooping flowers with "pants-like" spurs, *Dicentra* species are easily identified. **Flowers April–May.** Although it is potentially **poisonous,** the root of this plant was once used for skin ailments, but was taken internally in minute doses.

DOWNY RATTLESNAKE-PLANTAIN
Goodyera pubescens **p. 24**

The distinctive bluish green leaves with prominent white veins in a "rattlesnake" pattern earned this plant its common name, as did the use of the root for snakebites, based on the "doctrine of signatures" (see p. 6). The plant, like all orchids, should not be harvested. The spikes of tiny whitish flowers on a hairy stalk (see below) appear in summer. **Flowers July–Aug.**

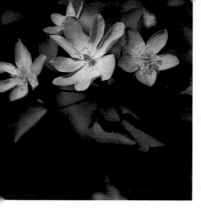

WINDFLOWER

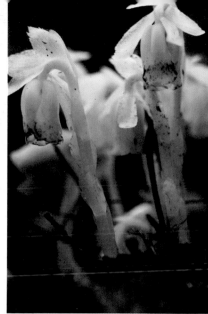

INDIAN-PIPE

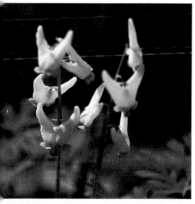

DUTCHMAN'S-BREECHES

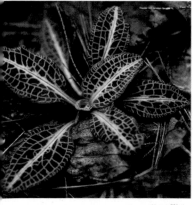

DOWNY RATTLESNAKE-PLANTAIN
leaves

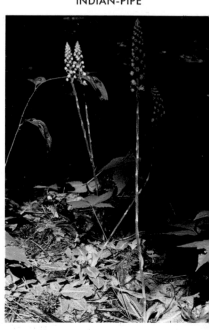

DOWNY RATTLESNAKE-PLANTAIN
in flower

PLATE 19
BOREAL FORESTS; UNDERSTORY PLANTS

These plants often grow in spruce-fir or pine forests of the Northeast.

WINTERGREEN, TEABERRY
Gaultheria procumbens   **p. 26**
"Wintergreen" refers to the evergreen nature of the leaves, but to most of us the name has become associated with a specific flavor produced by the compound methyl salicylate. This plant and Sweet or Black Birch were once commercial sources of wintergreen flavor, now largely replaced by synthetic methyl salicylate. This low-growing, creeping perennial of boreal forest and forest margins has bell-shaped, drooping white flowers, and edible red berries. **Flowers July–Aug.** Once the leaves of this plant *(top right)* are hit by a hard frost and turn purplish, they seem to have a sweeter, stronger flavor. Although it has not been confirmed scientifically, this may indicate a higher essential oil content.

PINK LADY'S-SLIPPER
Cypripedium acaule   **p. 138**
This showy orchid has a single pair of leaves at the base of the plant. **Flowers May–June.** Historically, the roots of Pink and Yellow lady's-slippers have been used as nerve sedatives. Harvest of these rare orchids should be strongly discouraged.

WILD SARSAPARILLA
Aralia nudicaulis   **p. 54**
Perhaps best described as nondescript, this member of the ginseng family spreads on creeping runners and often forms large colonies. It is common in pine woods in New England. The leaves, divided into 5 toothed leaflets, are on a single stalk. The umbel of tiny white flowers is on a separate stalk arising from the roots that is shorter than the leaves. **Flowers May–July.** The root was used medicinally.

BUNCHBERRY
Cornus canadensis   **p. 36**
This perennial of cool woods often forms large colonies in acidic soil. Its leaves are in a whorl of 6 topped by a single white bloom with 4 showy bracts. **Flowers May–July.** A bunch of red berries matures in fall, hence the common name. The leaves and roots were used medicinally.

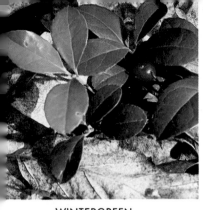

WINTERGREEN

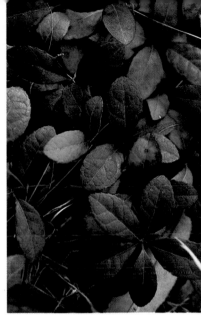

WINTERGREEN leaves

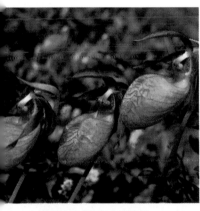

PINK LADY'S-SLIPPER

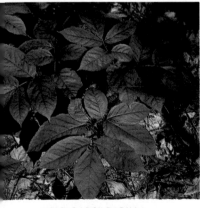

WILD SARSAPARILLA

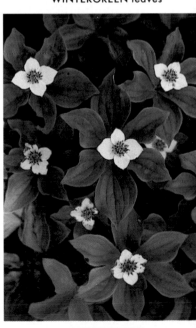

BUNCHBERRY

PLATE 20

DRY FORESTS WITH ACIDIC SOIL; UNDERSTORY PLANTS

GOLDTHREAD, CANKER ROOT
Coptis groenlandicum   **p. 38**
This diminutive, mat-forming member of the buttercup family has 3 shiny leaflets, resembling miniature strawberry leaves. The star-shaped white flowers are on separate stalks. **Flowers May–July.** The plant derives its name from the threadlike, bright yellow roots. The roots derive their color and astringency from the alkaloid berberine. The common name "Canker Root" refers to the use of the root in the treatment of canker sores.

WOOD LILY
Lilium philadelphicum   **p. 134**
This 3-ft.-tall perennial has leaves in whorls. The upturned, spotted, bright orange blossoms are a welcome sight in open woods with acidic soil in the North. **Flowers June–July.** The root was used in tea for digestive and lung disorders. American Indians applied the flowers to spider bites.

PIPSISSEWA
Chimaphila umbellata   **p. 44**
This perennial has toothed, lance-shaped leaves in whorls. It often appears in small colonies. The pinkish white, waxy, drooping flowers reveal their beauty in the close-up photograph at right. **Flowers June–Aug.** The leaves were once used for kidney and bladder ailments. This close-up photograph of the flower reveals its unusual detail.

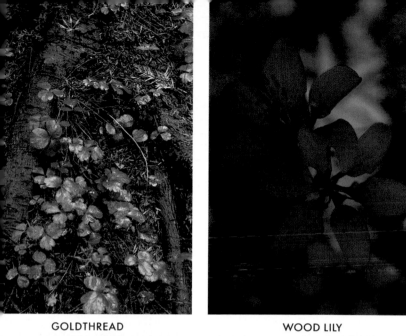

GOLDTHREAD

WOOD LILY

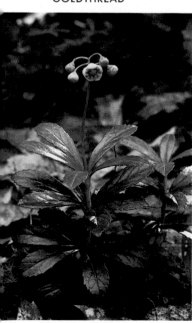

PIPSISSEWA

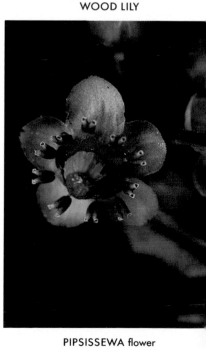

PIPSISSEWA flower

PLATE 21
COMMON LAWN "WEEDS" (1)

DANDELION
Taraxacum officinale **p. 130**
The flower stem of the common Dandelion is hollow and has milky juice. **Flowers March–Sept.** The leaves and the roots have been used medicinally, primarily as a diuretic for kidney and bladder ailments, as well as for liver and gall bladder disease. The leaves have been used as a laxative.

SPEEDWELLS
Veronica species **p. 174**
Of the 20 or so *Veronica* species that occur in our range, almost all are naturalized weeds from Europe and Asia. They are often found growing on lawns in the U.S. A typical *Veronica* flower is pictured here. Most species have blue veins on violet-blue flowers, and a whitish center. **Flowers Feb.–Aug.** The leaf tea was used in Europe as a "blood purifier" and diuretic.

BLUETS
Houstonia caerulea **p. 174**
The familiar Bluets of yards, open fields, and other areas are a delicate native plant common throughout most of our area. **Flowers March–July.** The leaf tea was used by American Indians to stop bedwetting.

PINEAPPLE-WEED
Matricaria matricarioides **p. 124**
This pineapple-scented annual, usually 6–8 in. high, has finely dissected leaves with threadlike segments. The familiar yellow "button" is a rayless composite flower. Found throughout much of our range. **Flowers May–Oct.** Introduced from Europe, where the plant tea is traditionally used for stomachaches, colds, and other minor ailments. See warning in text.

PURSLANE
Portulaca oleracea **p. 96**
A smooth, fleshy, often reddish, creeping annual, common on the edges of lawns and as a garden weed. Well known as a wild edible; medicinal uses include using the leaves as a poultice for burns and in tea for headaches; the plant has anti-inflammatory properties. The yellowish flowers of this species are seldom noticed. **Flowers June–Nov.** *Photo by Jim Duke.*

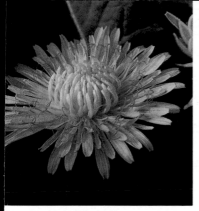

DANDELION

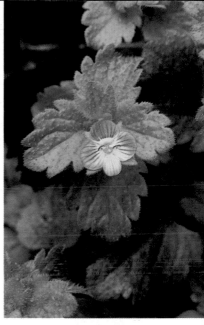

SPEEDWELL

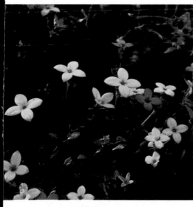

BLUETS

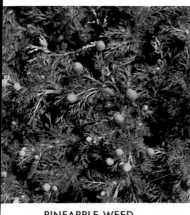

PINEAPPLE-WEED

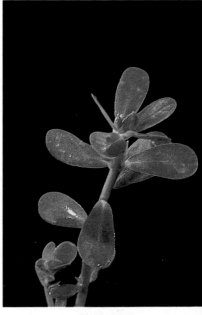

PURSLANE

PLATE 22

COMMON "WEEDS" OF ROADSIDES, FIELDS, AND LAWNS (2)

RED CLOVER
Trifolium pratense **p. 158**

 The 3 leaflets, arranged in a whorl, are often marked by a prominent, light-colored "V." The pink to red flowerheads are a familiar sight in fields and on lawn edges and roadsides throughout our area. **Flowers May–Sept.** This clover was originally introduced from Europe. Traditionally, the flower tea has been used to check spasms and as a mild sedative and "blood purifier." See warning in text.

CHICORY
Cichorium intybus **p. 198**

The azure blue flowers of Chicory are a common sight on the edges of lawns, in fields, and along roadsides from mid- to late summer. The dandelion-like leaves and roots have been used medicinally, in fact, like those of Dandelion. **Flowers June–Oct.**

YELLOW SWEET-CLOVER
Melilotus officinalis **p. 116**

A straggly biennial, occasionally growing to 6 ft. The yellow, pea-like blooms are fragrant only when crushed. This European plant is common along American roadsides. A tea made from the dried flowering plant (potentially **toxic**) was traditionally used for nervous headaches, nervous stomach, painful menstruation, aching muscles, and other ailments. **Flowers April–Oct.**

WHITE SWEET-CLOVER
Melilotus alba **p. 74**

Like Yellow Sweet-clover, White Sweet-clover is a weedy biennial introduced from Europe. It is often found in the same areas and has a parallel blooming period. Its yellow cousin, however, was more often used as a medicine. White Sweet-clover was once used in ointments for external ulcers. Animal studies have shown that components in the plant may lower blood pressure.

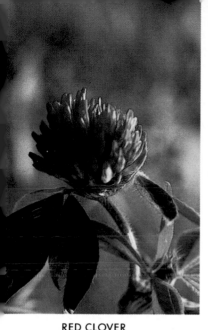

RED CLOVER

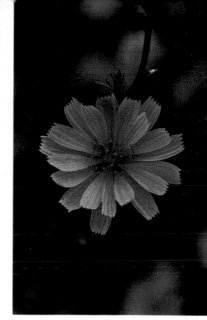

CHICORY

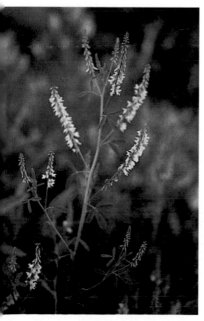

YELLOW SWEET-CLOVER

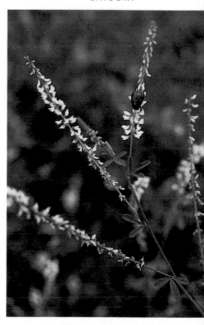

WHITE SWEET-CLOVER

PLATE 23

COMMON "WEEDS" OF ROADSIDES, FIELDS, AND LAWNS (3)

BUTTER-AND-EGGS
Linaria vulgaris   **p. 106**
The snapdragon-like flowers, in 2 shades of yellow, have given this plant the common name "Butter-and-eggs." Considered a folk laxative. An ointment made from the leaves was once used for piles and skin eruptions. A leaf "tea" made with milk has been used as an insecticide. **Flowers June–Oct.**

HEAL-ALL, SELF-HEAL
Prunella vulgaris   **p. 192**
This European plant is common throughout our range. When blooming, the square to cylindrical flowerheads are familiar to all. **Flowers May–Sept.** The leaf tea has been used as a gargle for sore throats and for other minor ailments. Its common name, implying a cure for "what ails you," may be proven valid by research that suggests antimutagenic and immune-system stimulating activity.

COLT'S FOOT
Tussilago farfara   **p. 130**
This European plant blooms early in spring, before the leaves appear. **Flowers March–April.** Common in the Northeast. In European tradition, the leaves and flowers, smoked or made into tea, were esteemed as one of the best treatments for lung ailments, asthma, and sore throats. Research suggests the leaf mucilage soothes inflamed mucous membranes and the plant is the source of a popular cough remedy in Europe, but see warning in text. Colt's Foot derives its common name from the resemblance of the leaf shape *(bottom left)* to the outline of a colt's hoof.

COMMON PLANTAIN
Plantago major   **p. 72**
The broad, wavy-margined leaves of this "weed" are more familiar to most people than the inconspicuous flower spikes. Several *Plantago* species are the source of psyllium seed, an ingredient in bulk laxatives available in every American pharmacy. The leaves of Common Plantain have been used in folk medicine throughout the world.

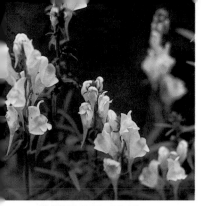

BUTTER-AND-EGGS

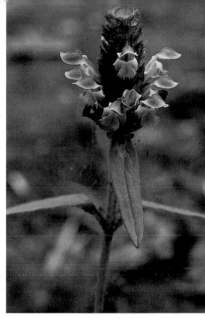

HEAL-ALL

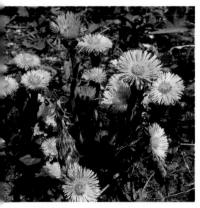

COLT'S FOOT flowers

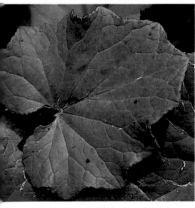

COLT'S FOOT leaves

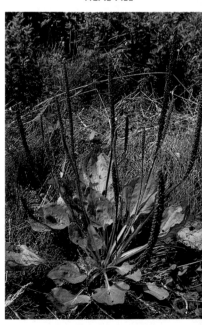

COMMON PLANTAIN

PLATE 24
ROADSIDES, FIELDS (4);
OFTEN CULTIVATED

COMMON EVENING-PRIMROSE
Oenothera biennis   **p. 92**
A biennial, growing from 1 to 8 ft. tall. The yellow blossoms open
after the sun has set, thus the common name. **Flowers June–Sept.**
The leaves and stems have been considered demulcent (soothing) and
mildly astringent. Recent research suggests the seed oil, a natural
source of gamma-linolenic acid, may be useful for atopic eczema,
asthma, migraines, premenstrual syndrome, metabolic disorders,
and other diseases.

BEE-BALM, OSWEGO TEA
Monarda didyma   **p. 162**
Found in thickets and fields, along stream banks, and often cultivated in herb gardens, this red-flowered American native is becoming increasingly familiar in gardens. **Flowers June–Sept.** The leaf
tea, like that of so many aromatic plants in the mint family, has been
historically valued as a treatment for colds, fevers, stomachaches,
insomnia, and other ailments.

WHITE CLOVER
Trifolium repens   **p. 74**
A common weed of lawns, roadsides, and waste places, this European
perennial was used by American Indians in leaf tea for colds, coughs,
fevers, and leukorrhea. In Europe the flower tea was used for rheumatism and gout. **Flowers April–Sept.**

WOOD STRAWBERRY
Fragaria vesca   **p. 38**
This wild strawberry differs from the cultivated species *(F. virginiana)* in that its leaves are more pointed and the fruits have seeds *on*
the surface, rather than embedded in the fruits. The leaves and roots
of *F. vesca* were once used for stomach ailments and as a "blood
purifier" and diuretic. A European plant, found in wood edges and
clearings. **Flowers May–Aug.**

LILY-OF-THE-VALLEY
Convallaria majalis   **p. 12**
This European plant, widely planted as an ornamental in the U.S.,
has escaped and become naturalized, often near old homesites, barns,
yards, etc. The root and flowers have been used medicinally. **Caution:** Improper administration could result in **toxic** effects. **Flowers
May–June.**

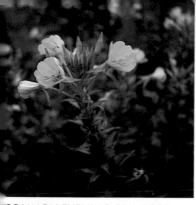

COMMON EVENING-PRIMROSE

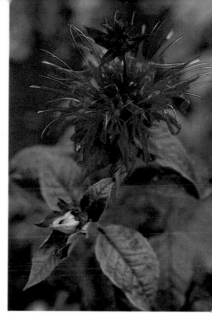

BEE-BALM (OSWEGO TEA)

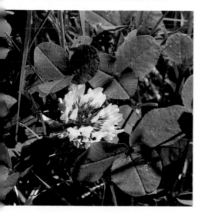

WHITE CLOVER

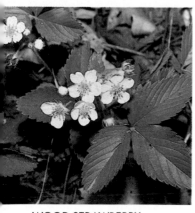

WOOD STRAWBERRY

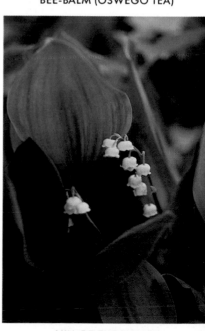

LILY-OF-THE-VALLEY

PLATE 25
ALIEN PLANTS OF OLD FIELDS AND PASTURES; OFTEN CULTIVATED

HORSERADISH
Armoracia rusticana   **p. 36**
A perennial herb with large, dock-like leaves. This member of the mustard family was introduced to cultivation from Europe and persists on old garden sites. The upper leaves, on flowering stalks, are much reduced and incised. The tiny, white, 4-petaled flowers are inconspicuous compared with the large basal leaves. **Flowers May–July.** The large root was used as a diuretic, antiseptic, and expectorant.

DAYLILY
Hemerocallis fulva   **p. 134**
A familiar garden perennial from e. Asia, Daylily has become widely naturalized in the U.S. It is now thought to be more common in the wild in the U.S. than it is in its native China. Although they may be toxic, the roots and young shoots are an ancient medicinal of Traditional Chinese Medicine, and have been used for over 2,000 years for mastitis, breast cancer, and a variety of other ailments. **Flowers May–Aug.**

VALERIAN
Valeriana officinalis   **p. 140**
Valerian, or Garden Heliotrope, is a perennial, introduced to American gardens from Europe at an early date. The plant escaped and became naturalized, especially in northern New England. **Flowers June–July.** The roots have proven mild sedative qualities and are widely used today in Europe.

YELLOW or CURLY DOCK
Rumex crispus   **p. 214**
This member of the buckwheat family is distinguished by its relatively large, lance-shaped leaves with distinctly wavy edges. Its root, which is yellow within, has been used for liver and kidney ailments and as a "blood purifier." See warning in text. **Flowers May–Sept.**

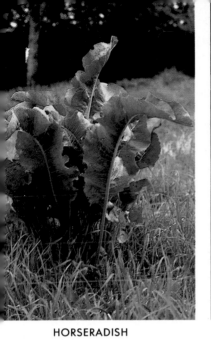

HORSERADISH

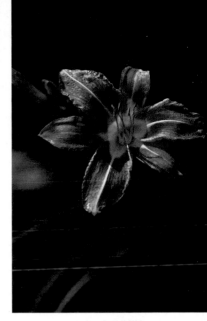

DAYLILY

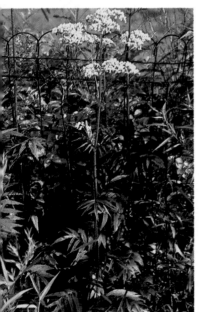

VALERIAN

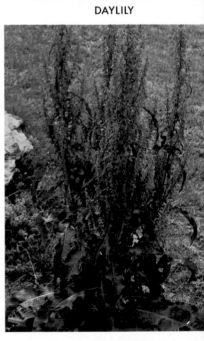

YELLOW DOCK

PLATE 26
WASTE-GROUND WEEDS; OFTEN CULTIVATED
AND ESCAPED FROM GARDENS

Early settlers of N. America brought many European plants with them by design or chance. These herbs are often considered "weeds," but may have hidden value.

BLESSED THISTLE
Cnicus benedictus **p. 120**

 An annual herb, sometimes cultivated in medicinal herb gardens and occasionally escaped in the Northeast. A tea made from the dried flowering plant is traditionally used in Europe to stimulate sweating and promote appetite and milk production; it is also used as a diuretic. See warning in text. **Flowers May–June.**

MILK THISTLE
Silybum marianum **p. 198**

Once considered a rank weed and an obscure food plant (young leaves with spines removed are edible), in recent years this thistle has gained prominence as a medicinal plant, especially in Europe. Extracts from the seeds are used as a liver-protectant. Clinical trials have found it especially useful in the treatment of *Amanita* mushroom poisoning; it is credited with saving a number of lives in Europe. This thistle is sometimes cultivated; it has escaped from gardens in some areas. It is common in Calif. **Flowers June–Sept.**

YARROW
Achillea millefolium **p. 64**

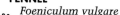 A common weed throughout the Northern Hemisphere, Yarrow has been used for dozens of medicinal applications by all cultures in its range. More than 100 biologically active compounds have been identified from the plant. One of the chief medicinal uses is as a vulnerary — an agent that stops bleeding of wounds. The Latin name *Achillea* honors Achilles. Legend states that he used a poultice of Yarrow flowers to stop the bleeding of his soldiers' wounds. **Flowers May–Sept.**

FENNEL
Foeniculum vulgare **p. 110**

 An herb with annual, biennial, and perennial varieties; often cultivated and escaped in some areas. Fennel is best identified by its green, threadlike leaves with a strong anise scent. The seeds have been used for stomach ailments and to relieve gas. **Flowers June–Sept.** Do not confuse with deadly members of the parsley family.

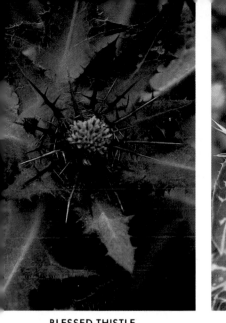

BLESSED THISTLE

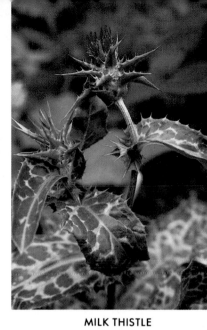

MILK THISTLE

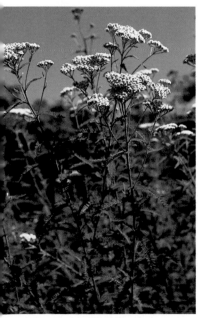

YARROW

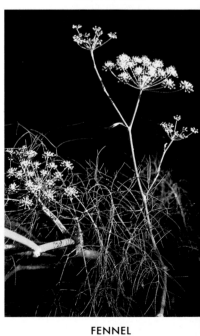

FENNEL

PLATE 27

WASTE-GROUND WEEDS

SICKLEPOD
Cassia obtusifolia   **p. 118**
An annual legume with long, sickle-shaped pods. Herbicides have
been developed to eradicate this weed from midwestern corn fields,
but it is both a food and medicinal plant. In Africa the leaves are
made into a high-protein paste. In China the seeds are used as medicine. **Flowers July–Sept.**

ANNUAL WORMWOOD, SWEET ANNIE
Artemisia annua   **p. 222**
A rank annual, native to Eurasia, and becoming increasingly common in the U.S. as it escapes from herb gardens. Often grown for its
fragrant dried leaves, which are used in wreaths and arrangements.
Preparations of this weedy annual are used in China as a malaria
treatment, when standard drugs are ineffectual. **Flowers July–Oct.**

HIGH MALLOW
Malva sylvestris   **p. 150**
The strongly lobed leaves (with 5–7 lobes) and dark-veined, rose-
purple flowers distinguish this mallow from other *Malva* species.
Flowers May–July.   The leaves and roots have been used for their
soothing and mildly astringent qualities. Other *Malva* species have
been used similarly.

QUEEN ANNE'S LACE, WILD CARROT
Daucus carota   **p. 58**

This biennial with finely dissected leaves is a very common weed.
Note the flat white cluster of flowers, with 1 deep purple floret. **Caution:** Proper identification is *essential* to make sure this plant is not
mistaken for one of the deadly poisonous members of the carrot family (Umbelliferae). The roots of Wild Carrot were once used in tea as
a diuretic. **Flowers April–Oct.**

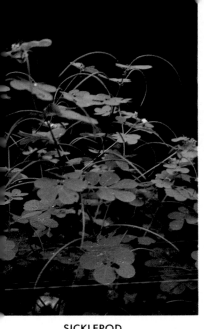

SICKLEPOD

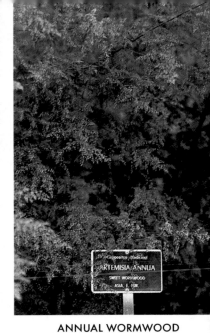

ANNUAL WORMWOOD

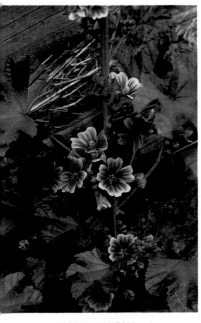

HIGH MALLOW

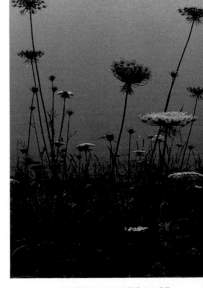

QUEEN ANNE'S LACE

PLATE 28

MOSTLY CULTIVATED PLANTS

Many cultivated plants, be they flowers, vegetables, culinary herbs, or illegal drugs, have a history of medicinal use.

CORN
Zea mays **p. 312**
No American vegetable has gained more importance in the diets of the world's population than corn. A tea made from corn silk, consisting of the stigmas of the flowers, has been valued as a diuretic.

MARIJUANA
Cannabis sativa **p. 206**
Although it grows on its own in some parts of the country where it was once commercially cultivated as a fiber plant (hemp), Marijuana is most often cultivated as an illegal intoxicant. The leaves and flower buds, with obvious biological activity, promise useful drugs of the future, as sources of an antinauseant for chemotherapy patients and as a treatment for glaucoma.

COMFREY
Symphytum species **p. 180**
While *Symphytum officinale* is listed as the species used in most herb books, a number of the 25 species of Comfrey *(Symphytum)* are cultivated in American gardens. Also called All-Heal, Comfrey has been used for many medicinal purposes. Comfrey was extremely popular in the 1970s and early 1980s, but studies showing **toxic** pyrrolizidine alkaloids, especially in the root, have tempered the enthusiasm for Comfrey. Recent studies show that leaves harvested during the blooming period (May–Sept.) are very low in alkaloid content. **Caution:** Consult an expert on identification of Comfrey leaves, lest they be mistaken for the **highly toxic** leaves of Foxglove.

FOXGLOVE
Digitalis purpurea **p. 172**
A biennial from Europe, often cultivated as an ornamental for its showy purple or white flowers, Foxglove has become naturalized in some areas. The plant is the source of heart-affecting glycosides used in pharmaceuticals to treat heart disease. **Caution:** The leaves are **deadly poisonous.** In recent years people have died after eating the leaves of first-year Foxglove plants, having mistaken them for Comfrey leaves. **For use by physicians only.**

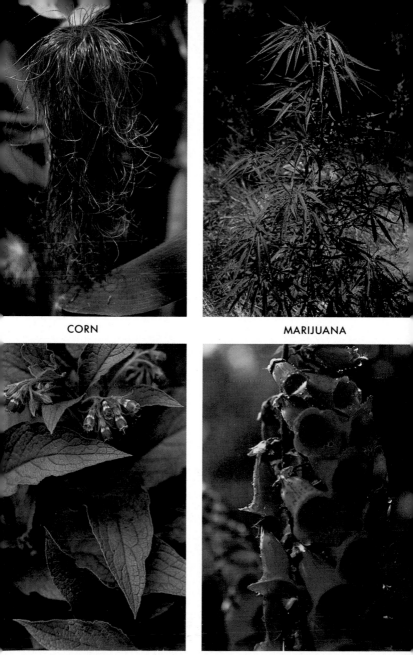

CORN

MARIJUANA

COMFREY

FOXGLOVE

PLATE 29

OFTEN CULTIVATED AND NATURALIZED; ROADSIDES, FIELDS, WASTE PLACES

These plants belong to the mint family. See also Pl. 30.

HOREHOUND
Marrubium vulgare **p. 70**

A perennial with tiny white flowers in whorls above leaf axils. **Flowers May–Sept.** The malodorous, bitter leaves are a well-known ingredient in cough syrups and throat lozenges. A European plant, common as a weed in pastures and often cultivated in herb gardens.

MOTHERWORT
Leonurus cardiaca **p. 162**

Unlike most plants in the mint family, Motherwort has leaves that are strongly cleft or divided, not simple. The tiny pinkish flowers with furry upper lips are in whorls, in leaf axils. **Flowers May–Aug.** Motherwort is sometimes grown in herb gardens. Traditionally, the leaf tea is used to regulate menses and aid in childbirth (hence the common name).

BLUE GIANT HYSSOP
Agastache foeniculum **p. 190**

The leaves have an anise-like or fennel-like scent, hence the species name, *foeniculum*. This 3-ft.-tall native perennial occurs in the northern prairies and dry thickets. It is often cultivated in herb gardens and has escaped, becoming established outside its natural range. **Flowers June–Sept.** The leaf tea has been used for fevers, colds, and coughs, and as an agent to strengthen a weak heart. Interestingly, an Asian species of *Agastache* is used in Traditional Chinese Medicine to treat angina pains.

CATNIP
Nepeta cataria **p. 70**

Best known for its intoxicating effect on cats, Catnip is native to Europe, but is often cultivated and has become widely established in the U.S. **Flowers June–Sept.** A tea of the flowering tops and leaves was once a popular folk remedy for colds, fevers, headaches, irregular menses, insomnia, and chicken pox.

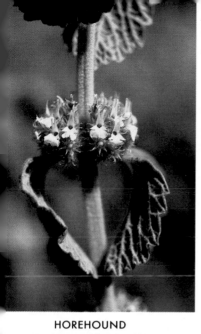

HOREHOUND

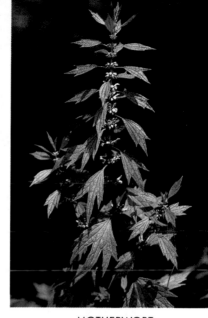

MOTHERWORT

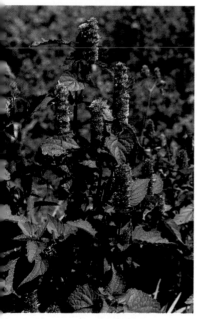

BLUE GIANT HYSSOP

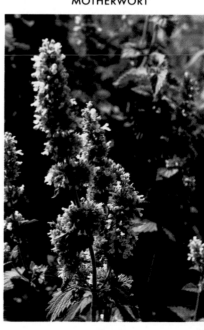

CATNIP

PLATE 30

MINTS AND RELATIVES;
OFTEN CULTIVATED AND NATURALIZED;
ROADSIDES, FIELDS, WASTE PLACES

SPEARMINT
Mentha spicata   p. 188
Often cultivated and naturalized, this European mint has a distinct
scent. The leaves are usually more wrinkled and less rounded than
those of Peppermint, and the stems are greenish rather than distinctly purple. **Flowers June to frost.**

PEPPERMINT
Mentha piperita   p. 188
Peppermint has a stronger scent than Spearmint. Spearmint smells
like chewing gum; Peppermint smells like toothpaste. **Flowers June
to frost.**

LEMON BALM
Melissa officinalis   p. 68
The leaves of this plant, similar in appearance to those of Catnip, are
best identified by the strong, pleasant lemony scent.

CREEPING THYME
Thymus species   p. 232
Most often seen in herb gardens, Creeping Thyme has sometimes
escaped from cultivation, though it is scarce in the wild. **Flowers
July–Aug.** The leaf tea was used for nervous disorders and stom-
achaches. See warning in text.

HYSSOP
Hyssopus officinalis   p. 190
Grown in herb gardens; sometimes escaped and naturalized in the
Northeast. The entire (toothless), opposite, stalkless leaves have a
peppery scent when stroked firmly. **Flowers June–Oct.** Leaf tea was
once used as a gargle for sore throats.

GROUND IVY
Glechoma hederacea   p. 192
A scentless, creeping perennial with rounded, scallop-edged leaves.
Flowers March–July. A folk remedy for cancers, backaches, etc. See
warning in text.

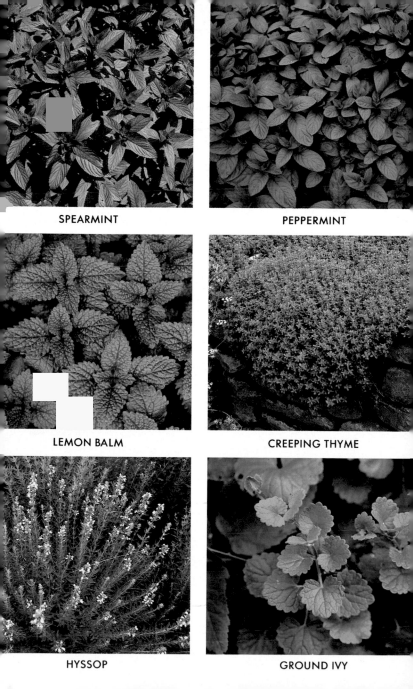

SPEARMINT

PEPPERMINT

LEMON BALM

CREEPING THYME

HYSSOP

GROUND IVY

PLATE 31

SHRUBS OR VINES OF OLD
FIELDS, WASTE PLACES

ELDERBERRY
Sambucus canadensis **p. 240**

 The white flowers of this common shrub are in flat, umbrella-like clusters. **Flowers June–July.** The purple-black, edible fruits develop Aug.–Sept. **Caution:** Though the fruits are edible and the flowers are used in medicinal teas and fried as fritters, most plant parts are considered **toxic.** The fruits should only be consumed cooked, and the flowers, dried or cooked.

SMOOTH SUMAC
Rhus glabra **p. 250**

 As both "smooth" and *glabra* (which means "smooth") imply, the twigs and leaf stalks of this sumac lack hairs. The 11–31 leaflets are toothed. The whitish flowers are not as showy as the fuzzy red fruit clusters. The fruits, bark, and leaves have been used in medicine. **Caution:** Do not confuse this plant with Poison Sumac, which has white berries and toothless leaves, and usually grows in or near swamps.

POISON IVY
Toxicodendron radicans **p. 300**

Poison Ivy is a plant of many forms; it may creep along the ground, develop a thick, hairy woody stem and climb up trees (as shown here), or grow as an erect shrub to 6 ft. tall. This is one of the most persistent, common, noxious plants in our range. The highly variable leaflets are glossy to hairy and toothed, lobed, or without teeth. Leaf preparations were once used in the treatment of paralytic and liver diseases. **Warning:** Never ingest Poison Ivy.

BLACK RASPBERRY
Rubus occidentalis **p. 234**

This familiar shrub produces purple-black fruits, with rows of white hairs between each drupelet. Originally a European plant, it has been widely cultivated. The astringent root tea was once used to treat diarrhea, dysentery, stomach pain, and other ailments. **Flowers April–July.**

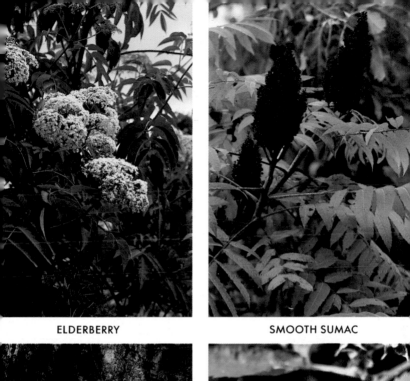

ELDERBERRY

SMOOTH SUMAC

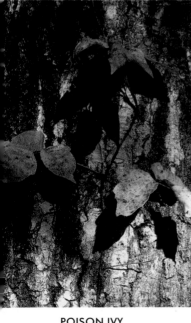

POISON IVY

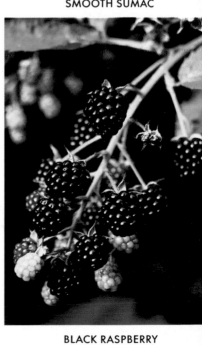

BLACK RASPBERRY
(BLACKBERRY)

PLATE 32
FENCEROWS, WASTE PLACES; VINES

HOPS
Humulus lupulus **p. 204**
This twining vine sometimes escapes from cultivation. It has oval to 3-lobed, toothed leaves. The inconspicuous male and female flowers occur on separate plants. The fruits (hops) are best known for their use in flavoring beer, but are a well-known herbal sedative as well. See warning in text.

KUDZU
Pueraria lobata **p. 170**
A noxious, robust, trailing or climbing vine with 3-parted leaves. The grape-scented purple flowers are in a loose raceme. **Flowers July–Sept.** In China, the root, flowers, seeds, stems, and root starch are used for a wide range of ailments. Perhaps this pernicious, invasive weed of the South could best be controlled by harvesting its economic and medicinal potential. *Photo by Jim Duke.*

VIRGINIA CREEPER
Parthenocissus quinquefolia **p. 302**
A climbing or creeping vine with 5-parted palmate leaves. Very common in thickets throughout our range. Though considered potentially **toxic,** the plant and root tea were used as medicine.

PASSION-FLOWER
Passiflora incarnata **p. 170**
The white to blue flowers, with numerous threads radiating from the center, are on a climbing vine with deeply cleft leaves. **Flowers July–Oct.** The whole plant has traditionally been used in tea as a nerve sedative. **Blue Morning Glory** *(Ipomoea hederacea)* is pictured along with the Passion-flower.

GREENBRIERS, CATBRIERS
Smilax species **p. 296**
Catbriers are a group of entangling, climbing vines with sharp prickles. The flowers are inconspicuous. The berries are blue-black or red. The prickles, leaves, and roots have been used medicinally.

JAPANESE HONEYSUCKLE
Lonicera japonica **p. 298**
This evergreen trailing, twining vine has become a troublesome weed in the South. The flowers are white but quickly fade to yellow, earning the plant the name "Gold and Silver Flower" in China. The leaves and flowers are used in Traditional Chinese Medicine.

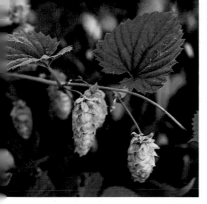

HOPS

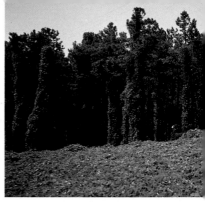

KUDZU

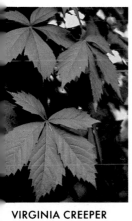

VIRGINIA CREEPER

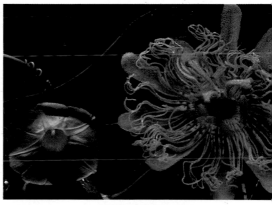

PASSION-FLOWER

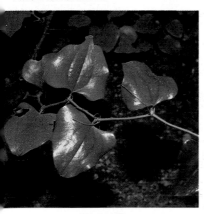

GREENBRIER

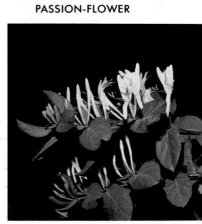

JAPANESE HONEYSUCKLE

PLATE 33
WASTE PLACES; POISONOUS PLANTS

See also Pl. 16.

JIMSONWEED
Datura stramonium   **p. 182**
The large, coarse, wavy-toothed leaves and trumpet-shaped, slightly spiraled blooms make this plant easy to identify. **Flowers May–Sept.** The 4-parted, chambered, spiny seedpods are distinctive, too. Although this plant produces useful alkaloids, it is **violently toxic.** Do not ingest any part of it.

CASTOR-OIL-PLANT
Ricinus communis   **p. 208**
This large, rank plant (to 12 ft. tall) is often cultivated for ornamental effect in the South, where it has escaped. It produces **highly poisonous** seeds (ingesting a single seed has resulted in fatalities). The seed oil, without the violent toxic ricin, is a well-known home remedy. **Flowers July–Sept.**

POKEWEED
Phytolacca americana   **p. 56**
This large, red-stemmed perennial produces greenish white flowers in elongate clusters. **Flowers July–Sept.** Found throughout much of our range (except extreme northern limits). The purple-black berries are relished by birds, but are generally considered **toxic** to humans. The roots, leaves, and fruits have been used medicinally but are **poisonous.**

WOODY NIGHTSHADE
Solanum dulcamara   **p. 182**
This common woody vine is found around barnyards and waste places. Each leaf has 1 or 2 earlike lobes at the base. The purple (rarely white), 5-parted flowers have backcurving petals. The plant was formerly used for skin eruptions, cancers, warts, and other ailments but is **toxic. Flowers May–Sept.**

HORSE-NETTLE
Solanum carolinense   **p. 182**
A common weed with sharp-spined stems and coarse-toothed leaves; grows to 4 ft. Pale violet or whitish, 5-parted flowers. **Flowers May–Oct.** The orange fruits, resembling tiny tomatoes, are considered **poisonous.** Once used in folk medicine.   *Photo by Jim Duke.*

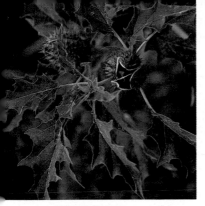

JIMSONWEED

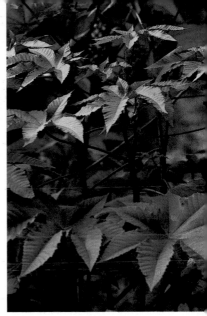

CASTOR-OIL-PLANT

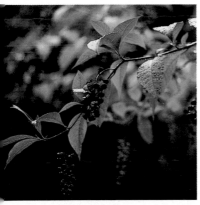

POKEWEED

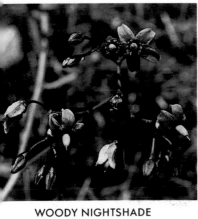

WOODY NIGHTSHADE

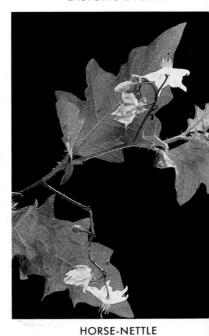

HORSE-NETTLE

PLATE 34
OPEN FIELDS; SUMMER-BLOOMING PLANTS

COMMON MILKWEED
Asclepias syriaca   **p. 154**
A milky-juiced, downy perennial, to 4 ft. The relatively large leaves, pink-purple flowers in globe-shaped clusters, and warty seedpods distinguish this species from other milkweeds. **Flowers June–Aug.** The root was once used in tea as a laxative and the latex (juice) has been used as an application to warts. **Caution:** Like most milkweeds, Common Milkweed is potentially **toxic.**

BLACK-EYED SUSAN
Rudbeckia hirta   **p. 126**
A familiar wildflower with lance-shaped leaves and yellow ray flowers surrounding a dark brown cone. **Flowers June–Oct.** The root was used to treat colds and expel worms; it was also used externally as a wash for sores, snakebites, swelling, and other ailments, although a few individuals might break out in a rash after touching this plant.

BLUE VERVAIN
Verbena hastata   **p. 172**
This 2- to 4-ft.-tall perennial has a grooved, 4-angled stem. The blue-violet flowers are in branched, pencil-like spikes. **Flowers July–Sept.** The leaves have traditionally been used for "female" diseases, coughs, fevers, dysentery, stomach cramps, and other ailments.

WILD SENNA
Cassia marilandica   **p. 118**
A weedy perennial, 3–6 ft. Leaves compound, with 4–8 pairs of leaflets. Note the small, club-shaped gland at the base of the leaf stalk. The yellow flowers are arranged in loose clusters. **Flowers July–Aug.** The leaves and seedpods have traditionally been used as a laxative.

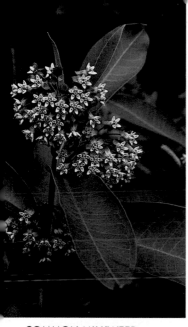

COMMON MILKWEED

BLACK-EYED SUSAN

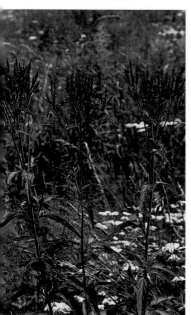

BLUE VERVAIN

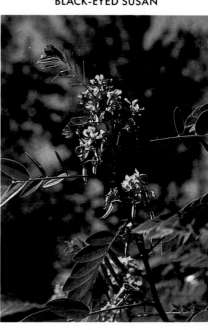

WILD SENNA

PLATE 35

ROADSIDES, WASTE PLACES;
OFTEN CULTIVATED AND NATURALIZED

These yellow composites (members of the daisy family) usually flower in late summer.

ELECAMPANE
Inula helenium   **p. 122**
A European plant; sometimes escaped from cultivation, then naturalized. The yellow blooms, up to 4 in. across, have long, thin ray flowers. **Flowers July–Sept.** The root is used in tea as a folk remedy for lung ailments.

SUNFLOWER
Helianthus annuus   **p. 132**

The wild ancestor of the common Sunflower has smaller blooms than cultivated forms (shown here). **Flowers July–Oct.** The whole plant has been used medicinally. See warning in text.

COMMON TANSY
Tanacetum vulgare   **p. 124**
A European plant, often grown in herb gardens; escaped and naturalized in the Northeast. Easily identified by its fernlike leaves and buttonlike, yellow, rayless blooms. **Flowers June–Sept.** The whole plant is used medicinally, though it is considered unsafe. (The oil can be *lethal* — see text.)

GERMAN or WILD CHAMOMILE
Chamomilla recutita
[*Matricaria chamomilla*]   **p. 84**
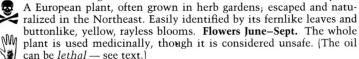
Well known as an herb garden plant and ingredient in tea, this annual can be distinguished from related plants by its hollow receptacle. **Flowers July–Oct.** (or earlier, if cultivated). The flowers are considered mildly sedative.

JERUSALEM ARTICHOKE
Helianthus tuberosus   **p. 132**
A close relative of Sunflower; this plant grows 5–10 ft. tall. Thick, oval leaves; sandpapery above, with a winged leaf stalk. The edible tubers (shown here) contain inulin, suggested by some as dietarily useful for diabetics. **Flowers Aug.–Oct.**

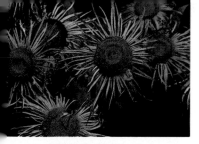

ELECAMPANE

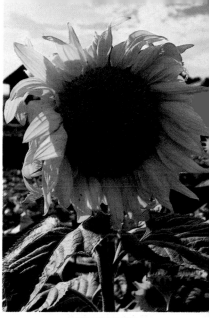

SUNFLOWER

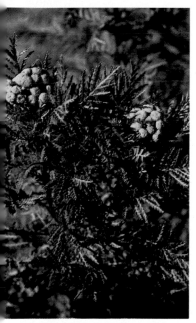

COMMON TANSY

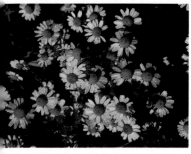

GERMAN or WILD CHAMOMILE

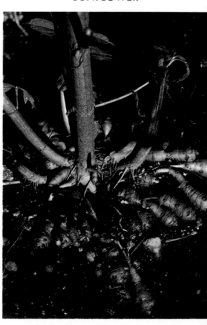

JERUSALEM ARTICHOKE tubers

PLATE 36

GLADES, PRAIRIES, WASTE GROUND, OPEN WOODS (1)

CREAM WILD INDIGO
Baptisia leucophaea   **p. 116**

A coarse, hairy perennial; 1–2 ft. Flowers cream yellow, in project-ing, slightly drooping clusters. **Flowers April–June.** The plant is un-der investigation as an immune-system stimulant, but it is poten-tially **toxic.**

BLUE FALSE INDIGO
Baptisia australis   **p. 194**

A smooth, bluish green perennial, 3–5 ft. The showy, blue-violet blooms are in an elongate raceme. **Flowers April–June.** The plant is under investigation as an immune-system stimulant.

GUMWEED
Grindelia lanceolata   **p. 122**

A common, weedy, late-summer bloomer in much of its range, this plant is characterized by a swollen, bulblike receptacle beneath the flowers with small, narrow, loosely spreading sticky bracts. **Flowers July–Sept.** The dried flowerheads were once used in tea as an asthma treatment.

FRAGRANT or STINKING SUMAC
Rhus aromatica   **p. 250**

A highly variable shrub. The strongly scented leaves have blunt-toothed margins. The tiny yellow blooms appear in early spring, be-fore or with the leaves. The hairy red fruits are oily to touch. The astringent root bark was used in medicine. See warning in text.

COMMON ST. JOHNSWORT
Hypericum perforatum   **p. 114**

A European plant, very commonly naturalized in dry soils through-out the U.S. When the leaves are held to light, translucent "perfo-rations" are visible, hence the species name *"perforatum."* The yel-low petals have black dots on their margins. **Flowers June–Sept.** Used medicinally for external wounds, ulcers, bruises, and other ail-ments, but may cause photodermatitis.

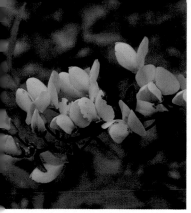

CREAM WILD INDIGO

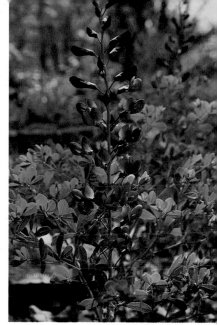

BLUE FALSE INDIGO

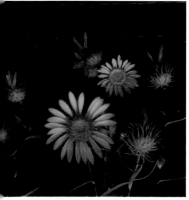

GUMWEED

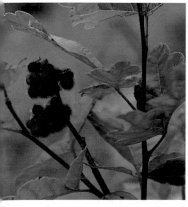

FRAGRANT or STINKING SUMAC

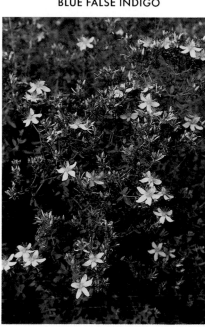

COMMON ST. JOHNSWORT

PLATE 37
GLADES (2)

Glades are open spaces in woods. These habitats are dry most of the year, but moist in spring. See also Plates 36 and 38.

PRICKLY-PEAR CACTUS
Opuntia humifusa   **p. 88**
Our most widespread cactus; the only one found in the East. **Flowers May–Aug.** Prickly-pear's yellow-orange blossoms are short-lived. Its fruits and leaves (shown below) have been used medicinally. The peeled pads ("leaves") have been used as a poultice on wounds, and in tea for lung ailments. The fruit juice has been applied to warts.

FALSE ALOE, RATTLESNAKE-MASTER
Manfreda virginica   **p. 104**
The succulent leaves, radiating from the roots in a basal rosette, are sometimes mottled with purple dots (in form *tigrina*). The greenish white to yellow flowers are in a tall (to 6 ft.), mostly leafless spike. **Flowers June–July.** The root has been used as a diuretic and was nibbled as a laxative, a treatment for severe diarrhea, and to expel worms.

CALAMINT
Satureja arkansana   **p. 190**
A creeping perennial; 4–8 in. high. This small, relatively inconspicuous plant is most often noticed after the strong-scented leaves are trampled, filling the air with their pennyroyal-like scent. Note the oil glands on the leaves in the close-up photograph *(bottom left)*. The leaves at the base of the plant are oval, while those on the flowering stems are linear. The blue-violet flowers are about ⅜ in. long. **Flowers April–July.**

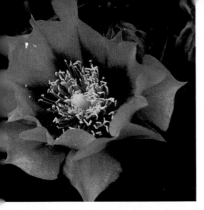

PRICKLY-PEAR CACTUS flowers

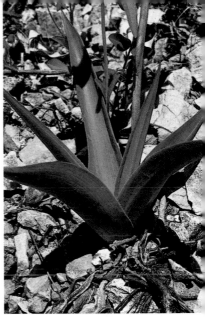

FALSE ALOE

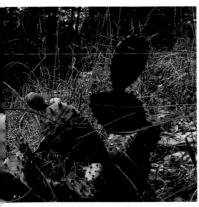

PRICKLY-PEAR CACTUS

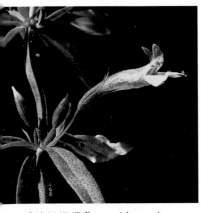

CALAMINT flower (close-up)

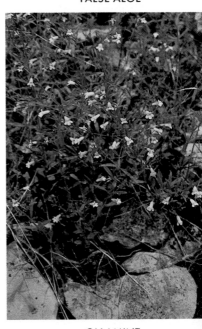

CALAMINT

PLATE 38

GLADES (3)

INDIAN PAINTBRUSH
Castilleja coccinea   **p. 138**

⚠ A well-known wildflower with showy red (sometimes yellow) bracts. This annual is most common in the southwestern part of our area. **Flowers April–July.** A weak flower tea was once used for rheumatism and "female" diseases. May be **toxic.**

HOARY PUCCOON
Lithospermum canescens   **p. 136**

A perennial covered with soft white hairs, hence the common name "hoary." The orange-yellow flowers, in curled flat clusters, have stamens concealed in the throat of the corolla. **Flowers April–June.** The leaf tea was once used as an external wash for fevers accompanied by convulsions.

NEW JERSEY TEA, RED ROOT
Ceanothus americanus   **p. 248**

This small shrub, to 2 ft. in height, has oval, toothed leaves with 3 prominent parallel veins. The white flowers are in showy clusters on non-woody stems. **Flowers April–Sept.** The leaf tea was once a popular tea substitute (beverage). The roots and leaves have been used medicinally.

LYRE-LEAVED SAGE, CANCERWEED
Salvia lyrata   **p. 192**

The cleft, round-toothed leaves are in a basal rosette. The violet-blue flowers are in whorled spikes. **Flowers April–June.** The leaves were once used externally as a folk remedy for cancer and warts.

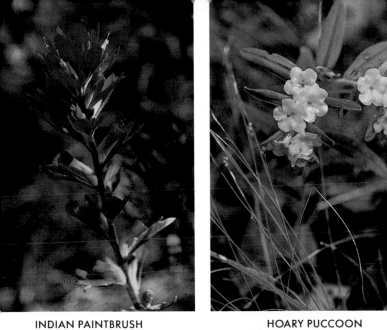

INDIAN PAINTBRUSH

HOARY PUCCOON

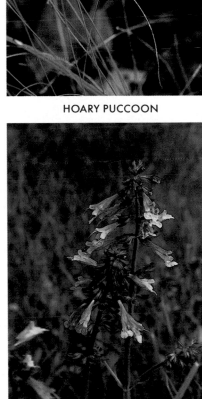

NEW JERSEY TEA

LYRE-LEAVED SAGE

PLATE 39

DRY, ROCKY OPENINGS, ROADSIDES, MOIST GRAVEL BANKS

AMERICAN BEAUTY BUSH
Callicarpa americana   **p. 244**
This shrub occurs only in the southern part of our area (Md. to n. Ark.), though Asian species of this genus are grown as ornamentals as far north as Boston. This species is easily recognized by the sticky, aromatic, opposite leaves and whorls of magenta fruits. **Fruits Sept.– Oct.** The root, leaves, and berries are used medicinally.

PRICKLY POPPY
Argemone albiflora   **p. 12**
The blue-green stems and thistle-like leaves have numerous sharp spines. If the stems or leaves are broken they exude a yellow juice. The white flowers are poppy-like. **Flowers May–Sept.** The seeds, leaves, and stem juice have been used medicinally, but the plant is generally considered **poisonous.**

YUCCA, SOAPWEED
Yucca glauca   **p. 18**
Yuccas are easily recognized by their sword-shaped, stiff, sharp-tipped leaves. The bell-like flowers of this species are in an erect spike. **Flowers May–July.** The root has been used to reduce inflammation and stop bleeding. See warning in text.

COMMON MULLEIN
Verbascum thapsus   **p. 114**
A common weed, naturalized from Europe. It grows along roadsides but also in sand pits and gravel pits, and seems to thrive in the poorest of soils. A biennial, it produces a rosette of large, gray-green, very fuzzy leaves the first year, and an attractive spike of light yellow flowers the second year. **Flowers July–Sept.** The leaves and flowers are used medicinally, but see warning in text.

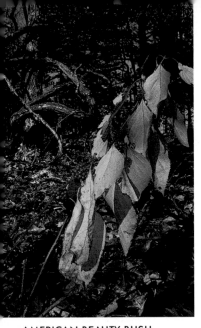

AMERICAN BEAUTY BUSH

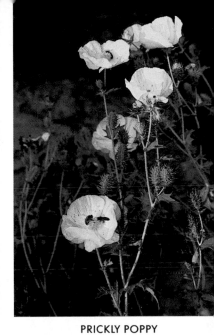

PRICKLY POPPY

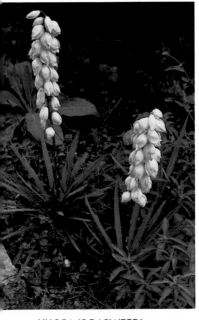

YUCCA (SOAPWEED)

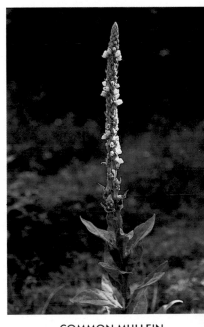

COMMON MULLEIN

PLATE 40

PRAIRIES, GLADES, OPEN WOODS;
MOSTLY DRY SOILS

PURPLE CONEFLOWER
Echinacea purpurea   **p. 200**

Distinguished from other purple coneflowers by its oval, coarsely toothed leaves, flatter (less cone-shaped) disk, and the orange-tipped bristles on the flowerheads. **Flowers June–Sept.** The leaves and root are used, especially in West German products, as stimulants to the immune system, for the treatment of colds, flu, and other common ailments.

PALE PURPLE CONEFLOWER
Echinacea pallida   **p. 200**

This coneflower grows from 2 to 4 ft. tall. The showy purple ray flowers may be 4 in. long. **Flowers May–Aug.** The range of this purple coneflower is more eastern than that of its close relative below.

NARROW-LEAVED PURPLE CONEFLOWER
Echinacea angustifolia   **p. 200**

Long considered the most important medicinal species of purple coneflower, *E. angustifolia* is smaller than *E. pallida*; it grows to 20 in. tall. The ray petals are shorter, usually no longer than the width of the disk. This species occurs in the western prairies. Hybrids occur where the ranges of *E. angustifolia* and *E. pallida* meet.

WILD QUININE
Parthenium species   **p. 78**

The large, dock-like leaves and fuzzy, white, nearly rayless, button-like flowers distinguish this highly variable plant group. The 4 species of *Parthenium* in our range are separated on technical details; *P. integrifolium* is shown here. **Flowers May–July.** The root has historically been used as an adulterant to purple coneflowers *(Echinacea)*, but was also used for bladder and kidney ailments.

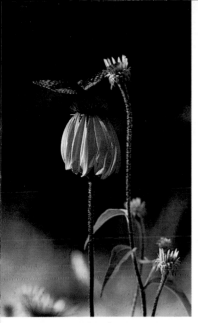

PURPLE CONEFLOWER

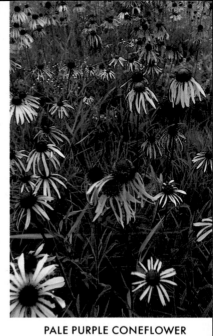

PALE PURPLE CONEFLOWER

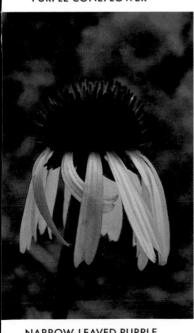

NARROW-LEAVED PURPLE
CONEFLOWER

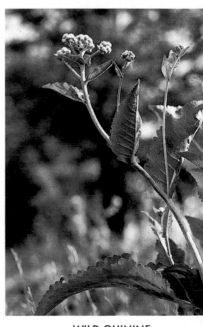

WILD QUININE

PLATE 41

DRY, OPEN HABITATS;
SUMMER-BLOOMING PLANTS

ROUGH BLAZING-STAR
Liatris aspera   **p. 196**
The purple to rose flowers on crowded, 3- to 4-ft.-tall spikes are a
common sight on midwestern prairies. **Flowers Aug.–Sept.** The root
was used to treat kidney and bladder ailments and gonorrhea. Other
Liatris species were used similarly.

BUTTERFLYWEED, PLEURISY-ROOT
Asclepias tuberosa   **p. 136**
The showy orange blossoms are a common sight, especially along dry
roadsides in the South. **Flowers June–Sept.** The large, tuberous root
has been valued as a treatment for pleurisy and other lung ailments,
but may be **toxic** in large quantities.

SWEET GOLDENROD
Solidago odora   **p. 124**
This species of goldenrod has strongly anise-scented leaves that can
be used to make a pleasant beverage tea. The plant was exported to
China from the U.S. in the late 1700s for that purpose. The flowers
are arranged on 1 side of the flower stems. The leaves are apparently
toothless, but have rough prickles that will catch your fingers if you
rub them backwards along the leaf edge. When held to the light, the
leaves appear to have translucent dots. **Flowers July–Sept.** The
leaves were once used to treat colds and rheumatism. See warning in
text.

HORSEMINT
Monarda punctata   **p. 112**
This biennial or short-lived perennial has yellowish, purple-dotted
blooms in whorls atop the plant. The flower clusters have yellowish
to purplish leaflike bracts beneath. The leaves were once used as a
commercial source of thymol, an antiseptic formerly derived from
oil of thyme but now produced synthetically. **Flowers July–Oct.**

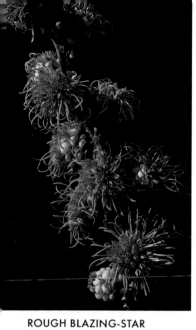

ROUGH BLAZING-STAR

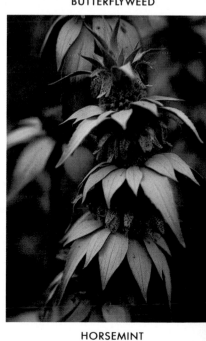

BUTTERFLYWEED

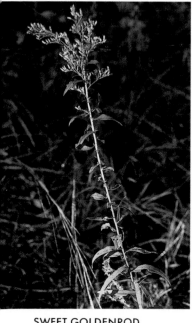

SWEET GOLDENROD

HORSEMINT

PLATE 42
DRY FIELDS OR FOREST MARGINS

EYEBRIGHT
Euphrasia species　　　　　　　　　　　　　　　**p. 66**

The tiny, semiparasitic plants in this group occur in subarctic regions of the Northern Hemisphere. Some species are found in the northern tier of states in the U.S. and Canada. These plants have traditionally been used for eye ailments, probably based on the doctrine of signatures (see p. 6): the flower bears some resemblance to an eye. The plants have mild astringent properties. **Flowers June–Sept.**

LOBELIA, INDIAN-TOBACCO
Lobelia inflata　　　　　　　　　　　　　　　　**p. 184**

An annual, to 24 in. The small, whitish to pale blue flowers produce inflated seedpods, hence the species name *"inflata."* **Flowers June–Oct.** The whole plant has been used to induce vomiting and sweating, as well as to allay spasms. For nearly 2 centuries controversy has raged over use of this herb and its potential toxicity.

SPIDERWORTS
Tradescantia species　　　　　　　　　　　　　**p. 168**

Spiderworts have 3-petaled flowers with many stamens. Each stamen is covered with prominent, large-celled hairs, used for a variety of biological tests. The root and leaves have been used medicinally. Various species of spiderwort are used interchangeably; pictured here is *Tradescantia ohiensis.* **Flowers April–June.**

WILD BERGAMOT, PURPLE BEE-BALM
Monarda fistulosa　　　　　　　　　　　　　　**p. 186**

Perennial; 2–3 ft. in height, with narrow lavender flowers crowded in a terminal head. Sometimes cultivated in herb gardens. The leaves make a pleasant-flavored tea that was used for colds, fevers, stomachaches, insomnia, etc. **Flowers May–Sept.**

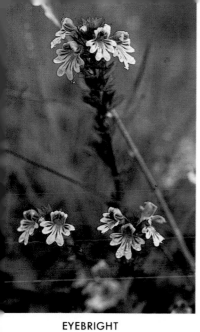

EYEBRIGHT

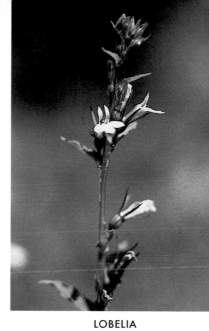

LOBELIA

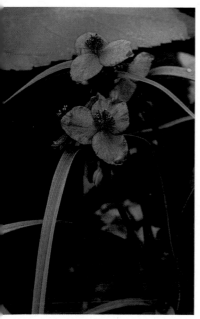

SPIDERWORT

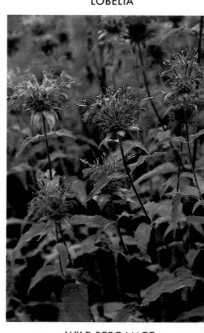

WILD BERGAMOT

PLATE 43
FIELDS AND FOREST EDGES; NORTHEAST

COMMON JUNIPER
Juniperus communis   **p. 226**
Grows as a shrub (to 6 ft.) in our area, but as a small tree (to 20 ft.) in Europe. The needles, in whorls of 3, have 2 white bands on the upperside that are mostly broader than the green margins. The bluish, rounded fruits (Aug.–Oct.) are used in medicine and as a flavoring in gin. See warning in text.

SHEEP LAUREL
Kalmia angustifolia   **p. 230**
A slender evergreen shrub, to 5 ft., with opposite, leathery leaves. The rose-pink flowers are axillary (rather than terminal, as in Mountain Laurel, *K. latifolia* — see p. 230). **Flowers May–July.** Minute amounts of the twigs, leaves, and flowers have been used for medicinal purposes; however, the plant is considered **highly toxic.** It is also known as Lambkill.

HAIRY SARSAPARILLA
Aralia hispida   **p. 54**
Shrub, to 3 ft., with ill-scented leaves; stems covered with many sharp, stiff bristles. The small, greenish white flowers are in globe-shaped umbels. The leaf tea was used to induce sweating. The root bark was considered diuretic and "tonic."

SPREADING DOGBANE
Apocynum androsaemifolium   **p. 152**
This plant differs from its close relative Indian Hemp (*A. cannabinum*, p. 52) in that its leaves are mostly sessile (stalkless), and the flowers are both in leaf axils and terminal. **Flowers June–July. Caution:** Although the milky sap from their stems has been used as an external remedy, both this species and *A. cannabinum* are considered **poisonous.**

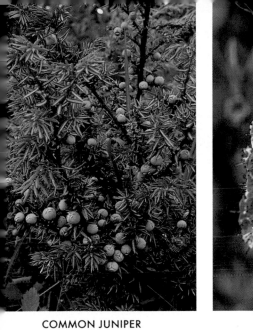

COMMON JUNIPER

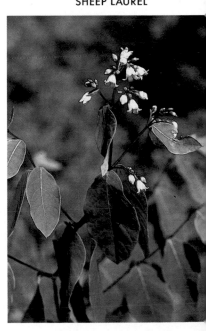

SHEEP LAUREL

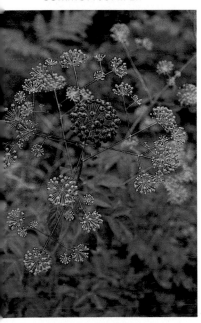

HAIRY SARSAPARILLA

SPREADING DOGBANE

PLATE 44
DRY OR MOIST OPEN WOODS; SMALL, SHOWY
SPRING-FLOWERING TREES OR SHRUBS

FLOWERING DOGWOOD
Cornus florida **p. 270**
Dogwood bark, twigs, and berries were used medicinally. Inner-bark preparations were used as a quinine substitute; the twigs were used as chewing sticks (toothbrushes). **Flowers April–May.** Pictured at right are the leaves and fruits. Dogwood's bitter fruits (Oct.–Nov.) were soaked in brandy, which was sipped as a digestive tonic.

OHIO BUCKEYE
Aesculus glabra **p. 264**
 The palmate leaves, 4–15 in. long, with 5 toothed leaflets, and the yellowish blooms characterize this horsechestnut. **Flowers April–May.** The nuts were once used medicinally, but are considered **poisonous** without elaborate processing.

CATALPAS
Catalpa species **p. 266**
The large heart-shaped leaves and large, showy flower clusters make catalpas popular as ornamental trees. **Flowers June–July.** The bark, seeds, leaves, and seedpods were used medicinally.

REDBUD
Cercis canadensis **p. 284**
A small tree with heart-shaped leaves; the red-purple flowers appear in early spring, before the leaves. **Flowers late March–May.** The bark is highly astringent.

GREAT RHODODENDRON
Rhododendron maximum **p. 230**
A common large evergreen shrub or small tree of the East; it often forms thickets. The showy clusters of rose-pink flowers are its chief feature. **Flowers June–July.** The leaves, once used medicinally, are considered **toxic.**

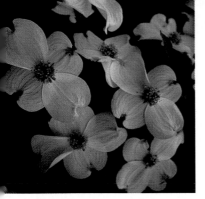

FLOWERING DOGWOOD

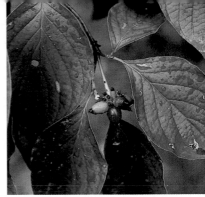

FLOWERING DOGWOOD
leaves and fruits

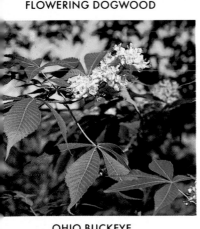

OHIO BUCKEYE

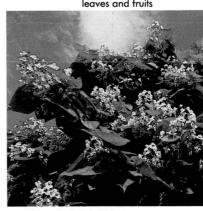

CATALPA

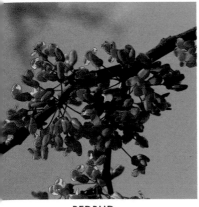

REDBUD

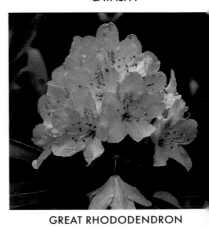

GREAT RHODODENDRON

PLATE 45

SMALL TREES OF DRY, OPEN WOODS, MOSTLY IN THE SOUTH

HOPTREE, WAFER ASH
Ptelea trifoliata **p. 272**
A small tree, to 20 ft., with 3-parted, black-dotted leaves. Each waferlike fruit consists of a papery wing surrounding 2 seeds. **Fruits July–Sept.**

FRINGETREE
Chionanthus virginica **p. 270**
A small tree, to 20 ft., with oval, opposite leaves to 8 in. long. The white, slender-petaled flowers are in drooping clusters. **Flowers May–June.** The root and trunk bark have been used as a treatment for jaundice and other liver ailments. See warning in text.

SASSAFRAS
Sassafras albidum **p. 278**
When Europeans first settled N. America, Sassafras was a major export; in fact, the Plymouth colony was in part founded on speculation of Sassafras exports. The root bark, twigs, trunk bark, and leaves of this tree have been used medicinally, but are now banned, rightly or wrongly, by the FDA as a carcinogen. The yellow flowers of Sassafras unfold from the ends of the twigs in early spring, before the leaves emerge. **Flowers March–May.** The leaves *(bottom right)* come in 3 shapes — oval, mittenlike, and 3-lobed.

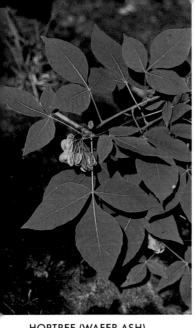

HOPTREE (WAFER ASH)

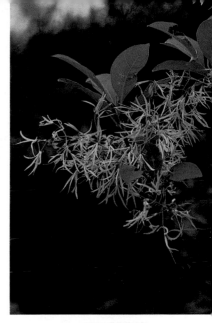

FRINGETREE

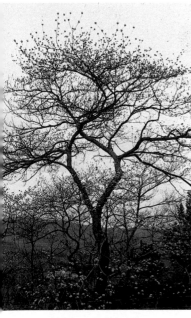

SASSAFRAS flowers

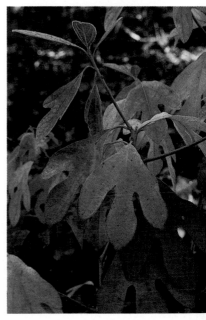

SASSAFRAS

PLATE 46
SOUTHERN TREES OR SHRUBS; WOODS OR VARIOUS HABITATS

COMMON PAWPAW
Asimina triloba   **p. 284**

The deep maroon to chocolate-colored, 3-petaled, drooping flowers appear before or with the leaves. **Flowers April–May.** The large, oblong to lance-shaped, toothless leaves grow to 1 ft. in length. In late summer, the succulent, slightly curved, oval, green to brown fruits ripen. The leaves, seeds, and fruits have been used medicinally. **Caution:** The seeds are considered insecticidal and **toxic;** the leaves may cause a rash.

SYCAMORE
Platanus occidentalis   **p. 280**
Sycamore is one of the largest deciduous trees in N. America, growing to 150 ft. in height. Without seeing the leaves or fruit, it is often easy to identify this tree by its multicolored peeling bark, which is smooth and light-colored, especially on upper portions of the trunk. The inner bark was once used as a folk medicine.

DEVIL'S WALKING-STICK
Aralia spinosa   **p. 238**
The largest N. American member of the ginseng family, Devil's Walking-stick may grow to 30 ft. tall, with a trunk 6 in. in diameter. Sharp curved spines surround joints on the trunk, especially of younger specimens. The large compound leaves are topped in summer by an enormous panicle of tiny white blooms. The purple-red berries shown here form by Sept. or Oct.

SOUTHERN PRICKLY-ASH
Zanthoxylum clava-herculis   **p. 238**
This small tree or large shrub is characterized by large, triangular corky knobs on the bark. The bark and berries are used in traditional medicine.

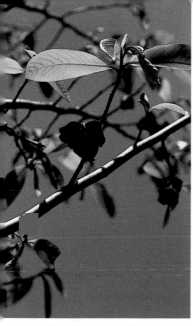

COMMON PAWPAW

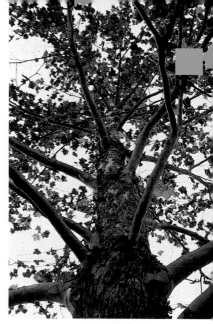

SYCAMORE

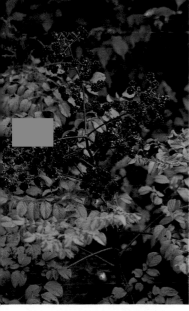
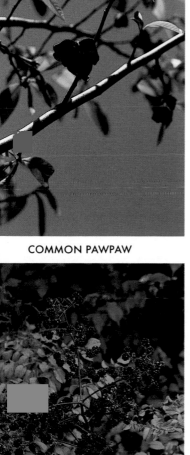

DEVIL'S WALKING-STICK

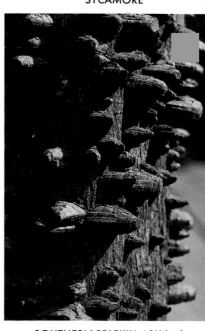

SOUTHERN PRICKLY-ASH bark

PLATE 47

WOODY PLANTS OF DRY SOILS, WASTE PLACES

WHITE PINE
Pinus strobus **p. 260**

The most common pine species of the Northeast, White Pine has long been used as a major source of lumber and wood pulp; the timber has been used for ship masts, as well as houses and other buildings. The twigs, bark, leaves, and pitch have been used medicinally for sores, cuts, bruises, rheumatism, and many other ailments.

BLACK WALNUT
Juglans nigra **p. 276**

This large tree (to 120 ft.) produces the famous walnut wood of commerce, as well as the familiar edible nuts. Although the tree is less well known as an "herb," its inner bark, fruits, and leaves have been used medicinally, as a remedy for toothaches, as well as an insecticide for bed bugs. The leaves are pinnate, with slightly alternate leaflets, uneven or heart-shaped at the base.

TREE-OF-HEAVEN, STINKTREE
Ailanthus altissima **p. 272**

This tree, native to China, was introduced from England in the late 19th century as an ornamental. It quickly established itself. In cities like New York and Boston it grows in harsh conditions where no other plants seem able to survive. It can easily be identified by the prominent glands on the teeth at the base of the leaflets. The trunk and root bark are used in Traditional Chinese Medicine.

COMMON BARBERRY
Berberis vulgaris **p. 236**

The unripe berries (shown here) turn red when mature (Aug. through winter). This alien shrub has been widely planted as an ornamental and has become naturalized in many areas. The root bark, high in the yellow alkaloid berberine, has been used for rheumatism, sciatica, arthritis, and many other ailments. See warning in text.

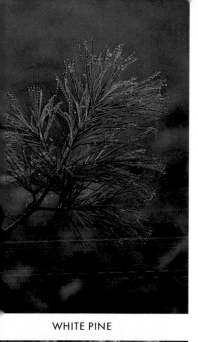

WHITE PINE

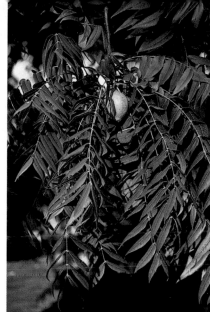

BLACK WALNUT

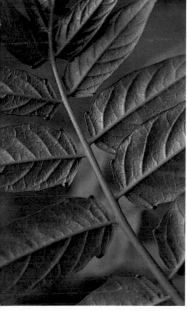

TREE-OF-HEAVEN (STINKTREE)

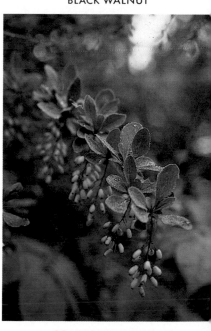

COMMON BARBERRY

PLATE 48
TREES OF DRY HABITATS

BLACK or WILD CHERRY
Prunus serotina **p. 290**

 Best known for its highly valued and beautiful wood, this tree has white flowers in slender, drooping racemes. **Flowers April–June.** The aromatic inner bark is traditionally used in tea or syrups to treat coughs, fevers, colds, sore throats, and other ailments. **Caution:** The bark contains cyanide-like compounds and can be **toxic** in large quantities. See text.

PRINCESS-TREE, PAULOWNIA
Paulownia tomentosa **p. 266**

 Another plant native to China, introduced here as an ornamental; it has made itself quite at home, especially in the South. The wood is highly valued by the Japanese and is exported at a high price. The panicles of large, fuzzy, purple-blue, trumpet-shaped flowers set this tree apart from any native tree. **Flowers April–June.** The bark is used in Traditional Chinese Medicine. See warning in text.

HONEY LOCUST
Gleditsia triacanthos **p. 274**

 This tree usually has distinctive and formidable branched spikes, often 6 in. long or more; a thornless variety (form *inermis*) also occurs in our area and is cultivated. The flowers attract many bees. **Flowers May–July.** The flat, leguminous seedpods and the inner bark were once used as medicine, but all parts of the plant may be **toxic.**

COMMON PERSIMMON
Diospyros virginiana **p. 284**

 Best known for its edible fruits (astringent before they are ripe). The inner bark is also highly astringent. Both the inner bark and the fruits have been used medicinally; see warning in text. The shiny, elliptical leaves have small, greenish yellow, urn-shaped flowers in their axils in spring (May–June). The roundish, pulpy fruits ripen after a heavy frost.

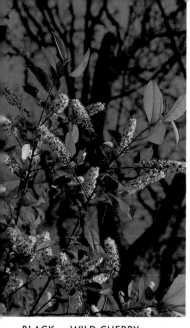

BLACK or WILD CHERRY

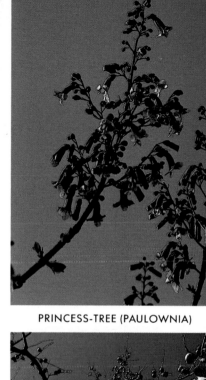

PRINCESS-TREE (PAULOWNIA)

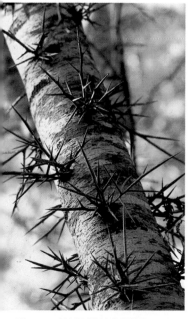

Thorns of HONEY LOCUST

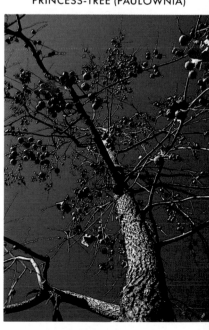

COMMON PERSIMMON

COMMON LOW-GROWING WILDFLOWERS;
PETALS IN 4'S OR 5'S

BLUETS   **Flowering plant**
Houstonia caerulea L.   **C. Pl. 21**   Madder Family
[*Hedyotis caerulea* (L.) Hook.]
Small perennial; 2–8 in. Leaves narrow, opposite; to ½ in. long. Flowers sky blue to white; *4-parted*, with a *yellow center*; March–July.
Where found: Fields, yards. N.S. to Ga.; Ark. to Wisc.
Uses: Cherokees used leaf tea to stop bed-wetting.

COMMON SPEEDWELL   **Leaves, root**
Veronica officinalis L.   **C. Pl. 21**   Figwort Family
Creeping, *hairy* herb; to 7 in. Leaves elliptical, narrow at base; evenly toothed. Blue-violet flowers in *glandular-haired racemes*; May–Aug.
Where found: Waste places. Much of our area. Alien.

 Uses: In Europe, astringent root or leaf tea traditionally used to promote urination, sweating, and menstruation; "blood purifier"; also used for skin and kidney ailments, coughs, asthma, lung diseases, gout, rheumatism, and jaundice. Considered expectorant, diuretic, tonic. **Warning:** One component, aucubin, though liver-protective, anti-oxidant, and antiseptic, can be **toxic** to grazing animals.

THYME-LEAVED SPEEDWELL   **Leaves**
Veronica serpyllifolia L.   Figwort Family
Creeping, much-branched, *smooth* perennial; 2–8 in. Leaves *oval to oblong; short-stalked*. Flowers small, violet-blue (to whitish); 4-petaled, with pale blue and dark stripes. April–Sept.   **Where found:** Lawns, roadsides. Nfld. to Ga.; Ark. to Minn. Alien.
Uses: Leaf juice used by American Indians for earaches; leaves poulticed for boils; tea used for chills and coughs.

JOHNNY-JUMP-UP, HEART'S EASE   **Leaves**
Viola tricolor L.   Violet Family
Angled-stemmed annual; 4–12 in. Leaves toothed, roundish on lower part of plant, oblong above; stipules large, leaflike; *strongly divided*. Pansy-like flowers in patterns of purple, white, and yellow; May–Sept.   **Where found:** Field weed. Escaped from gardens. Alien.
Uses: In Europe, leaf tea a folk medicine for fevers, mild laxative; gargle for sore throats; considered diuretic, expectorant, mild sedative, "blood purifier"; used for asthma, heart palpitations, skin eruptions such as eczema. Rat experiments confirm possible use for skin eruptions. **Warning:** Contains saponins; may be **toxic** in larger doses.

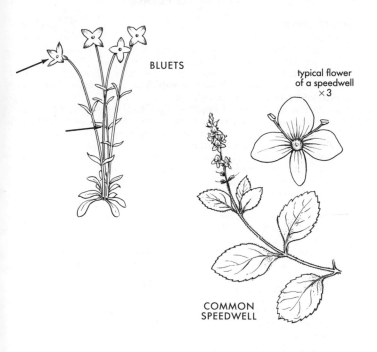

BLUETS

typical flower
of a speedwell
× 3

COMMON
SPEEDWELL

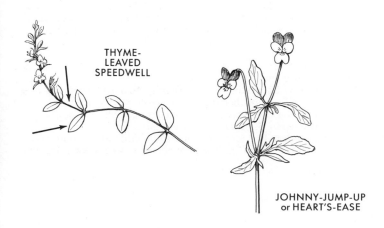

THYME-
LEAVED
SPEEDWELL

JOHNNY-JUMP-UP
or HEART'S-EASE

LOW-GROWING PLANTS WITH SHOWY FLOWERS; 5 OR MORE PETALS

PASQUEFLOWER   **Whole plant**
Anemone patens L.   Buttercup Family
Perennial; 2–16 in. Leaves arising from root; *silky, dissected into linear segments.* Showy flowers, 1–1½ in. wide; March–June. "Petals" (sepals) purple or white, in a *cup-shaped receptacle.* Seeds with *feathery plumes.* **Where found:** Moist meadows, prairies, woods. Iowa to Colo., Wash., Alaska.

☠ **Uses:** As few as 5 drops of highly diluted tincture in water used in homeopathic practice for eye ailments, skin eruptions, rheumatism, leukorrhea, obstructed menses, bronchitis, coughs, asthma. **Warning: Poisonous.** Extremely irritating.
Remarks: The homeopathic doses reported here and elsewhere in this plant identification guide are so dilute as to be harmless (*i.e.,* without side effects), if not biologically inactive, by the medical establishment's standards.

SHARP-LOBED HEPATICA, LIVERLEAF   **Leaves**
Hepatica acutiloba DC.   **C. Pl. 12**   Buttercup Family
Perennial; 4–8 in. Leaves usually evergreen, *3-lobed;* lobes *pointed.* Flowers lavender, blue, white, or pink; Feb.–June. "Petals" (6–10) are actually sepals. **Where found:** Rich woods. W. Me. to Ga.; La., Ark., Mo. to Minn.
Uses: American Indians used leaf tea for liver ailments, poor indigestion, laxative; externally, as a wash for swollen breasts. In folk tradition, tea used for fevers, liver ailments, coughs. Thought to be mildly astringent, demulcent, diuretic. A "liver tonic" boom resulted in the consumption of 450,000 pounds of the dried leaves (domestic and imported) in 1883 alone.

ROUND-LOBED HEPATICA   **Leaves**
Hepatica americana (DC.) Ker   **C. Pl. 12**   Buttercup Family
Similar to *H. acutiloba,* but leaf lobes are *rounded.* Flowers March–June. **Where found:** Dry woods. N.S. to Ga., Ala.; Mo. to Man.
Uses: Same as for *H. acutiloba* (see above).

BLUE-EYED GRASS   **Root, leaves**
Sisyrinchium angustifolium Mill.   Iris Family
Perennial; 4–18 in. Differs from the other 10 or so *Sisyrinchium* species in our range in that the leaves are narrow (¼ in. wide), much flattened, and deep green. Flowers at tip of *long, flat stalk;* May–July. **Where found:** Meadows. Most of our area.
Uses: American Indians used root tea for diarrhea (in children); plant tea for worms, stomachaches. Several species were used as laxatives.

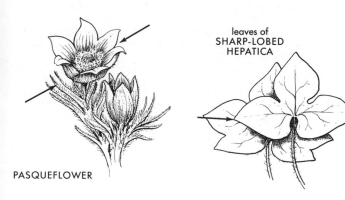

PASQUEFLOWER

leaves of
SHARP-LOBED
HEPATICA

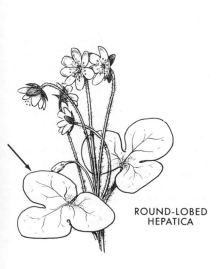

ROUND-LOBED
HEPATICA

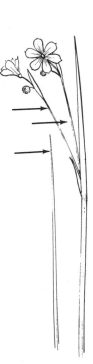

BLUE-EYED GRASS

MISCELLANEOUS FLOWERS WITH 5 PETALS

STIFF GENTIAN, AGUE-WEED
Roots

Gentiana quinquefolia L.
Gentian Family

Perennial; 6–30 in. *Stem 4-ridged.* Leaves oval, clasping. Tubular flowers, in *tight, often 5-flowered clusters;* Aug–Oct. **Where found:** Rich woods, moist fields.

Uses: Tea or root tincture was once used as bitter tonic to stimulate digestion, weak appetite. Also used for headaches, hepatitis, jaundice, constipation.

VIRGINIA WATERLEAF
Whole plant, root

Hydrophyllum virginianum L.
Waterleaf Family

Perennial; 1–3 ft. Leaves *deeply divided,* with *5–7 lobes;* lower segments 2-parted, with marks like water stains. Flowers bell-like, *stamens protruding;* violet to whitish; May–Aug. **Where found:** Rich woods. Que. and w. New England to Va.; Tenn., n. Ark., e. Kans. to Man.

Uses: American Indians used root tea as an astringent for diarrhea, dysentery. Tea (or roots chewed) for cracked lips, mouth sores.

FLAX
Seeds

Linum usitatissimum L.
Flax Family

Delicate annual; 8–22 in. Leaves linear; 3-veined. Flowers with 5 *slightly overlapping* blue petals (½–¾ in. across); June–Sept. **Where found:** Waste places. Throughout our area. Alien.

⚠️ **Uses:** Source of linseed oil and linen. Said to be soothing and softening to irritated membranes. Seeds once used for skin and mouth cancers; colds, cough, lung and urinary ailments, fevers; laxative; poulticed (mixed with lime water) to relieve pain of burns, gout, inflammation, rheumatism, boils. Oil, a folk remedy used for pleurisy and pneumonia, has been promoted like Evening-primrose oil. A folk cancer remedy, possibly containing some antitumor compounds found in Mayapple (p. 46). **Warning:** Contains a cyanide-like compound. Oil may be emetic and purgative.

GREEK VALERIAN, JACOB'S LADDER
Root

Polemonium reptans L.　　　**C. Pl. 17**　　　Phlox Family

Perennial; 8–24 in. Leaves paired; sessile. Flowers loose clusters of violet-blue bells; *stamens not protruding;* April–June. **Where found:** Moist bottoms. N.Y. to Ga.; Miss., Okla. to Minn.

Uses: American Indians used root in prescriptions for piles, to induce vomiting, treat eczema, enhance action of Mayapple (p. 46). The Indian name for this plant, which translates as "smells like pine," refers to the root fragrance. Root tea once used to induce sweating, astringent; for pleurisy, fevers, scrofula, snakebites, bowel complaints, and bronchial afflictions.

Related species: *P. vanbruntia* (not shown) is larger and has protruding stamens.

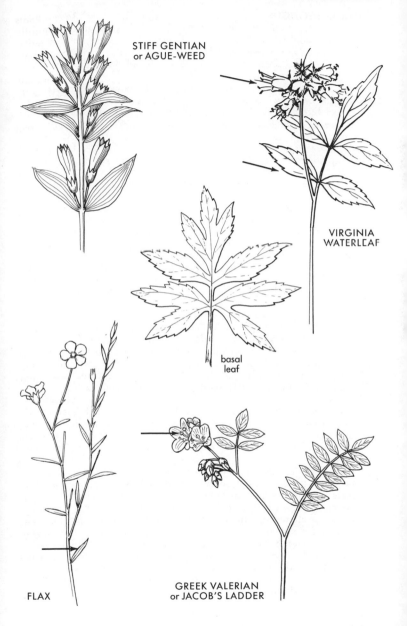

STIFF GENTIAN
or AGUE-WEED

VIRGINIA
WATERLEAF

basal
leaf

FLAX

GREEK VALERIAN
or JACOB'S LADDER

FLOWERS WITH 5 PETALS; CURLED CLUSTERS

HOUND'S TONGUE **Leaves, root**
Cynoglossum officinale L. Forget-me-not Family
Downy biennial; 1–3 ft., with a mousy odor. Leaves lance-shaped.
Flowers purplish, enclosed by a soft-hairy calyx; Aug–Sept. Flat
fruits covered with soft spines. **Where found:** Roadsides, pastures.
Much of our area. Alien.

  Uses: Leaf and root tea once used to soothe coughs, colds, irritated
membranes; astringent in diarrhea, dysentery. Leaf poultice used for
insect bites, piles. **Warning:** Contains the potentially carcinogenic
alkaloids, cynoglossine and consolidine, both CNS-depressant. May
cause dermatitis.

WILD COMFREY **Leaves, root**
Cynoglossum virginianum L. Forget-me-not Family
Rough, hairy perennial; 1–2 ft. Basal leaves in a rosette; stalked stem
leaves clasping. Violet-blue flowers on spreading racemes; May–
June. Flowers are somewhat like those of Borage. **Where found:** Open
woods. Sw. Conn., N.J., Pa. to Fla.; Texas to Mo., s. Ill.

Uses: Cherokees used root tea for "bad memory," cancer, itching of
genitals, milky urine. In 19th-century texts, authors suggest use as a
substitute for Comfrey (*Symphytum officinale*); leaves smoked like
Tobacco. **Warning:** Do not confuse the leaves of either Comfrey with
those of Foxglove (*Digitalis*, p. 172); fatal poisoning may result.

VIPER'S BUGLOSS **Whole plant, root**
Echium vulgare L. Forget-me-not Family
Bristly perennial; 1–2½ ft. Leaves lance-shaped. Flowers violet-blue,
on curled branches. *One flower blooms at a time* on each curled
branch; June–Sept. Upper lip longer than lower; stamens *red*, protruding. **Where found:** Waste places. Much of our area. Alien.

 Uses: Leaf tea a folk medicine, used to promote sweating, diuretic,
expectorant, soothing; used for fevers, headaches, nervous conditions, pain from inflammation. Root contains healing allantoin.
Warning: Contains a **toxic** alkaloid. Hairs may cause rash.

COMFREY **Leaves, root**
Symphytum officinale L. **C. Pl. 28** Borage Family
Large-rooted perennial; 1–3 ft. Leaves large, *rough-hairy;* broadly
oval to lance-shaped. Bell-like flowers in furled clusters; purple-blue,
pink, or white; May–Sept. **Where found:** Escaped. Alien. Often cultivated.

 Uses: Root tea and weaker leaf tea considered tonic, astringent, demulcent, for diarrhea, dysentery, bronchial irritation, coughs, vomiting of blood, "female maladies"; leaves and root poulticed to "knit
bones," promote healing of bruises, wounds, ulcers, sore breasts, etc.
Contains allantoin, which promotes healing. **Warning:** Root use discouraged due to high levels of liver-toxic (or cancer-causing) pyrrolizidine alkaloids. Leaf tea (at least some types), although less carcinogenic than beer, was recently banned in Canada. There is also a
danger that the leaves of Comfrey (*Symphytum*) may be confused
with the first-year leaf rosettes of Foxglove (*Digitalis*), with **fatal results.** Consult an expert on identification first.

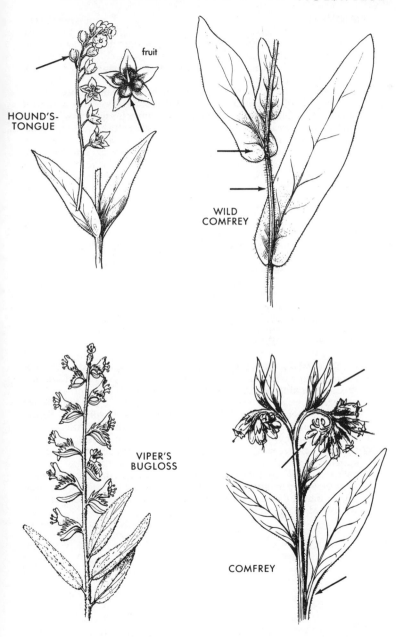

VIOLET/BLUE

HOUND'S-TONGUE

fruit

WILD COMFREY

VIPER'S BUGLOSS

COMFREY

5-PARTED FLOWERS; NIGHTSHADE FAMILY

JIMSONWEED
Leaves, root, seed

Datura stramonium L.   **C. Pl. 33**   Nightshade Family

Annual; 2–5 ft. Leaves coarse-toothed. Flowers white to pale violet, 3–5 in.; *trumpet-shaped*; May–Sept. Seedpods shiny, chambered, with *prickles*; seeds lentil-shaped. **Where found:** Waste places. Throughout our area.

Uses: Whole plant contains atropine and other alkaloids, used in eye diseases (to dilate pupils); causes dry mouth, depresses action of bladder muscles, impedes action of parasympathetic nerves; used in Parkinson's disease; also contains scopolamine, used in patches behind ear for vertigo. Leaves once smoked as antispasmodic for asthma. Folk cancer remedy. **Warning: Violently toxic.** Causes severe hallucinations. Many fatalities recorded. Those who collect this plant may end up with swollen eyelids. Licorice (*Glycyrrhiza*) has been suggested as an antidote.

HORSE-NETTLE
Leaves

Solanum carolinense L.   **C. Pl. 33**   Nightshade Family

Perennial; 1–4 ft. Stems *sharp-spined.* Leaves oval to elliptical; lobed to coarse-toothed. Flowers violet to white stars; May–Oct. Fruits orange-yellow; Aug.–Sept. **Where found:** Sandy soil. Old fields, farmlands, waste places. New England to Fla.; Texas to s. S.D.

Uses: Properly administered, berries were once used for epilepsy; diuretic, pain-killing, antispasmodic, aphrodisiac. Berries fried in grease were used as an ointment for dog's mange. American Indians gargled wilted leaf tea for sore throats; poulticed leaves for poison-ivy rash; drank tea for worms. **Warning: Toxic.** Fatalities reported in children.

WOODY NIGHTSHADE, BITTERSWEET
Leaves, stems, berries

Solanum dulcamara L.   **C. Pl. 33**   Nightshade Family

Woody climbing vine. Leaves oval, often with 1 or 2 *prominent lobes at base.* Flowers violet (or rarely white) stars with yellow protrusions (stamens); petals curved back; May–Sept. Fruits ovoid, red; Sept.–Nov. **Where found:** Waste places. Throughout our area. Alien.

Uses: Externally, plant used as a folk remedy for felons, warts, and tumors. Science confirms significant anti-cancer activity. Used as a starting material for steroids. Formerly used as narcotic, diuretic, sweat inducer; used for skin eruptions, rheumatism, gout, bronchitis, whooping cough. **Warning: Toxic.** Contains steroids, toxic alkaloids, and glucosides. Will cause vomiting, vertigo, convulsions, weakened heart, paralysis.

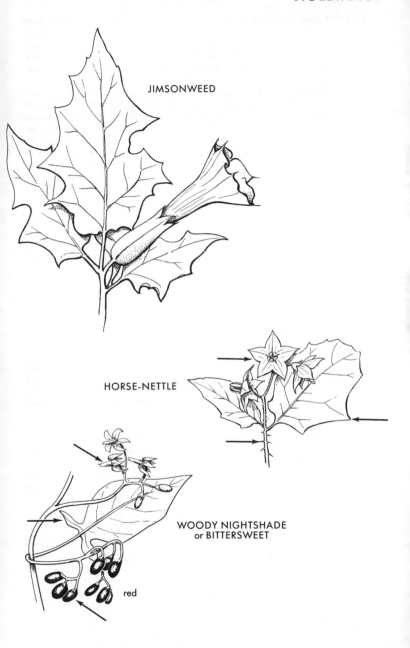

JIMSONWEED

HORSE-NETTLE

WOODY NIGHTSHADE
or BITTERSWEET

red

LIPPED FLOWERS WITH SPLIT COROLLAS; LOBELIAS

LOBELIA, INDIAN-TOBACCO
Lobelia inflata L. **C. Pl. 42**

Whole plant
Bluebell Family

Hairy annual; 6–18 in. Leaves oval, toothed; *hairy beneath.* Inconspicuous white to pale blue flowers, in racemes; to ¼ in.; June–Oct. Seed pods *inflated.* **Where found:** Fields, waste places, open woods. N.S. to Ga.; La., Ark., e. Kans. to Sask.

Uses: American Indians smoked leaves for asthma, bronchitis, sore throats, coughs. Traditionally used to induce vomiting (hence the nickname "pukeweed") and sweating; sedative; used for asthma, whooping cough, fevers, to enhance or direct action of other herbs. Lobeline, one of 14 alkaloids in the plant, is used in commercial "quit-smoking" lozenges and chewing gums — said to appease physical need for nicotine without addictive effects. **Warning:** Considered **toxic,** due to its strong emetic, expectorant, and sedative effects. This plant has rightly or wrongly been implicated in deaths from improper use as a home remedy.

GREAT LOBELIA
Lobelia siphilitica L. **C. Pl. 2**

Leaves, roots
Bluebell Family

Perennial; 1–5 ft. Leaves oval, toothed. Blue-lavender flowers; corolla throat *white-striped;* Aug.–Oct. **Where found:** Moist soil, stream banks. Me. to N.C.; Miss., Ark., e. Kans. to Minn.

Uses: American Indians used root tea for syphilis; leaf tea for colds, fevers, "stomach troubles," worms, croup, nosebleeds; gargled leaf tea for coughs; leaves poulticed for headaches, hard-to-heal sores. Formerly used to induce sweating and urination. Considered similar to, but weaker than, *L. inflata.* **Warning:** Potentially **poisonous.**

PALE-SPIKE LOBELIA
Lobelia spicata Lam.

Leaves
Bluebell Family

Perennial; 2–4 ft. Stem *smooth* above, *densely hairy* at base. Leaves lance-shaped to slightly oval; barely toothed or without teeth. Flowers pale blue or whitish; June–Aug. **Where found:** Fields, glades, meadows, thickets. Most of our area.

Uses: American Indians used a tea of the plant as an emetic. A wash made from the stalks was used for "bad blood," or neck and jaw sores. The root tea was used to treat trembling by applying the tea to scratches made in the affected limb. **Warning:** Toxicity unknown, but may have poisonous attributes.

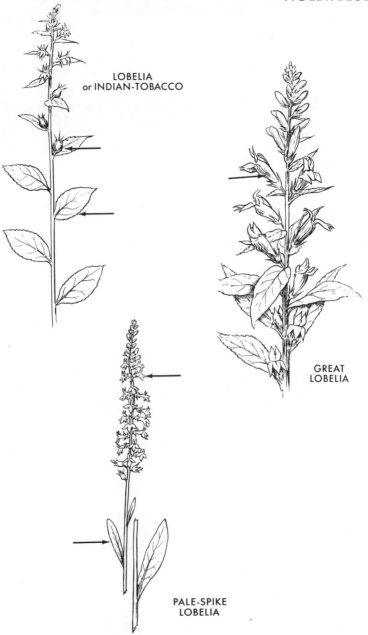

LOBELIA
or INDIAN-TOBACCO

GREAT
LOBELIA

PALE-SPIKE
LOBELIA

MISCELLANEOUS MINT RELATIVES WITH SQUARE STEMS AND PAIRED LEAVES

WILD BERGAMOT, PURPLE BEE-BALM   Leaves
Monarda fistulosa L.   **C. Pl. 42**   Mint Family
Perennial; 2–3 ft. Leaves paired; triangular to oval or lance-shaped.
Flowers lavender; *narrow, lipped tubes in crowded heads;* May–
Sept. Bracts slightly purple-tinged. **Where found:** Dry wood edges,
thickets. Que. to Ga.; La., e. Texas, Okla. to N.D., Minn.
Uses: American Indians used leaf tea for colic, flatulence, colds, fevers, stomachaches, nosebleeds, insomnia, heart trouble; in measles to induce sweating; poulticed leaves for headaches. Historically, physicians used leaf tea to expel worms and gas.

PERILLA   Leaves, seeds
Perilla frutescens (L.) Britt.   **C. Pl. 7**   Mint Family
Annual; 1–3 ft. Leaves oval, *wrinkled, long-toothed; often purplish,*
with a *peculiar fragrance.* Flowers whitish to lavender or pale violet,
in axillary and terminal clusters; July–Sept. **Where found:** Moist
open woods. Mass. to Fla.; Texas to Iowa. Asian alien.
Uses: Leaf tea used in Asian traditional medicine for abdominal
pains, diarrhea, vomiting, coughs, to "quiet a restless fetus," relieve
morning sickness, irritability during pregnancy, fevers, colds. Considered diaphoretic, sedative, and spasmolytic. A favorite culinary herb of some Oriental cultures. **Warning:** Avoid during pregnancy.
May be **toxic** to lungs. Once used as a fish poison.

MAD-DOG SKULLCAP   Leaves
Scutellaria lateriflora L.   Mint Family
Perennial; 1–3 ft. Leaves opposite; oval to lance-shaped, toothed.
Flowers violet-blue, *hooded,* lipped; May–Sept. Easily distinguished
from other Scutellaria's — flowers are in 1-sided *racemes from leaf
axils.* **Where found:** Rich woods, moist thickets. Much of our area.
Uses: Known as Mad-dog Skullcap because tea was once used as folk
remedy for rabies. A strong tea was traditionally used as a sedative,
nerve tonic, and antispasmodic for all types of nervous conditions,
including epilepsy, insomnia, anxiety, neuralgia, etc. Scutellarin, a
flavonoid compound in the plant, has confirmed sedative and antispasmodic qualities. Other *Scutellaria* species may have similar
properties. **Warning:** Large doses are of unknown toxicity.

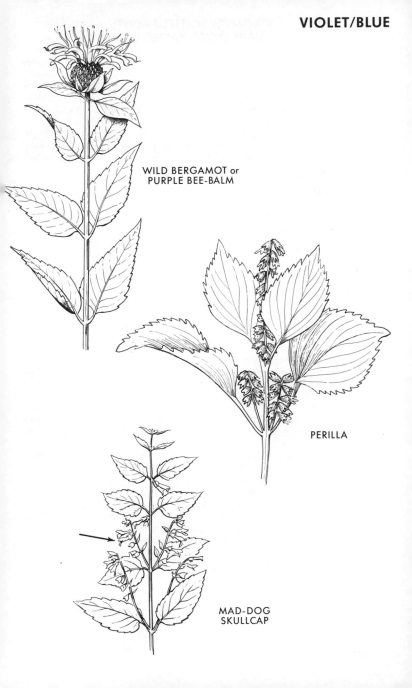

WILD BERGAMOT or
PURPLE BEE-BALM

PERILLA

MAD-DOG
SKULLCAP

STRONGLY SCENTED MINTS;
SQUARE STEMS, PAIRED LEAVES

WATERMINT
Leaves
Mentha aquatica L.   Mint Family
Perennial; to 2 ft. Leaves opposite, round to oval; *hairs curved*. Pale lavender flowers in *crowded globular terminal clusters* (or 1–3 clusters below); calyx hairy. Flowers Aug.–Oct. **Where found:** Wet ground. N.S. to Del. Alien.

Uses: Leaf tea traditionally used for fevers, stomachaches, headaches, and other minor ailments. **Warning:** Essential oil of this mint, probably like all essential oils, is antiseptic, but can be **toxic** to humans in a concentrated form.

PEPPERMINT
Leaves
Mentha piperita L.   **C. Pl. 30**   Mint Family
Perennial; 12–36 in. Stem purplish (not greenish, as in Spearmint); smooth, with few hairs. Leaves opposite, stalked; distinct *odor of peppermint*. Flowers pale violet; in *loose, interrupted terminal spikes*; June–frost. **Where found:** Wet places. Escaped from cultivation. Throughout. European alien.

Uses: Leaf tea traditionally used for colds, fevers, indigestion, gas, stomachaches, headaches, nervous tension, insomnia. Extracts experimentally effective against *herpes simplex*, Newcastle disease, and other viruses. The oil stops spasms of smooth muscles. Animal experiments show that azulene, a minor component of distilled peppermint oil residues, is anti-inflammatory and has anti-ulcer activity. Enteric-coated peppermint capsules are used in Europe for irritated bowel syndrome. **Warning:** Oil is **toxic** if taken internally; causes dermatitis. Menthol, the major chemical component of Peppermint oil, may cause allergic reactions.

SPEARMINT
Leaves
Mentha spicata L.   **C. Pl. 30**   Mint Family
Creeping perennial; 6–36 in. Leaves opposite; *without stalks* (or very short stalks); with a distinct *odor of spearmint*. Flowers pale pink-violet; in slender, elongated spikes; June–frost. **Where found:** Wet soil. Much of our area. Escaped. European alien.

Uses: Spearmint and spearmint oil are used as carminatives (to relieve gas), and primarily to disguise the flavor of other medicines. Spearmint has been traditionally valued as a stomachic, antiseptic, and antispasmodic. The leaf tea has been used for stomachaches, diarrhea, nausea, colds, headaches, cramps, fevers, and is a folk cancer remedy. **Warning:** Oil is **toxic** if taken internally; causes dermatitis.

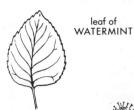

leaf of
WATERMINT

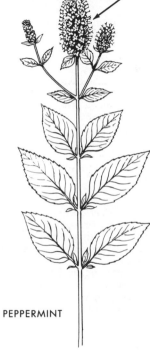

PEPPERMINT

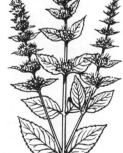

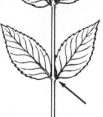

SPEARMINT

BLUE GIANT HYSSOP, ANISE-HYSSOP

Leaves, roots

Agastache foeniculum (Pursh) O. Kuntze   **C. Pl. 29**   Mint Family
Perennial; to 3 ft. Smooth-stemmed, branched above. Leaves *strongly anise-scented*, minute downy beneath. Bluish flowers in whorls; June–Sept. Stamens in *2 protruding pairs; pairs crossing.*
Where found: Prairies, dry thickets. Ont. south to Ill., Iowa; west to Colo., S.D., Wash. Cultivated; escaped eastward.
Uses: Leaf tea used for fevers, colds, coughs; induces sweating, strengthens weak heart.
Related species: The Chinese use *A. rugosa* leaf tea for angina pains. Root tea used for coughs, lung ailments.

AMERICAN PENNYROYAL

Leaves

Hedeoma pulegioides (L.) Pers.   Mint Family
Aromatic, soft-hairy annual; 6–18 in. Leaves small, lance-shaped; toothed or entire. Bluish flowers in leaf axils; July–Oct. Calyx 2-lipped, with 3 short and 2 longer teeth. **Where found:** Dry woods. Que. to Ga.; Ala. to Okla.; Neb. to Mich.

Uses: Leaf tea traditionally used for colds, fevers, coughs, indigestion, kidney and liver ailments, headaches; to promote sweating, induce menstruation, expectorant; insect repellent. **Warning:** Ingesting essential oil can be **lethal;** contact with essential oil (a popular insect repellant) can cause dermatitis.

HYSSOP

Leaves

Hyssopus officinalis L.   **C. Pl. 30**   Mint Family
Bushy, aromatic perennial; 1–2 ft. Leaves opposite; *lance-shaped to linear; stalkless, entire* (not toothed). Purple, bluish, or pink flowers in whorls of leaf axils, forming small spikes; June–Oct. **Where found:** Dry soils. Locally abundant. Alien.
Uses: Traditionally, leaf tea was gargled for sore throats. Tea thought to relieve gas, stomachaches, loosen phlegm; used with Horehound (p. 70) for bronchitis, coughs, and asthma. Experimentally, extracts are useful against *herpes simplex.*

CALAMINT

Leaves

Satureja arkansana (Nutt.) Briq.   **C. Pl. 37**   Mint Family
Creeping perennial; 4–8 in. Leaves oval at base of plant; stem leaves linear. Leaves *strongly pennyroyal-scented.* Flowers purplish, 2-lipped; April–July. **Where found:** Rocky glades. W. N.Y. to Ark., Texas; north to Ill., Ind.
Uses: Used as a substitute for American Pennyroyal (see above).

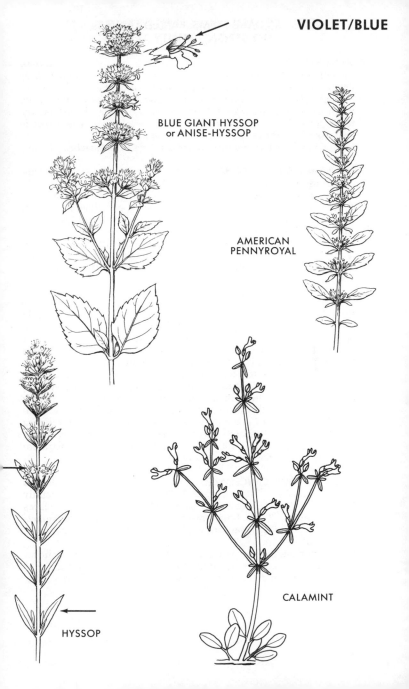

VIOLET/BLUE

BLUE GIANT HYSSOP
or ANISE-HYSSOP

AMERICAN
PENNYROYAL

HYSSOP

CALAMINT

DOWNY WOODMINT   **Leaves**
Blephilia ciliata (L.) Bentham   Mint Family
Perennial; 10–26 in. Leaves oblong-oval to lance-shaped, *downy beneath; stalkless,* on flowering stems. Flowers pale bluish purple, in terminal and axillary whorls; June–Aug. Calyx 2-lipped, with bristly teeth; lower lip of corolla narrower than lateral lobes. **Where found:** Dry woods, clearings. Vt. to Ga.; e. Texas to Minn.
Uses: Cherokees used poultice of fresh leaves for headaches.

GROUND IVY, GILL-OVER-THE-GROUND   **Leaves**
Glechoma hederacea L.   **C. Pl. 30**   Mint Family
Creeping, ivy-like perennial. Leaves scallop-edged, round to kidney-shaped; sometimes tinged with purple. Two-lipped violet flowers, in whorls of leaf axils; March–July. **Where found:** Roadsides, lawns. Throughout our area. Alien.
⚠ **Uses:** Traditionally, leaf tea used for lung ailments, asthma, jaundice, kidney ailments, "blood purifier." Externally, a folk remedy for cancer, backaches, bruises, piles. **Warning:** Reportedly **toxic** to horses.

HEAL-ALL, SELF-HEAL   **Whole plant**
Prunella vulgaris L.   **C. Pl. 23**   Mint Family
Low perennial; to 1 ft. Leaves oval to lance-shaped; mostly smooth; opposite, on a weakly squared stem. Purple flowers crowded on a terminal head; hooded, with a fringed lower lip; May–Sept. **Where found:** Waste places, lawns. Throughout our area. Eurasian alien.
Uses: Traditionally, leaf tea was used as a gargle for sore throats and mouth sores, also for fevers, diarrhea; externally, for ulcers, wounds, bruises, sores. In China a tea made from the flowering plant is considered cooling, and was used to treat heat in the liver and aid in circulation; used for conjunctivitis, boils, and scrofula; diuretic for kidney ailments. Research suggests the plant possesses antibiotic, hypotensive, and antimutagenic qualities. Contains the antitumor and diuretic compound ursolic acid.

LYRE-LEAVED SAGE, CANCERWEED   -   **Roots, leaves**
Salvia lyrata L.   **C. Pl. 38**   Mint Family
Perennial; to 1 ft. Leaves mostly basal; oblong, cleft (dandelion-like); edges rounded. Purple-blue flowers, to 1 in., in whorled spikes; April–June. **Where found:** Sandy soils, lawns. Pa. to Fla.; Texas to se. Kansas., Ill.
Uses: American Indians used root in salve for sores. Whole plant tea used for colds, coughs, nervous debility; with honey for asthma; mildly laxative and diaphoretic. Folk remedy for cancer and warts.

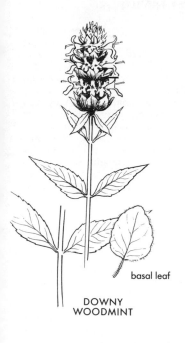

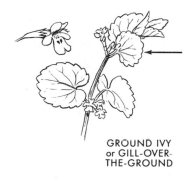

GROUND IVY
or GILL-OVER-
THE-GROUND

basal leaf

DOWNY
WOODMINT

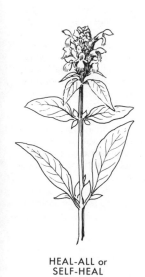

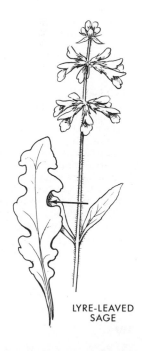

HEAL-ALL or
SELF-HEAL

LYRE-LEAVED
SAGE

LEGUMES (PEA FAMILY)

ALFALFA   **Flowering plant**
Medicago sativa L.   Pea Family
Deep-rooted perennial; 1–3 ft. Leaves cloverlike, but leaflets elongate. Violet-blue flowers in loose heads, ¼–½ in. long; April–Oct. Pods loosely spiral-twisted. **Where found:** Fields, roadsides. Throughout our area. Often cultivated, escaped. Alien.

⚠ **Uses:** Nutritious fresh or dried leaf tea traditionally used to promote appetite, weight gain; diuretic, stops bleeding. Experimentally, antifungal and estrogenic. Unsubstantiated claims include use for cancer, diabetes, alcoholism, arthritis, etc. A source of commercial chlorophyll and carotene, both with valid health claims. Contains the anti-oxidant tricin. **Warning:** Consuming large quantities of Alfalfa saponins may cause breakdown of red blood cells, causing bloating in livestock (thus weight gain). Recent reports suggest that Alfalfa sprouts (or the canavanine therein, especially in seeds) may be associated with lupus (systemic lupus erythematosus), causing recurrence in patients in which the disease had become dormant.

BLUE FALSE INDIGO   **Root**
Baptisia australis (L.) R. Brown   **C. Pl. 36**   Pea Family
Smooth perennial; 3–5 ft. Leaves thrice-divided, cloverlike; leaflets obovate (wider at tips). Deep blue to violet flowers, to 1 in. long; on erect racemes; April–June. **Where found:** Open woods, forest margins, thickets. Pa. to Ga.; Texas to Okla., Neb., s. Ind.

⚠ **Uses:** American Indians used the root tea as an emetic and purgative; cold tea given to stop vomiting. Root poulticed as an anti-inflammatory. Held in mouth to treat toothaches. Like other *Baptisia* species, *B. australis* is currently under investigation as a potential stimulant of the immune system. **Warning:** Considered potentially **toxic.**

WILD LUPINE   **Leaves**
Lupinus perennis L.   Pea Family
Perennial; 1–2 ft. Leaves long-stalked; divided into 7–11 oblong-lance-shaped segments. Flowers blue, *pea-like*; in a showy raceme; April–July. **Where found:** Dry soils, open woods. Sw. Me., N.Y. to Fla.; W. Va., Ohio, Ind., Ill.

☠ **Uses:** American Indians drank cold leaf tea to treat nausea and internal hemorrhage. A fodder used to fatten horses and make them "spirited and full of fire." **Warning:** Seeds are **poisonous.** Some lupines are toxic, others are not. Even botanists may have difficulty distinguishing between toxic and nontoxic species.

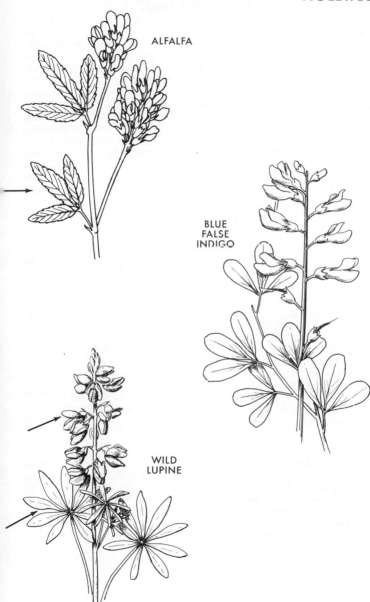

ALFALFA

BLUE
FALSE
INDIGO

WILD
LUPINE

FLAT-TOPPED CLUSTERS OR SPIKES;
COMPOSITE FAMILY

WILD LETTUCE   **Leaves**
Lactuca biennis (Moench) Fernald   Composite Family
Smooth biennial; 2–15 ft. Leaves irregularly divided; coarsely toothed. Flowers bluish to creamy white (rarely yellow); July–Sept. **Where found:** Damp thickets. Nfld. to Va. mountains; Tenn. to Iowa and westward.
Uses: American Indians used root tea for diarrhea, heart and lung ailments; for bleeding, nausea, pains. Milky stem juice used for skin eruptions. Leaves applied to stings; tea sedative, nerve tonic, diuretic. **Warning:** May cause dermatitis or internal poisoning.
Remarks: Variable genus; highly technical taxonomy.

ROUGH BLAZING-STAR   **Root**
Liatris aspera Michx.   **C. Pl. 41**   Composite Family
Perennial; 6–30 in. Leaves alternate, linear. Rose-purple flowers with 25–30 florets, in crowded, *sessile or short-stalked* heads on a *crowded spike*; Aug.–Sept. Note wide, rounded bracts. **Where found:** Dry soils, prairies. Ohio to N.C.; La., Texas to N.D.
Uses: Root tea of most *Liatris* species was used as a folk remedy for kidney and bladder ailments, gonorrhea, colic, painful or delayed menses; gargled for sore throats; root used externally in poultice for snakebites. Thought to be diuretic, tonic.

DEER'S TONGUE   **Leaves**
Trilisa odoratissima (Walter ex J.F. Gmel.) Cass.   Composite Family
Smooth perennial; 2–5 ft. Leaves elliptic, to 1 ft.; toothed or entire; *vanilla-scented when dry.* Flowers lavender or pink; July–Oct. **Where found:** Pine barrens. N.C. to Fla., Ala., Miss.
Uses: Folk remedy for coughs, malaria, neuroses; induces sweating; diuretic, tonic, demulcent. One million pounds used each year to flavor tobacco products. High in coumarins, experimentally effective for high-protein edema. **Warning:** Coumarins are implicated in liver disease and hemorrhage.

IRONWEED   **Root**
Vernonia glauca (L.) Willd.   Composite Family
Blue-green perennial; 2–5 ft. Leaves on stem only (not at base); *oval to lance-shaped; narrowly sharp-pointed* at tip and base. Flowers July–Oct. Seed crowns *yellowish* (brown-purple in other *Vernonias*). **Where found:** Rich woods. N.J. to Ga.; Ala. to Pa.
Uses: American Indians used the root as a "blood tonic," to regulate menses, relieve pain after childbirth; also for bleeding, stomachaches.
Related species: Other Vernonias have been used similarly.

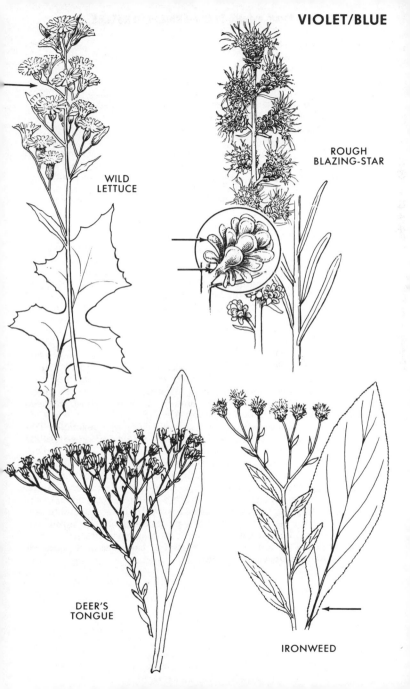

VIOLET/BLUE

WILD LETTUCE

ROUGH BLAZING-STAR

DEER'S TONGUE

IRONWEED

DAISY-LIKE FLOWERS OR THISTLES

NEW ENGLAND ASTER   **Root**
Aster novae-angliae L.   Composite Family
Hairy-stemmed perennial; 3–7 ft. The *most showy wild aster in our area*. Leaves *lance-shaped*, without teeth; clasping stem. Flowers *deeper violet* than most asters, with up to 100 rays; Aug.–Oct. Bracts sticky. **Where found:** Moist meadows, thickets. S. Canada, Me. to uplands of N.C., Ark.; Kans., Colo. to N.D.
Uses: American Indians used root tea for diarrhea, fevers.

CHICORY   **Roots, leaves**
Cichorium intybus L.   **C. Pl. 22**   Composite Family
Biennial or perennial; 2–4 ft. Basal leaves dandelion-like; upper ones reduced. Flowers blue (rarely white or pink), *stalkless*; rays square-tipped; June–Oct. **Where found:** Roadsides. Throughout our area. Alien.
Uses: One ounce root in 1 pint of water used as a diuretic, laxative; folk use in jaundice, skin eruptions, fevers. Extract diuretic, cardiotonic; lowers blood sugar, slightly sedative, and mildly laxative. Homeopathically used for liver and gall bladder ailments. Leaf extracts weaker than root extracts. Experimentally, root extracts are antibacterial. In experiments, animals given chicory root extracts exhibit a slower and weaker heart rate (pulse). It has been suggested that the plant should be researched for use in heart irregularities. Root extracts in alcohol solutions have proven anti-inflammatory effects in experiments.

MILK THISTLE   **Seeds, whole plant**
Silybum marianum (L.) Gaertn.   **C. Pl. 26**   Composite Family
Annual or biennial thistle; to 6 ft. Leaves *mottled* or *streaked with white veins; sharp-spined,* clasping. Flowers purple tufts; receptacle densely bristle-spined. Flowers June–Sept. **Where found:** Escaped from cultivation, common in Calif. Alien (Europe).
Uses: Young leaves (with spines removed) eaten as a vegetable. Traditionally, tea made from whole plant used to improve appetite, allay indigestion, restore liver function. Used for cirrhosis, jaundice, hepatitis, liver poisoning from chemicals or drug and alcohol abuse. Silymarin, a seed extract, dramatically improves liver regeneration in hepatitis, cirrhosis, mushroom poisoning, and other liver diseases. German research suggests that silybin, a flavonoid component of the seed, is clinically useful in treating severe *Amanita* mushroom poisoning. While used clinically in Europe, its use in the U.S. is not well known. Research suggests seed extracts may have therapeutic possibilities in liver cirrhosis. Commercial preparations of the seed extracts are manufactured in Europe.

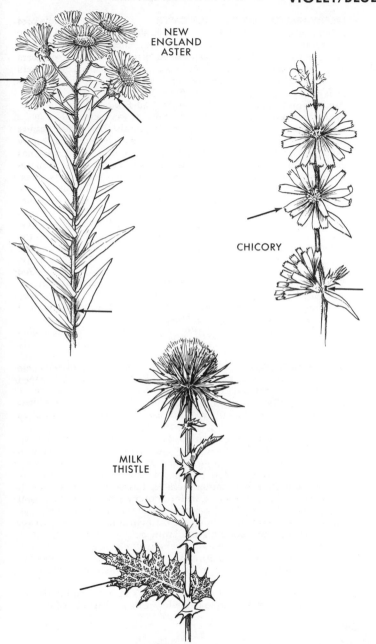

VIOLET/BLUE

NEW
ENGLAND
ASTER

CHICORY

MILK
THISTLE

PURPLE CONEFLOWERS

NARROW-LEAVED PURPLE CONEFLOWER   Root, whole plant
Echinacea angustifolia DC.   **C. Pl. 40**   Composite Family
Tap-rooted perennial; 6–20 in. Leaves lance-shaped; stiff-hairy.
Flowers with prominent cone-shaped disk surrounded by pale to
deep purple spreading rays; June–Sept. *rays about as long as width
of disk* (to 1¼ in.). **Where found:** Prairies. Texas, w. Okla., w. Kans.,
Neb.; west to e. Colo., e. Mont., N.D., Man., Sask.
Uses: Plains Indians are said to have used *Echinacea* for more medicinal purposes than any other plant group. Root (chewed, or in tea)
used for snakebites, spider bites, cancers, toothaches, burns, hard-to-
heal sores and wounds, flu, and colds. Science confirms many traditional uses, plus cortisone-like activity; also insecticidal, bactericidal, and immunostimulant activities. Considered a nonspecific immune system stimulant. More than 200 pharmaceutical preparations
are made from *Echinacea* plants in W. Germany, including extracts,
salves, and tinctures; used for wounds, herpes sores, canker sores,
throat infections; preventative for influenza, colds. A folk remedy for
brown recluse spider bites. This application should be investigated.
Remarks: Hybrids occur where the range of this species overlaps that
of Pale Purple Coneflower (*E. pallida*, below).

PALE PURPLE CONEFLOWER   Root
Echinacea pallida Nutt.   **C. Pl. 40**   Composite Family
Similar to *E. angustifolia* (above), but larger — to 40 in. Rays strongly
drooping, to 4 in. long. Flowers May–Aug. **Where found:** Prairies,
glades. Ark. to Wisc., Minn.; e. Okla., Kans., Neb.
Uses: Same as for *E. angustifolia*, though some consider this plant
less active.

PURPLE CONEFLOWER   Root, whole flowering plant
Echinacea purpurea (L.) Moench.   **C. Pl. 40**   Composite Family
Perennial; 2–3 ft. Leaves oval, *coarsely toothed.* Bristle tips of flower
disks *orange.* Rays purple to white. Flowers June–Sept. **Where found:**
Open woods, thickets; cultivated in gardens. Mich., Ohio to La., e.
Texas, Okla.
Uses: Same as for *E. angustifolia*. Widely used in Europe, but not
native there. Most commercial W. German *Echinacea* preparations
utilize extracts of above-ground parts and roots of *E. purpurea*. Extracts are used to stimulate nonspecific defense mechanisms at infections and chronic inflammations. It has been asserted that the
components thought responsible for immune-system stimulating activity were not absorbed by oral ingestion, and could be effective
only in an injectable form. A recent German study, however, showed
significant immune-system stimulating activity with orally administered extracts of *E. purpurea*, *E. angustifolia*, and *E. pallida*, both
in mice and laboratory experiments. Perhaps additional components
are involved in immuno-stimulating activity than those previously
known.
Remarks: Wild Quinine root is often used as an adulterant to the root
(sold in dried form) of Purple Coneflower (*E. purpurea*). See p. 78.

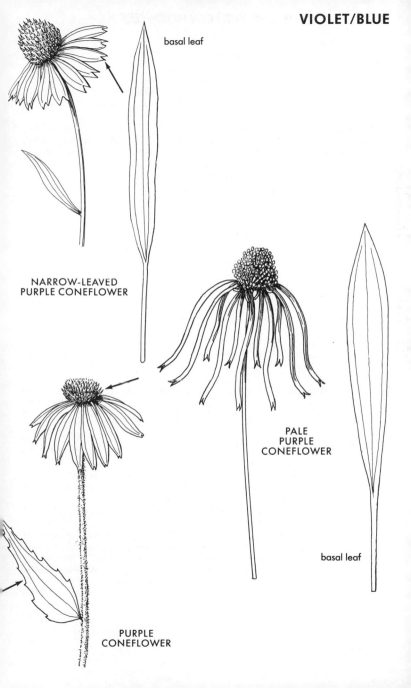

VIOLET/BLUE

basal leaf

NARROW-LEAVED
PURPLE CONEFLOWER

PALE
PURPLE
CONEFLOWER

basal leaf

PURPLE
CONEFLOWER

PLANTS WITH GREEN HOODLIKE FLOWERS

DRAGON or GREEN ARUM   Root
Arisaema dracontium (L.) Schott   **C. Pl. 16**   Arum Family
Perennial; 1–3 ft. Leaf solitary; divided into 5–15 lance-shaped leaflets along a horseshoe-shaped frond. Spathe sheathlike, *narrow; spadix much longer.* Flowers May–July. **Where found:** Rich, moist
woods. Sw. Que., Vt., s. N.H. to Fla.; Texas, e. Kans., Neb., Wisc.,
Mich.

Uses: American Indians used dried, aged root for "female disorders."
Root considered edible once it has been dried, aged, and elaborately
processed. **Warning:** Whole fresh plant contains intensely burning,
irritating calcium oxalate crystals.
Related species: The Chinese use related *Arisaema* species for epilepsy, hemiplegia (paralysis); externally, as a local anesthetic or in
ointment for swellings and small tumors.

JACK-IN-THE-PULPIT   Root
Arisaema triphyllum (L.) Schott   **C. Pl. 16**   Arum Family
Perennial; 1–2 ft. 1–2 leaves, 3 leaflets each; green beneath. Spathe
cuplike, with a curving flap; green to purplish brown, often striped.
Flowers April–early July. Berries clustered, scarlet. **Where found:**
Moist woods. Most of our area.

Uses: American Indians used the dried, aged root for colds and dry
coughs, and to build blood. Externally, the root was poulticed for
rheumatism, scrofulous sores, boils, abscesses, and ringworm. Dried
root tea traditionally considered expectorant, diaphoretic, and purgative. Historically used for asthma, bronchitis, colds, cough, laryngitis, and headaches. Externally for rheumatism, boils, and swelling
from snakebites. **Warning:** Intensely irritating. Calcium oxalate crystals found in whole fresh herb.
Related species: *A. atrorubens* (not shown) is generally larger; leaves
grayish green beneath. Both species are treated as one by most modern authorities. The Chinese used related species to treat snakebites.

SKUNK CABBAGE   Root
Symplocarpus foetidus (L.) Nutt.   **C. Pl. 11**   Arum Family
Strongly skunk-scented perennial; 1–2 ft. Leaves broad, oval. Flowers appear before leaves, Feb.–May; greenish to purple, hooded,
sheathing spathe, with a *clublike* organ within. **Where found:** Wet,
rich woods. N.S. to Ga.; Tenn., Ill. to Iowa.

Uses: American Indians used root for cramps, convulsions, whooping coughs, toothaches; root poulticed for wounds, underarm deo-
dorant; leaf poulticed to reduce swelling, ate dried root to stop epileptic seizures. Subsequently used by physicians as antispasmodic
for epilepsy, spasmodic coughs, asthma; externally in lotion for itching, rheumatism; diuretic; emetic in large doses. **Warning:** Eating
leaves causes burning, inflammation. Roots considered **toxic.**

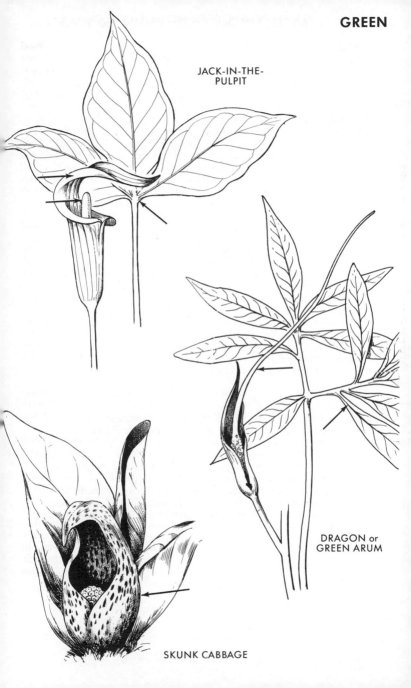

GREEN

JACK-IN-THE-PULPIT

DRAGON or
GREEN ARUM

SKUNK CABBAGE

MISCELLANEOUS GREEN-FLOWERED VINES

WILD YAM   **Roots**
Dioscorea villosa L.   **C. Pl. 15**   Yam Family
Perennial twining vine; *stem smooth*. Leaves *alternate* (lower ones
in whorls of 3–8), heart-shaped, hairy beneath; veins conspicuous.
Flowers not showy; male and female flowers separate; May–Aug.
Where found: Wet woods. Conn. to Tenn.; Texas to Minn.

 Uses: American Indians used root tea to relieve labor pains. Fresh
dried root (tea) formerly used by physicians for colic, gastrointestinal
irritations, morning sickness, asthma, spasmodic hiccough, rheumatism, and "chronic gastritis of drunkards." Contains diosgenin,
used to manufacture progesterone and other steroid drugs. Of all
plant genera, there is perhaps none with greater impact on modern
life but whose dramatic story is as little known as *Dioscorea*. Most
of the steroid hormones used in modern medicine, especially those
in contraceptives, were developed from elaborately processed chemical components derived from yams. Drugs made with yam-derived
components (diosgenins) relieve asthma, arthritis, eczema, regulate
metabolism and control fertility. Synthetic products manufactured
from diosgenins include human sex hormones (contraceptive pills),
drugs to treat menopause, dysmenorrhea, premenstrual syndrome,
testicular deficiency, impotence, prostate hypertrophy, and psycho-
sexual problems, as well as high blood pressure, arterial spasms, migraines, and other ailments. Widely prescribed cortisones and hydro-
cortisones were indirect products of the genus *Dioscorea*. They are
used for Addison's disease, some allergies, bursitis, contact dermatitis, psoriasis, rheumatoid arthritis, sciatica, brown recluse spider
bites, insect stings, and other diseases and ailments. **Warning:** Fresh
plant may induce vomiting and other undesirable side effects.

HOPS   **Fruits (strobiles)**
Humulus lupulus L.   **C. Pl. 32**   Hemp Family
Rough-prickly, twining perennial. Leaves mostly with 3–5 lobes,
sinuses (notches) rounded; yellow resinous granules beneath. Male
and female flowers on separate plants; July–Aug. Fruits (strobiles)
inflated. **Where found:** Waste places. Throughout our area. Alien.

 Uses: Tea of fruits traditionally used as sedative, antispasmodic, diuretic; for insomnia, cramps, coughs, fevers; externally, for bruises,
boils, inflammation, rheumatism. Experimentally antimicrobial, relieves spasms of smooth muscles, acts as sedative (disputed). **Warning:** Handling plant often causes dermatitis. Dislodged hairs may irritate eyes.

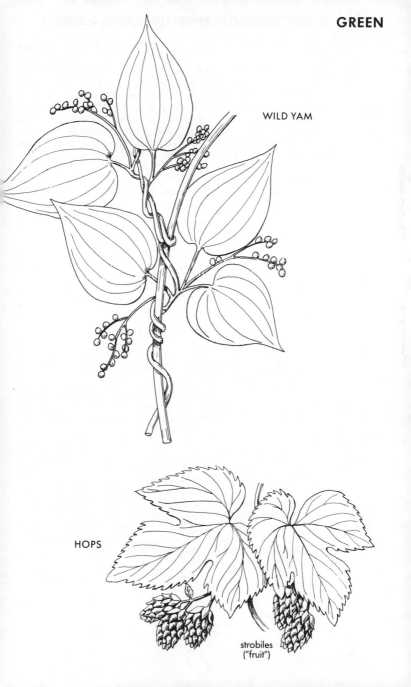

GREEN

WILD YAM

HOPS

strobiles
("fruit")

MISCELLANEOUS PLANTS WITH GREEN FLOWERS

MARIJUANA   **Leaves, seeds, flowering tops**
Cannabis sativa L.   **C. Pl. 28**   Hemp Family
Annual weed; 5–14 ft. Leaves *palmate, with 5–7 lobes*. Leaflets lance-shaped, toothed. Flowers greenish, sticky; Aug.–Sept. **Where found:** Escaped or cultivated (illegally) throughout our area. Alien.
Uses: Leaves smoked; illegal intoxicant. Legitimate use of chemical components to treat glaucoma; also relieves nausea following chemotherapy. Antibiotic for gram-positive bacteria. Many folk uses. Much maligned, but potentially a very useful medicinal plant. A legitimate fiber (hemp) and oilseed plant in many other countries.

BLUE COHOSH   **Root**
Caulophyllum thalictroides (L.) Michx.   **C. Pl. 17**   Barberry Family
Perennial; 1–2 ft. Smooth-stemmed; stem and leaves covered with *bluish film*. Leaves divided into 3 (occasionally 5) *leaflets with 2–3 lobes*. Flowers greenish yellow, in terminal clusters; April–June, before leaves expand. **Where found:** Moist rich woods. N.B. to S.C.; Ark., N.D. to Man.
Uses: Root tea used extensively by American Indians to aid labor, treat profuse menstruation, abdominal cramps, urinary tract infections, lung ailments, fevers; emetic. A folk remedy for rheumatism, cramps, epilepsy, and inflammation of the uterus. Historically prescribed by physicians for chronic uterine diseases. Said to cause abortion by stimulating uterine contractions. Roots possess estrogenic activity and check muscle spasms. Studies by scientists in India suggest the root may possess some contraceptive potential. Extracts shown to be anti-inflammatory (in rats). An alkaloid in the root, methylcytisine, has effects similar to those of nicotine, increasing blood pressure, stimulating the small intestine, and causing hyperglycemia. It also contains glycosides, which are believed to be responsible for its uterine-stimulant activity. **Warning:** Root powder strongly irritating to mucous membranes. Avoid during pregnancy.

WILD IPECAC   **Leaves, root**
Euphorbia ipecacuanhae L.   Spurge Family
Large-rooted perennial with underground stems; 3–12 in. tall. Stem smooth, succulent. Leaves inserted at joints; rounded to linear, green to purple. Solitary flowers on long stalks; "cups" have 5 glands, with narrow, white, yellow, green, or purple appendages. Flowers April–May. **Where found:** Sandy soil. Mostly coastal. N.J. to Fla.

Uses: American Indians used leaf tea for diabetes; root tea as a strong laxative and emetic, for pinworms, rheumatism; poulticed root on snakebites. **Warning:** Extremely strong laxative. Juice from fresh plant may cause blistering.

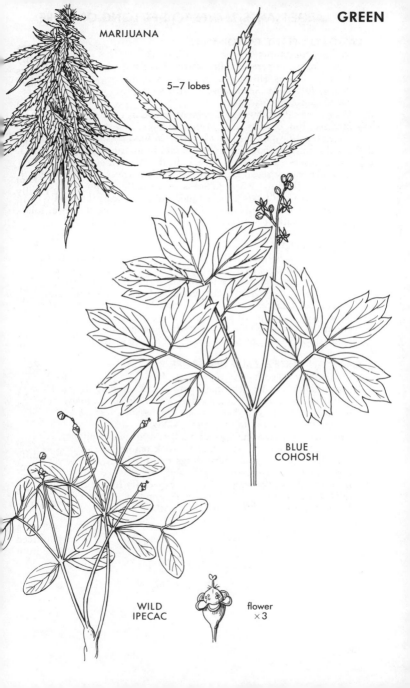

GREEN

MARIJUANA

5–7 lobes

BLUE
COHOSH

WILD
IPECAC

flower
×3

LARGE PLANTS; LEAVES TO 1 FT. LONG OR MORE

CASTOR-OIL-PLANT, CASTOR BEAN   Seed oil
Ricinus communis L.   **C. Pl. 33**   Spurge Family
Large annual or perennial (in South); 5–12 ft. Leaves large, palmate, with 5–11 lobes. Flowers in clusters — female ones above, male ones below; July–Sept. Seed capsule with soft spines. **Where found:** Escaped exotic cultivar; alien.

Uses: Seed oil famous since ancient Egyptian time as a purgative or laxative; folk remedy used to induce labor. Nauseous taste may induce vomiting. Oil used as a laxative in food poisoning or before X-ray diagnosis of bowels. Used externally for ringworm, itch, piles, sores, abscesses; hairwash for dandruff. Oil even suggested as a renewable energy resource. Poulticed boiled leaves a folk remedy to produce milk flow. **Warning: Seeds are a deadly poison** — 1 seed may be fatal to a child. After oil is squeezed from seeds, the deadly toxic protein, ricin, remains in seed cake. Oil is used in industrial lubricants, varnishes, plastics, etc. May induce dermatitis.

COLUMBO ROOT   Root
Swertia caroliniensis (Walt.) Ktze.   Gentian Family
Smooth biennial; 3–8 ft. Leaves *in 4's;* large, lance-shaped or oblong. Flowers greenish yellow, with *brown-purple dots;* 4-parted, with a *large, glandular greenish dot on each division.* Flowers June–July. **Where found:** Limey slopes, rich woods. N.Y. to Ga.; La. to Wisc.
Uses: Root tea formerly used for colic, cramps, dysentery, diarrhea, stomachaches, lack of appetite, nausea; general tonic.
Related species: Asian species have been used similarly.

AMERICAN WHITE or FALSE HELLEBORE   Root
Veratrum viride Ait.   **C. Pl. 5**   Lily Family
Perennial; 2–8 ft. Leaves large, broadly oval, *strongly ribbed.* Flowers yellowish, turning dull green; small, *star-shaped,* in a many-flowered panicle; April–July. **Where found:** Wet wood edges, swamps. New England to Ga. mountains; Tenn. to Wisc.

Uses: Historically valued as an analgesic for pain, epilepsy, convulsions, pneumonia, heart sedative; weak tea for sore throats, tonsillitis. Used in pharmaceutical drugs to slow heart rate, lower blood pressure; for arteriosclerosis, forms of nephritis. Powdered root used in insecticides. **Warning: All parts, especially root, are highly or fatally toxic.** Leaves have been mistaken for Pokeweed (p. 56) or Marsh-marigold (p. 88), then eaten, with fatal results.

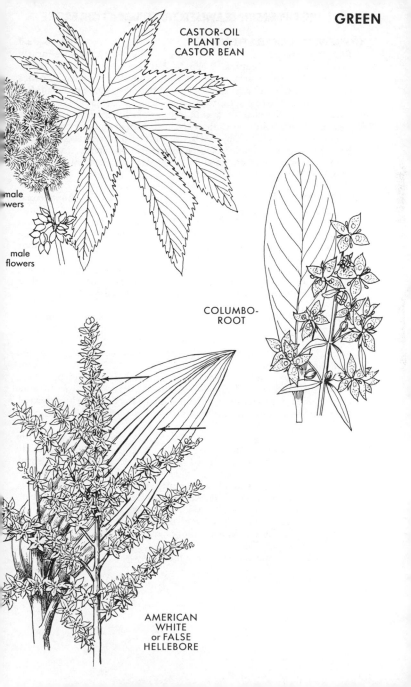

GREEN

CASTOR-OIL
PLANT or
CASTOR BEAN

male
flowers

male
flowers

COLUMBO-
ROOT

AMERICAN
WHITE
or FALSE
HELLEBORE

HORSEWEED, CANADA FLEABANE
Erigeron canadensis L.

Whole plant
Composite Family

Bristly annual or biennial weed; 1–7 ft. Leaves numerous, lance-shaped. Tiny (to ¼ in.), greenish white flowers on many branches from leaf axils; disk yellow, with short rays. Flowers July–Nov. **Where found:** Waste places, roadsides. Throughout our area.

 Uses: Plant tea used as a folk diuretic, astringent for diarrhea, "gravel" (kidney stones), diabetes, painful urination, hemorrhages of stomach, bowels, bladder, and kidneys; also for nosebleeds, fevers, bronchitis, tumors, piles, coughs. Africans used it for eczema and ringworm. Essential oil used for bronchial ailments and cystitis. **Warning:** May cause contact dermatitis.

ALUMROOT
Heuchera americana L.

Root, leaves
Saxifrage Family

Variable perennial; 1–2 ft. Leaves toothed, roundish to somewhat maple-shaped; base heart-shaped. Flowers small, greenish white; on short stalks; April–June. **Where found:** Woods, shaded rocks. S. Ont., Conn. to Ga.; Okla. to Mich.

Uses: Similar to those of alum; styptic, astringent. Leaf tea used for diarrhea, dysentery, piles; gargled for sore throats. Root poulticed on wounds, sores, abrasions. Other Heucheras are used similarly.

DITCH STONECROP
Penthorum sedoides L.

Seeds, whole plant
Saxifrage Family

Perennial; 1–3 ft. Leaves lance-shaped, finely toothed. Yellowish green flowers on 2–3 spreading, terminal stalks; July–Sept. **Where found:** Muddy soil. Most of our area.

Uses: American Indians used seeds in cough syrups. Historically, plant tincture was used as a demulcent, laxative, and tonic, for mucous membrane irritations, vaginitis, diarrhea, dysentery, pharyngitis, tonsillitis, piles, chronic bronchitis, and nervous indigestion.

FIGWORT
Scrophularia marilandica L.

Leaves, root
Figwort Family

Perennial; 3–6 ft. Stems angled, grooved. Leaves oval, rounded or heart-shaped at base; toothed. Flowers like a *miniature scoop*; stamens 4, with an additional wide, sterile, *purple* stamen (yellow in *S. lanceolata*, not shown). Flowers June–Oct. **Where found:** Rich woods. Sw. Me. to n. Ga.; La., Okla. to Minn.

Uses: American Indians used root tea for irregular menses, fevers, piles; diuretic, tonic. Poultice a folk cancer remedy. Folk remedy to allay restlessness, anxiety, sleeplessness in pregnant women. Other species used similarly. **Warning:** Of unknown toxicity.

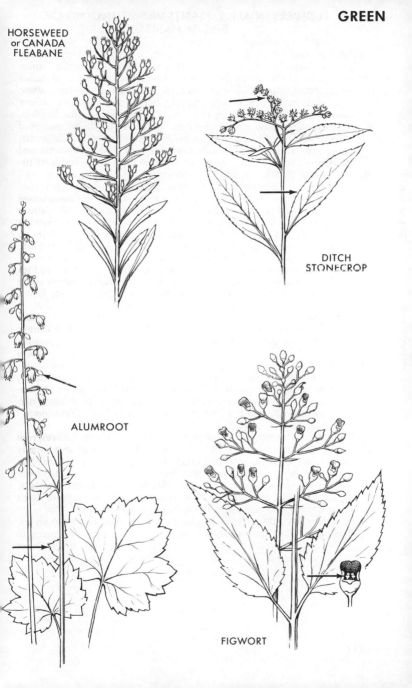

GREEN

HORSEWEED
or CANADA
FLEABANE

DITCH
STONECROP

ALUMROOT

FIGWORT

FLOWERS IN AXILS; PLANTS WITH STINGING OR BRISTLY HAIRS

STINGING NETTLE   **Whole plant**
Urtica dioica L.   **C. Pl. 6**   Nettle Family
Perennial; 12–50 in. *Stiff stinging hairs.* Leaves mostly oval; bases
barely *heart-shaped.* Flowers greenish, in branched clusters; June–
Sept. Male and female flowers on separate plants or branches. **Where
found:** Waste places. Scattered over much of our area. Alien.

Uses: Traditionally, leaf tea used in Europe as a "blood purifier,"
"blood builder," diuretic, astringent; for anemia, gout, glandular diseases, rheumatism, poor circulation, enlarged spleen, mucous discharges of lungs, internal bleeding, diarrhea, dysentery. Its effect in-
volves the action of white blood cells, aiding coagulation and
formation of hemoglobin in red blood corpuscles. Iron-rich leaves
have been cooked as a potherb. Studies suggest CNS-depressant, antibacterial, and mitogenic activity; inhibits effects of adrenaline.
This plant should be studied further for possible uses against kidney
and urinary system ailments. Recently, Germans have been using
the root in treatments for prostate cancer. Russians are using the
leaves in alcohol for cholecystitis (inflammation of the gall bladder)
and hepatitis. Some people keep potted Stinging Nettle in the
kitchen window, alongside an Aloe plant, in the belief that an occasional sting alleviates arthritis. **Warning:** Fresh plants **sting.** Dried
plant (used in tea) does not sting. One fatality has been attributed,
rightly or wrongly, to the sting of a larger tropical nettle.
Related species: Other *Urtica* species occurring in N. America are
said to be used interchangeably.

COCKLEBUR   **Leaves, root**
Xanthium strumarium L.   Composite Family
Variable weedy annual; to 5 ft. Leaves oval to heart-shaped, some-
what lobed or toothed, on long stalks. Flowers inconspicuous, green.
Fruits oval, with *crowded hooked prickles;* Sept.–Nov. **Where found:**
Waste places. Scattered.

Uses: Root historically used for scrofulous tumors (strumae —
hence the species name). This plant and the related species *X. spi-
nosum* (not shown) were formerly used for rabies, fevers, malaria;
considered diuretic, fever-reducing, sedative. American Indians used
leaf tea for kidney disease, rheumatism, tuberculosis, and diarrhea;
also as a blood tonic. Chinese used it similarly. **Warning:** Most cocklebur species are **toxic** to grazing animals, and are usually avoided by
them. Seeds contain toxins, but seed oil has served as lamp fuel.
Remarks: Taxonomy confusing.

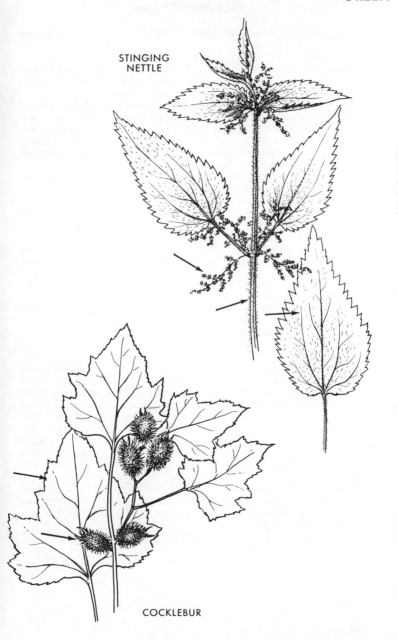

STINGING
NETTLE

COCKLEBUR

SLENDER, MOSTLY TERMINAL FLOWER CLUSTERS; BUCKWHEAT FAMILY

COMMON SMARTWEED, MILD WATER PEPPER
Leaves

Polygonum hydropiper L.   Buckwheat Family

Reddish-stemmed annual; to 2 ft. Leaves lance-shaped, lacking sheath bristle; very *acrid* and *peppery to taste*; margin wavy. Greenish flowers in arching clusters (most Polygonums have pink flowers); June–Nov. **Where found:** Moist soils, shores. Much of our area.

Uses: American Indians used leaf tea as a diuretic for painful or bloody urination, fevers, chills; poulticed leaves for pain, piles; rubbed them on a child's thumb to prevent sucking. Leaf tea a folk remedy for internal bleeding, menstrual or uterine disorders. Leaves contain rutin, which helps strengthen fragile capillaries and thus helps prevent bleeding. **Warning:** Plant can irritate skin.

Related species: Many other Polygonums have been used in American, European, and Asian folk or traditional medicine.

SHEEP-SORREL
Leaves, root

Rumex acetosella L.   Buckwheat Family

Slender, smooth, *sour-tasting* perennial; 4–12 in. Leaves *arrow-shaped*. Tiny flowers in green heads, interrupted on stalk; turning reddish or yellowish; April–Sept. **Where found:** Acid soils. Throughout our area.

Uses: Leaf tea of this common European alien traditionally used for fevers, inflammation, scurvy. Fresh leaves considered cooling, diuretic; leaves poulticed (after roasting) for tumors, wens (sebaceous cysts); folk cancer remedy. Root tea used for diarrhea, excessive menstrual bleeding. **Warning: May cause poisoning** in large doses, due to high oxalic acid and tannin content.

YELLOW or CURLY DOCK
Roots, leaves

Rumex crispus L.   **C. Pl. 25**   Buckwheat Family

Perennial; 1–5 ft. Leaves large, lance-shaped; *margins distinctly wavy*. Flowers green, on spikes; May–Sept. Winged, heart-shaped seeds; June–Sept. Roots yellowish in cross-section. **Where found:** Waste ground. Throughout our area.

Uses: Herbalists consider dried root tea an excellent "blood purifier," for "bad blood," chronic skin diseases, chronic enlarged lymph glands, tendency for skin sores, rheumatism, liver ailments, sore throats. May cause or relieve diarrhea, depending on dose, harvest time, and concentrations of anthraquinones (laxative) and/or tannins (antidiarrheal). Anthraquinones can arrest growth of ringworm and other fungi. **Warning:** Large doses may cause gastric disturbance, nausea, diarrhea, etc.

GREEN

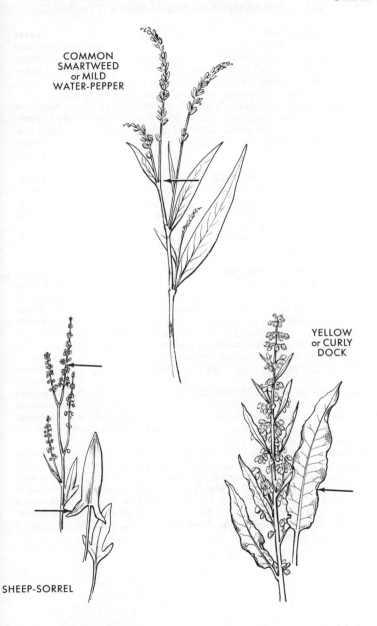

COMMON SMARTWEED or MILD WATER-PEPPER

YELLOW or CURLY DOCK

SHEEP-SORREL

FLOWERS IN TERMINAL CLUSTERS AND IN UPPER AXILS: AMARANTH AND GOOSEFOOT FAMILIES

SMOOTH PIGWEED   Leaves
Amaranthus hybridus L.   Amaranth Family
Smooth-stemmed annual; 1–6 ft. Leaves to 6 in. long, hairy. Flower spikes green (or red-tinged); *lateral spikes erect or ascending;* Aug.–Oct. **Where found:** Throughout our area. Alien weed.
Uses: Leaf tea astringent, stops bleeding; used in dysentery, diarrhea, ulcers, intestinal bleeding. Reduces swelling. Many members of the pigweed (amaranth) family and goosefoot family serve as potherbs and/or cereal grains. The National Academy of Sciences is vigorously investigating both grain amaranths and the goosefoot relatives as food crops.

GREEN AMARANTH, PIGWEED   Leaves
Amaranthus retroflexus L.   Amaranth Family
Grayish, downy annual; 6–24 in. Leaves oval, stout-stalked. Flower spikes to 2½ in. long; blunt, chaffy, interspersed with bristly bracts; Aug.–Oct. **Where found:** Throughout our area. Alien weed.
Uses: Astringent. Used for diarrhea, excessive menstrual flow, hemorrhages, hoarseness.

LAMB-QUARTERS, PIGWEED   Leaves
Chenopodium album L.   Goosefoot Family
Annual weed; 1–3 ft. Stem *often mealy, red-streaked.* Leaves somewhat diamond-shaped, coarsely toothed; mealy white beneath. Flowers greenish, inconspicuous; in clusters; June–Oct. **Where found:** Gardens, fields, waste places. Throughout our area. Alien.
Uses: American Indians ate leaves to treat stomachaches and prevent scurvy. Cold tea used for diarrhea. Leaf poultice used for burns. Folk remedy for vitiligo, a skin disorder.

MEXICAN TEA, AMERICAN WORMSEED   Seeds, essential oil
Chenopodium ambrosioides L.   Goosefoot Family
Stout *aromatic* herb; 3–5 ft. Leaves *wavy-toothed.* Flowers greenish, in spikes, *among leaves;* Aug.–Nov. Seeds *glandular-dotted.* **Where found:** Waste places. Throughout our area.
Uses: Until recently, the essential oil distilled from flowering and fruiting plant was used against roundworms, hookworms, dwarf (not large) tapeworms, intestinal amoeba. Now largely replaced by synthetics. **Warning:** Oil is **highly toxic.** Still, a dash of the leaves is added as a culinary herb to Mexican bean dishes in the belief that it may reduce gas. May cause dermatitis or an allergic reaction. S. Foster has experienced vertigo from contact with essential oil released during harvest.

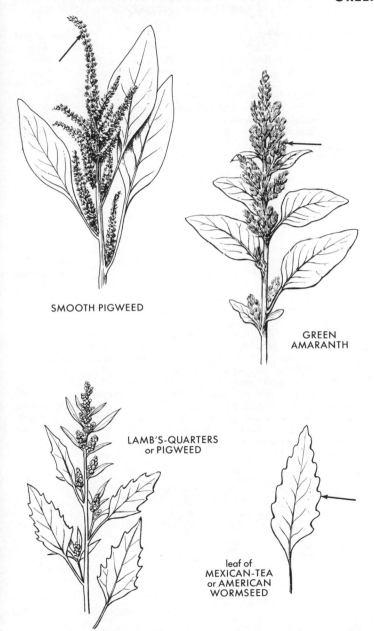

SMOOTH PIGWEED

GREEN
AMARANTH

LAMB'S-QUARTERS
or PIGWEED

leaf of
MEXICAN-TEA
or AMERICAN
WORMSEED

NODDING, INCONSPICUOUS FLOWERS WITH YELLOW POLLEN; RAGWEEDS

COMMON RAGWEED   Leaves, root
Ambrosia artemisiifolia L.   Composite Family
Annual; 1–5 ft. Leaves dissected, artemisia-like; highly variable —
as a rule alternate, but opposite as well. Drooping, *inconspicuous
green flowerheads on conspicuous erect spikes;* July–Oct. **Where
found:** Waste ground. Noxious weed. Throughout our area.
Uses: American Indians rubbed leaves on insect bites, infected toes,
minor skin eruptions, and hives. Tea used for fevers, nausea, mucous
discharges, intestinal cramping; very astringent, emetic. Root tea
used for menstrual problems and stroke. **Warning:** Pollen causes allergies. Ingesting or touching plant may cause allergic reactions. Pollen from the genus *Ambrosia* is responsible for approximately 90 percent of pollen-induced allergies in the U.S. Goldenrods (*Solidago*
species) are often pointed to as the source of late summer allergies,
but at the same time the showy goldenrods are blooming, the inconspicuous flowers of ragweeds are really guilty.

GIANT RAGWEED   Leaves, root
Ambrosia trifida L.   Composite Family
Annual; to 6–15 ft. Stems and leaves with stiff hairs, rough to touch.
Leaves opposite, deeply 3-lobed (sometimes 5-lobed or without
lobes); tips pointed. Lower leaves are most uniform in appearance.
Flowers similar to those of Common Ragweed. **Where found:** Alluvial waste places, sometimes forming vast, pure, pollen-producing
stands. Much of our area.
Uses: Astringent, stops bleeding. Leaf tea formerly used for pro-
lapsed uterus, leukorrhea, fevers, diarrhea, dysentery, nosebleeds;
gargled for mouth sores. American Indians used the crushed leaves
on insect bites. The root was chewed to allay fear at night. The pollen
of both this and Common Ragweed are harvested commercially,
then manufactured into pharmaceutical preparations for the treatment of ragweed allergies. **Warning:** Pollen causes allergies. Ingesting
or touching plant may cause allergic reactions. The composite family, to which the ragweeds and the allergy-inducing artemisias (see
following pages) belong, is *the worst* family as far as pollenosis is
concerned.

COMMON
RAGWEED

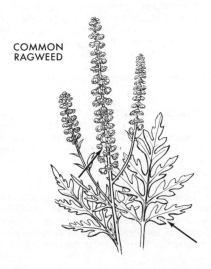

leaf of
GIANT RAGWEED

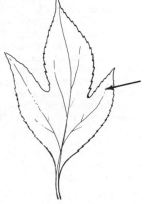

FLOWERS IN TERMINAL CLUSTERS; LEAVES SILVER-HAIRY, AT LEAST BENEATH; ARTEMISIAS

WORMWOOD
Artemisia absinthium L.

Leaves
Composite Family

Aromatic perennial; 1–4 ft. Leaves silver-green, strongly divided; *segments blunt,* with *silky silver hairs on both sides.* Flowers tiny, drooping; July–Sept. **Where found:** Waste ground. Escaped from cultivation in n. U.S. Alien.

Uses: Extremely bitter leaves nibbled to stimulate appetite. Tea a folk remedy for delayed menses, fevers, worm expellent, liver and gall bladder ailments. Formerly used for flavoring absinthe liqueurs. Contains the toxic principle thujone. Intoxication from absinthe liqueurs has been likened to that induced by marijuana. It is theorized that the active component of both plants may react with the same receptors of the central nervous system. **Warning:** Relatively small doses may cause nervous disorders, convulsions, insomnia, nightmares, and other symptoms. Flowers of artemisias may induce allergic reactions. Approved as a food additive (flavoring) with thujone removed.

WESTERN MUGWORT, WHITE SAGE, CUDWEED
Artemisia ludoviciana Nutt.

Leaves
Composite Family

Highly variable aromatic perennial; to 3 ft. Leaves *white-felty beneath;* lance-shaped, entire. Flowers in dense panicles; July–Sept. **Where found:** Weedy. Waste ground. Mich. to s. Ill., Texas; north to Mont. and westward. Naturalized east to New England.

Uses: Much used by American Indians as an astringent, to induce sweating, curb pain and diarrhea. Weak tea used for stomachaches, menstrual disorders. Leaf snuff used for sinus ailments, headaches, nosebleeds. Externally, wash used for itching, rashes, skin eruptions, swelling, boils, sores. Compress for fevers. Used in sweatbaths for rheumatism, fevers, colds, and flu. **Warning:** May cause allergies.

MUGWORT
Artemisia vulgaris L.

Leaves
Composite Family

Aromatic; 2–4 ft. Leaves *deeply cut, silvery-woolly beneath.* Flowerheads erect; July–Aug. **Where found:** Waste ground. S. Canada to Ga.; Kans., Mich.; occasional westward. Alien weed.

Uses: Leaf tea diuretic, induces sweating; checks menstrual irregularity, promotes appetite, "tonic" to nerves. Used for bronchitis, colds, colic, epilepsy, fevers, kidney ailments, sciatica. Experimentally, lowers blood sugar. Dried leaves used as "burning stick" (moxa), famous in Chinese medicine, to stimulate acupuncture points, treat rheumatism. **Warning:** May cause dermatitis.

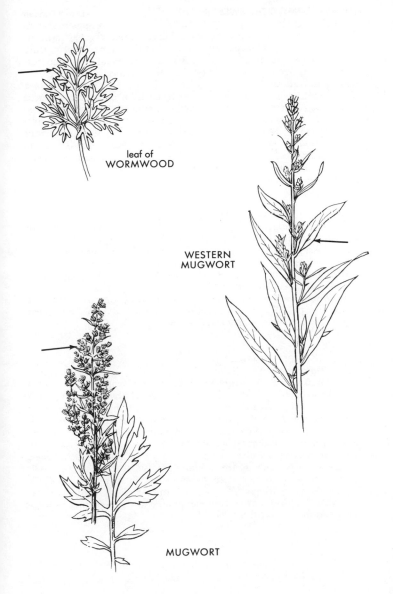

leaf of
WORMWOOD

WESTERN
MUGWORT

MUGWORT

FLOWERS IN TERMINAL CLUSTERS;
LEAVES NOT SILVER-HAIRY; ARTEMISIAS

ANNUAL WORMWOOD, SWEET ANNIE   Leaves, seeds
Artemisia annua L.   **C. Pl. 27**   Composite Family
Sweet-scented, bushy annual; 1–9 ft. Leaves thrice-divided, *fernlike;*
segments oblong to lance-shaped, sharp-toothed or cleft. Tiny, green-
yellow flowers, in clusters; July–Oct. **Where found:** Waste ground.
Throughout our area; becoming much more common, escaping from
cultivation. Alien.
Uses: Leaf tea (gather before flowering) used for colds, flu, malarial
fevers, dysentery, diarrhea. Externally, poulticed on abscesses and
boils. For quinine and/or chlorquinine-resistant malaria (of interest
to U.S. Army); clinical use of derivative compounds in China (tested
with 8,000 patients) shows near 100 percent efficacy. Seeds used for
night sweats, indigestion, flatulence. The compound responsible for
the antimalarial activity also demonstrates marked herbicidal activity. **Warning:** May cause allergic reactions or dermatitis.

TALL WORMWOOD, WESTERN SAGEBRUSH   Leaves
Artemisia caudata Michx.   Composite Family
[*A. campestris* L. var. *caudata* (Michx.) Hall & Clem.]
Smooth-stemmed biennial; 2–6 ft. Leaves divided into *linear seg-
ments, not toothed.* Flower stalks *very leafy.* Flowers tiny, greenish
yellow, in *drooping clusters;* July–Oct. **Where found:** Sands. Me. to
Fla.; Texas, N.D., and westward.
Uses: American Indians used leaf tea for colds, coughs, tuberculosis.
Externally, poultice of steamed herb used for bruises and sores. **Warn-
ing:** Allergic reactions may result from use.

WILD or RUSSIAN TARRAGON   Leaves, roots
Artemisia dracunculus Pursh   Composite Family
[*A. redowskii* Led., *A. glauca* var. *draculina* (S. Wat.) Fern.]
Variable — aromatic to odorless. To 5 ft. Leaves lance-shaped to linear (sometimes divided), without teeth. Whitish green flowers in
loose, spreading clusters; July–Oct. **Where found:** Prairies, dry soil.
Wisc., Mo., Texas, and westward. Rare eastward to New England.
Uses: American Indians used leaf or root tea for colds, dysentery,
diarrhea, headaches, difficult childbirth. Promotes appetite. Leaves
poulticed for wounds, bruises. Sometimes substituted for the cooking herb French Tarragon, which, not producing viable seed, must be
propagated vegetatively. The French Tarragon smells strongly of anise; Wild Tarragon may be odorless and flavorless. **Warning:** Allergic
reactions may result from use.

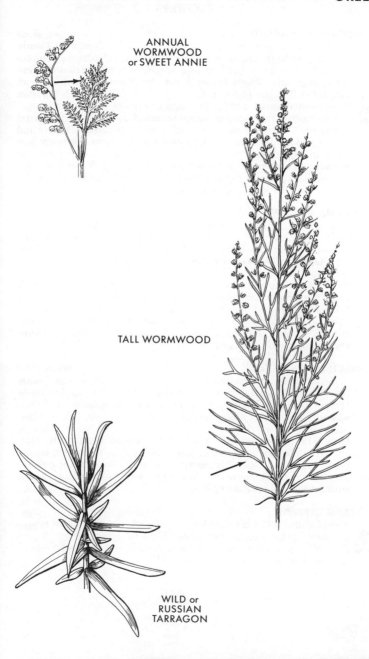

ANNUAL
WORMWOOD
or SWEET ANNIE

TALL WORMWOOD

WILD or
RUSSIAN
TARRAGON

MISCELLANEOUS PLANTS WITH GREEN-BROWN FLOWERS

VIRGINIA SNAKEROOT   **Root**
Aristolochia serpentaria L.   Birthwort Family
Delicate; 8–20 in. Leaves elongate, *strongly arrow-shaped.* Flowers
calabash-pipelike, purplish brown; at *base of plant,* often under leaf
litter; May–July. **Where found:** Woods. Sw. Conn. to Fla.; Texas to
Mo., Ohio. Too rare to harvest.

 Uses: Aromatic root nibbled (in minute doses) or in weak tea (1 teaspoon dried root in 1 cup of water) promotes sweating, appetite; expectorant. Used for fevers, stomachaches, indigestion, suppressed
menses, and snakebites. Tea gargled for sore throats. **Warning:** Irritating in large doses.
Remarks: Recent high prices following increasing demand and de-
creasing supplies may suggest this as a prospect for cultivation in the
forest — further justification for saving our forests.

DUTCHMAN'S-PIPE   **Leaves**
Aristolochia tomentosa Sims   Birthwort Family
Climbing woody vine. Leaves *heart-shaped,* blunt-tipped; lower surface with *dense soft white hairs.* Flowers *pipe-shaped;* calyx yellowish; May–June. **Where found:** Rich river banks. N.C., Fla., and Texas;
north to e. Kans., Mo., s. Ill., to s. Ind.
Uses: Like *A. serpentaria* (above), but much weaker in effect. Little
used. **Warning:** Potentially irritating in large doses.
Related species: *A. macrophylla* (not shown) has nearly smooth,
sharp-pointed leaves. Flowers brown-purple. Ironically, Virginia
farmers spray *A. macrophylla* as a weed. It contains the antiseptic,
antitumor compound aristolochic acid.

BEECH-DROPS   **Whole plant**
Epifagus virginiana (L.) Barton   Broomrape Family
A chlorophyll-lacking parasite found under Beech trees. Brownish,
cream-colored, yellowish, or reddish. Leaves scale-like. Flowers
whitish; Aug.–Oct. **Where found:** Ont. to Fla.; Miss., La., Ark. and
northward.
Uses: The highly astringent tea of the whole fresh plant (loses
strength upon drying) was once used for diarrhea, dysentery, mouth
sores, "obstinate ulcers" (external), cold sores. Folk cancer remedy;
also known as "cancer root." Recent scientific investigations for antitumor activity proved negative.

SKUNK CABBAGE   **Root**
Symplocarpus foetidus (L.) Nutt.   **C. Pl. 11**   Arum Family
Strongly skunk-scented perennial. Flowers appear before leaves,
Feb.–May; greenish to purple, hooded, *sheathing spathe,* with a *club-
like* organ within. Root **toxic.** See p. 202.

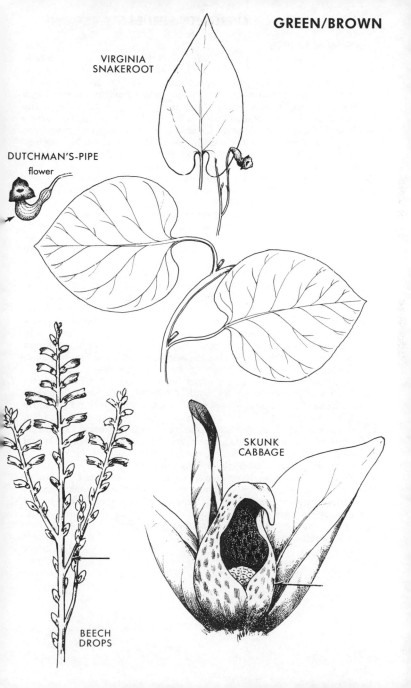

GREEN/BROWN

VIRGINIA
SNAKEROOT

DUTCHMAN'S-PIPE
flower

BEECH
DROPS

SKUNK
CABBAGE

EVERGREEN SHRUBS

COMMON JUNIPER   **Fruits**
Juniperus communis L.   **C. Pl. 43**   Pine Family
Shrub or small tree; 2–20 ft. Bark reddish brown, shredding off in
papery peels. Leaves (needles) taper to a spiny tip, in *whorls of 3's*
with *2 white bands above* (or 1 white band sometimes divided by a
green midrib, broader than green margin). Fruits on short stalk;
round to broadly oval, bluish black, usually with 3 seeds. **Where
found:** Rocky, infertile soils. Canada to Alaska, south to mountains
of Ga., e. Tenn.; north to Ill., Minn.; west to N.M., Calif. N. America,
Europe and Asia. N. American forms are small and shrublike,
whereas European forms are more tree-like.

 Uses: Fruits used to flavor gin and other alcoholic beverages; also
used commercially in some diuretic and laxative products. Fruits
eaten raw or in tea are a folk remedy used as a diuretic and urinary
antiseptic for cystitis, carminative for flatulence, antiseptic for intestinal infections; once used for colic, coughs, stomachaches, colds,
and bronchitis. Externally, used for sores, aches, rheumatism, arthritis, snakebites, and cancer. Volatile oil is responsible for diuretic
and intestinal antiseptic activity. Diuretic activity results from irritation of renal tissue. **Warning:** Considered **toxic.** Large or frequent
doses cause kidney failure, convulsions, and digestive irritation.
Avoid during pregnancy. Oil may cause blistering.

AMERICAN YEW   **Leaves (needles)**
Taxus canadensis Marsh.   Yew Family
Straggling evergreen shrub (rarely to 7 ft.). *Twigs smooth*, green; reddish brown on older branches. Needles 2-ranked, ⅜–1 in. long, nar-
rowing into abrupt fine points; *green on both sides*, but with light
green bands below; needles often develop a reddish tint in winter.
Female plants produce juicy, *cuplike red arils* (pulp) surrounding ½-
in. fruits. Seeds stony. **Where found:** Rich woods. Nfld. to w. Va.; ne.
Ky. to Iowa, Man.

Uses: American Indians used minute amounts of **toxic** leaf tea internally and externally, for rheumatism, bowel ailments, fevers,
colds, scurvy; to expel afterbirth, dispel clots; diuretic; twigs used as
fumigant in steam baths for rheumatism. Leaves (needles) said to be
antirheumatic and hypotensive. Yew sap was used by Celts to
produce poison arrows. A component of the plant is under investigation for anticancer activity. **Warning:** All plant parts (except perhaps the red aril) of this and other yews contain the toxic alkaloid
taxine and are considered **poisonous.** Ingesting as few as 50 leaves
(needles) has resulted in fatalities.

COMMON
JUNIPER

AMERICAN
YEW

note
cuplike
red arils
around
fruits

EVERGREEN SHRUBS WITH SWORDLIKE LEAVES; PALMS AND YUCCAS

SAW PALMETTO   **Fruits**
Serenoa repens (Bartr.) Small   Palm Family
Shrub; to 6 ft., with horizontal creeping stems above ground. Leaf
stalks armed with *sawlike teeth*. Leaves fanlike, with sword-shaped
leaf blades *radiating from a central point*. Flowers whitish green,
with 3–5 petals; May–July. Fruits black, fleshy, 1 in. long, surrounding 1 large seed; in large, branched clusters; Oct.–Nov. **Where found:**
Low pine woods, savannas, thickets. S.C., Ga., Fla., to Ala., Miss.
Uses: Fruit extracts, tablets, and tincture traditionally used to treat
prostate enlargement and inflammation. Also used for colds, coughs,
irritated mucous membranes, tickling feeling in throat, asthma,
chronic bronchitis, head colds, and migraine. A suppository of the
powdered fruits in cocoa butter was used as a uterine and vaginal
tonic. Considered expectorant, sedative, diuretic. Historical pharmacological studies suggest the plant may be useful in treatment of
prostate disorders.

YUCCA, ADAM'S NEEDLES   **Roots**
Yucca filamentosa L.   Lily Family
Perennial; to 9 ft. in flower. Leaves in a rosette; stiff, spine-tipped,
oblong to lance-shaped, with *fraying twisted threads on margins*.
Flowers whitish green bells, on *smooth*, branched stalks; June–Sept.
Where found: Sandy soils. S. N.J. to Ga.
Uses: American Indians used root in salves or poultices for sores,
skin diseases, and sprains. Pounded roots were put in water to
stupefy corralled fish so they would float to the surface for easy har-
vest. Could be used as yet another starting material for steroids.
Warning: Root compounds **toxic** to lower life forms.

YUCCA, SOAPWEED   **Roots**
Yucca glauca Nutt.   **C. Pl. 39**   Lily Family
Blue-green perennial; 2–4 ft. Leaves in a rosette; stiff, swordlike,
rounded on back, *margins rolled in*. Flowers whitish bells; May–
July. **Where found:** Dry soils. Iowa, N.D. to Mo., Texas.
Uses: American Indians poulticed root on inflammations, used it to
stop bleeding; in steam baths for sprains and broken limbs; as a hairwash for dandruff and baldness. In experiments with mice, water extracts have shown antitumor activity against B16 melanoma. One
human clinical study suggests that saponin extracts of root were effective in the treatment of arthritis (findings disputed). **Warning:** See
under *Y. filamentosa* (above).

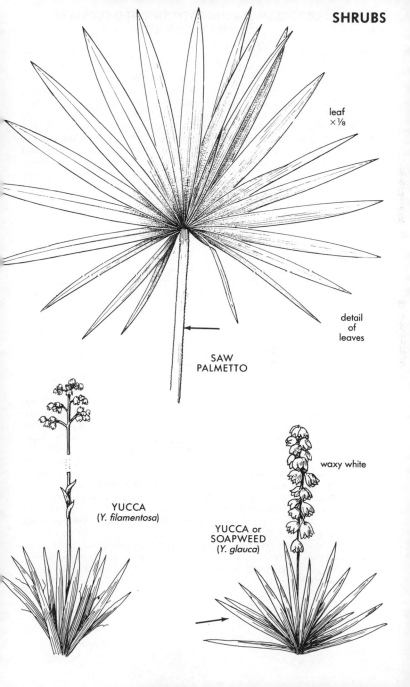

leaf
× ⅛

detail
of
leaves

SAW
PALMETTO

YUCCA
(*Y. filamentosa*)

waxy white

YUCCA or
SOAPWEED
(*Y. glauca*)

EVERGREEN SHRUBS WITH 5-PARTED FLOWERS; HEATH FAMILY

SHEEP LAUREL, LAMBKILL   **Twigs, leaves, flowers**
Kalmia angustifolia L.   **C. Pl. 43**   Heath Family
Slender shrub; 3–5 ft. Leaves opposite, leathery, elliptical to lance-shaped. Flowers deep rose-pink (or white), to ½ in. across; in *clusters on sides of twigs*; May–July. **Where found:** Dry soils. Nfld. to Va., Ga. mountains; north to Mich.

Uses: American Indians used minute amounts of flower, leaf, and twig tea for bowel ailments. Tiny amounts of leaf tea used for colds, backaches, stomach ailments; externally, for swelling, pain, and sprains. **Warning: Highly toxic. Do not ingest.**

MOUNTAIN LAUREL   **Leaves**
Kalmia latifolia L.   Heath Family
Shrub or small tree; 5–30 ft. Leaves evergreen, leathery; ovate, without teeth. Flowers pink (rose or white), about 1 in. wide; in *terminal clusters*; May–July. **Where found:** Rocky woods, clearings. New England, N.Y. to Fla.; La. to Ohio, Ind.
Uses: American Indians used leaf tea as an external wash for pain, rheumatism, in liniments for vermin. Historically, herbalists used minute doses to treat syphilis, fever, jaundice, heart conditions, neuralgia, and inflammation. **Warning:** Plant is **highly toxic;** even honey from flowers is reportedly toxic. **Avoid use.**

LABRADOR TEA   **Leaves**
Ledum groenlandicum L.   **C. Pl. 4**   Heath Family
Shrub; to 3 ft. Leaves fragrant; oblong or linear-oblong; *white* to *rusty-woolly* beneath; *edges turned under.* Small white flowers in terminal clusters; May–July. **Where found:** Peat soils, bogs. Lab. to N.J., Pa., Ohio, Mich., Wisc., Minn.; across Canada to Alaska.
Uses: American Indians used leaf tea for asthma, colds, stomachaches, kidney ailments, scurvy, fevers, rheumatism; "blood purifier"; externally, as a wash for burns, ulcers, stings, chafing, poison-ivy rash. Folk remedy for coughs, lung ailments, dysentery, indigestion; used externally for leprosy, itching and to kill lice.

GREAT RHODODENDRON   **Leaves**
Rhododendron maximum L.   **C. Pl. 44**   Heath Family
Thicket-forming evergreen shrub or small tree; 10–14 ft. Leaves large, *leathery*, without teeth; edges *rolled under.* Rose-pink (white), spotted flowers in very showy clusters; June–July. **Where found:** Damp woods. S. Me. to Ga.; Ala. to Ohio.
Uses: American Indians poulticed leaves to relieve arthritis pain, headaches; taken internally in controlled dosage for heart ailments. **Warning:** Leaves **toxic.** Ingestion may cause convulsions and coma. **Avoid use.**

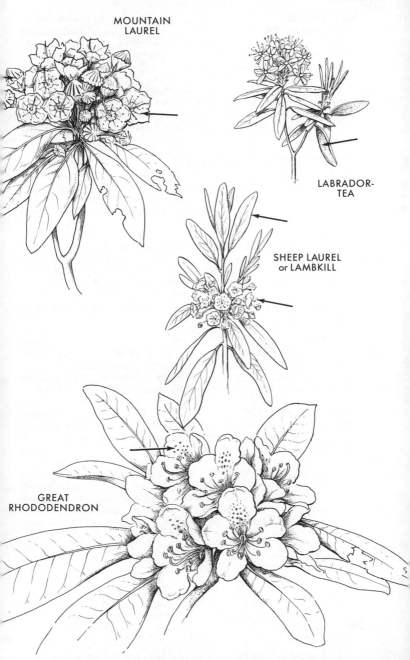

SHRUBS

MOUNTAIN
LAUREL

LABRADOR-
TEA

SHEEP LAUREL
or LAMBKILL

GREAT
RHODODENDRON

SEMI-EVERGREEN SHRUBS; LEAVES LEATHERY

YAUPON HOLLY   **Leaves, berries**
Ilex vomitoria Ait.   Holly Family
Evergreen shrub or small tree; 6–15 ft. Leaves to 2 in. long; elliptical,
leathery, *round-toothed*. Berries in clusters, red (rarely yellow);
Sept.–Nov. Calyx segments rounded, with few hairs on margins.
Where found: Sandy woods. Se. Va. to Fla.; Texas, Ark.

 Uses: American Indians used a very strong leaf tea as a ceremonial
cleansing beverage, drinking large amounts to induce vomiting or act
as purgative. This may be the only caffeine-containing plant native
to N. America. **Warning:** Many hollies are considered potentially
toxic.

CREEPING THYME, MOTHER-OF-THYME   **Leaves**
Thymus pulegioides L.   **C. Pl. 30**   Mint Family
Prostrate perennial subshrub; to 6 in. Leaves small (to ⅜ in. long),
oval, entire (not toothed); short-stalked. Flowers small, purple or
(rarely) white; clustered at ends of branches; July–Aug. **Where found:**
Scattered to rare. N.S. to N.C.; Ohio to Ind. European alien; escaped
from cultivation.

Uses: In European folk tradition, thyme leaf tea has been used for
nervous disorders, angina pectoris, flu, coughs, stomachaches;
"blood purifier"; also to relieve cramps. Experimentally, oil of thyme
is antispasmodic, expectorant, antimicrobial; lowers arterial pressure, increases heart rhythms, respiratory volume; lowers blood
pressure, alleviates toothaches. **Warning:** Oil is **toxic** and highly irritating to skin.

BEARBERRY, UVA-URSI   **Leaves**
Arctostaphylos uva-ursi (L.) Spreng   **C. Pl. 10**   Heath Family
Trailing shrub; to 1 ft. Bark finely hairy. Leaves *shiny, leathery,*
spatula-shaped. Flowers white, urn-shaped; May–July. Fruit a dry red
berry. **Where found:** Sandy soil, rocks. Arctic to n. U.S. See p. 26.

WINTERGREEN, TEABERRY   **Leaves**
Gaultheria procumbens L.   **C. Pl. 19**   Heath Family
Wintergreen-scented; to 6 in. Leaves oval, glossy. Flowers waxy,
drooping bells; July–Aug. Fruit a dry berry. See p. 26.

PARTRIDGEBERRY, SQUAW VINE   **Leaves**
Mitchella repens L.   **C. Pl. 11**   Madder Family
Leaves opposite, rounded. Flowers white (or pink), 4-parted; terminal, *paired;* May–July. Each flower produces a single dry red berry,
lasting over the winter. See p. 26.

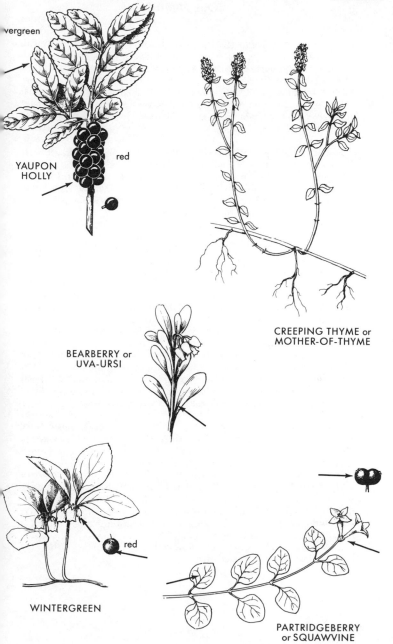

vergreen

YAUPON HOLLY

red

CREEPING THYME or MOTHER-OF-THYME

BEARBERRY or UVA-URSI

WINTERGREEN

red

PARTRIDGEBERRY or SQUAWVINE

SHRUBS WITH WHITE, 5-PETALED FLOWERS; ROSE FAMILY

NINEBARK   **Bark**
Physocarpus opulifolius (L.) Maxim.   **C. Pl. 9**   Rose Family
Shrub; to 9 ft. *Bark peels in thin strips* or layers. Leaves oval to obovate; irregularly toothed, with star-shaped hairs. Flowers white; May–July. Seedpods inflated, 2-valved; usually 3 pods per cluster. **Where found:** Stream banks. Que. to S.C.; Ala., Ark. to Minn.
Uses: American Indians used inner-bark tea for "female maladies," gonorrhea, tuberculosis; to enhance fertility; emetic, laxative. **Warning:** Potentially **toxic.**

LARGE-HIP, RUGOSA or WRINKLED ROSE   **Fruit, flowers**
Rosa rugosa Thunb.   **C. Pl. 10**   Rose Family
Coarse, *bristly stemmed* shrub; 2–6 ft. Leaves *strongly wrinkled;* 5–9 leaflets. Large, rose (or white) flowers to 3¼ in. across; June–Sept. Fruits (hips) red, to 1 in., crowned with sepals. **Where found:** Seaside, sand dunes. Northern U.S., Canada. Asian alien.
Uses: The Chinese use flower tea to "regulate vital energy (qi)," promote blood circulation; also for stomachaches, liver pains, mastitis, dysentery, leukorrhea, rheumatic pains; also thought to "soothe a restless fetus." Fruits (rose hips) make a pleasant tea.

RED RASPBERRY   **Leaves, root, fruits**
Rubus idaeus L.   Rose Family
Upright shrub; *canes do not root at tips.* Smooth, bristly stem, with or without hooked prickles. 3–7 oval leaflets. Flowers white; June–Oct. *Drupelets not separated by bands of hairs.* **Where found:** Cultivated throughout our area. European alien.
Uses: Astringent leaf tea a folk remedy for diarrhea, dysentery; used to strengthen pregnant women, aid in childbirth. Root also used. Animal studies suggest efficacy in childbirth, painful menstrual cramps. Active compound relaxes *and* stimulates the uterus. Fruit syrup (juice boiled in sugar) gargled for inflamed tonsils.

BLACK RASPBERRY   **Root, leaves, fruits**
Rubus occidentalis L.   **C. Pl. 31**   Rose Family
Shrub with *arching canes* that *root at tips. Stem glaucous,* with *curved prickles.* Leaves whitened beneath; sharply double-toothed. Flowers white; April–July. Fruits *purple-black;* July–Sept. *Rows of white hairs between drupelets.* **Where found:** Throughout our area. Alien.
Uses: Astringent root tea traditionally used for diarrhea, dysentery, stomach pain, gonorrhea, back pain, "female tonic," blood tonic for boils. Leaf tea a wash for sores, ulcers, boils.
Related species: The same parts of most blackberry plants (other *Rubus* species) have been used similarly.

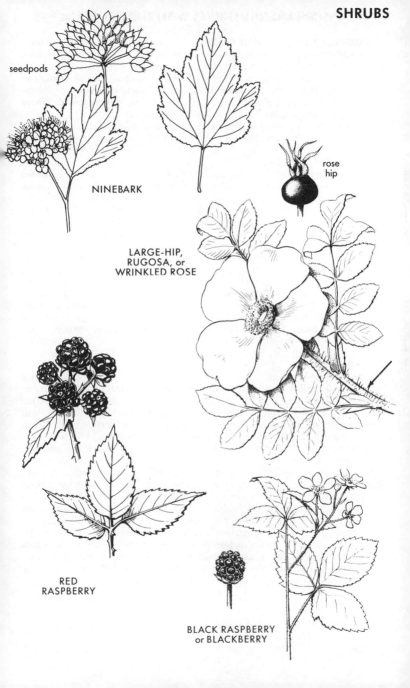

SHRUBS

seedpods

NINEBARK

rose hip

LARGE-HIP,
RUGOSA, or
WRINKLED ROSE

RED
RASPBERRY

BLACK RASPBERRY
or BLACKBERRY

MISCELLANEOUS SHRUBS WITH THORNY BRANCHES

AMERICAN or ALLEGHENY BARBERRY
Root bark

Berberis canadensis Mill.　　(not shown)　　Barberry Family
Shrub; 10–25 in. *Brownish to dull purple branches*; spines usually
3-parted. Leaves spatula-shaped, sparsely toothed; grayish white beneath, without prominent veins. Flowers bright yellow, 5–10 per raceme; May. *Petals notched.* Berries red, *round.* **Where found:** Rocky
woods. Mountains. Va. to Ga., Ala.; Mo. to Ind.
Uses: Root tea used for fevers. A Cherokee remedy for diarrhea. See
Common Barberry (below).

COMMON BARBERRY
Root bark

Berberis vulgaris L.　　**C. Pl. 47**　　Barberry Family
Branching shrub; to 9 ft. *Grayish branches*; spines 3-parted. Leaves
alternate or in rosettes from previous year's leaf axils; spatula-
shaped, with numerous *spiny teeth; veins beneath prominent.* Flowers 10–20 per raceme; April–June. Petals not notched. Fruits red, *elliptical.* Root bark yellow. **Where found:** Widely planted and escaped;
gone wild in s. New England. Alien.

Uses: Berry tea used to promote appetite, diuretic, expectorant, laxative; also relieves itching. Root-bark tea promotes sweating; astringent, antiseptic, "blood purifier"; used for jaundice, hepatitis (stimulates bile production), fevers, hemorrhage, diarrhea. Leaf tea for
coughs. Root-bark tincture used for arthritis, rheumatism, sciatica.
Contains berberine, which has a wide spectrum of biological activity
(see p. 240), including antibacterial activity; useful against infection. **Warning: Large doses harmful.**

HAWTHORNS
Flowers, fruits

Crataegus species　　Rose Family
Very complex group; 100–1,000 species in N. America. Highly variable; hybridize readily — species identification is difficult even for
the specialist. Spiny shrubs. Leaves simple, toothed; cut or lobed.
Flowers mostly white, usually with 5 petals; calyx tube bell-shaped,
5-parted. Flowers spring–early summer. Fruits dry red berries; each
berry has 1–5 hard seeds. **Where found:** Most abundant in e. and cen.
U.S.

Uses: Fruits and flowers famous in herbal folk medicine (American
Indian, Chinese, European) as a heart tonic. Studies confirm use in
hypertension with weak heart, angina pectoris, arteriosclerosis. Dilates coronary vessels, reducing blood pressure; acts as direct and
mild heart tonic. Prolonged use necessary for efficacy. Tea or tincture
used. Should be investigated further by scientists. Hawthorn products are very popular in Europe and China. **Warning:** Eye scratches
from thorns can cause blindness. Contains heart-affecting compounds that may affect blood pressure and heart rate.

SHRUBS or
SMALL TREES

COMMON
BARBERRY

red

typical
HAWTHORNS

red

flowers white
or pale pink

leaf

thorns

SHRUBS OR SMALL TREES WITH COMPOUND LEAVES; BRANCHES OR TRUNKS ARMED WITH SHORT SPINES

DEVIL'S-WALKING STICK, ANGELICA TREE   **Root, berries**
Aralia spinosa L.   **C. Pl. 46**   Ginseng Family
Woody; 6–30 ft. Main stem and leaf stalks with *many sharp (often stout) spines*. Leaves large (to 6 ft. long), twice-divided; leaflets numerous, oval, toothed. Tiny white flowers in umbels, in a very large panicle; July–Sept. **Where found:** Rich woods, alluvial soils. S. New England (cultivated) to Fla.; Texas north to Mich.
Uses: In folk tradition, fresh bark strongly emetic, purgative, thought to cause salivation. Tincture of berries used for toothaches, rheumatic pain. Root poulticed for boils, skin eruptions, swelling.
Warning: Handling roots may cause dermatitis. Large amount of berries **poisonous.**

NORTHERN PRICKLY-ASH   **Bark, berries**
Zanthoxylum americanum Mill.   Rue Family
[*Xanthoxylum americanum*]
Aromatic shrub *with paired short spines*. Compound leaves with 5–11 leaflets; oval, toothed, *lemon-scented* when crushed. Tiny, green-yellow flowers; April–May, before leaves. Fruits red-greenish berries, covered with lemon-scented dots; Aug.–Oct. **Where found:** Moist woods, thickets. Que. to Fla.; Okla. to Minn.
Uses: Bark tea or tincture historically used by American Indians and herbalists for chronic rheumatism, dyspepsia, dysentery, kidney trouble, heart trouble, colds, coughs, lung ailments, and nervous debility. When chewed, bark induces copious salivation. Once popular to stimulate mucous surfaces, bile, and pancreas activity. Bark chewed for toothaches. Berry tea used for sore throats, tonsillitis; also used as a diuretic.

SOUTHERN PRICKLY-ASH   **Bark, berries**
Zanthoxylum clava-herculis L.   **C. Pl. 46**   Rue Family
Small tree or shrub; larger than *Z. americanum* — to 30 ft. Bark with large, *triangular, corky knobs*. Fruits Aug.–Oct. **Where found:** Poor soils. S. Va. to Fla.; Texas to s. Ark., se. Okla.
Uses: Same as for *Z. americanum*; also a folk cancer remedy.

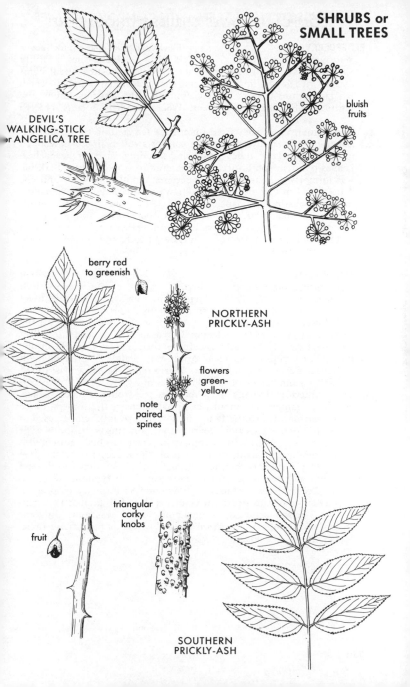

SHRUBS or SMALL TREES

DEVIL'S WALKING-STICK or ANGELICA TREE

bluish fruits

berry red to greenish

NORTHERN PRICKLY-ASH

flowers green-yellow

note paired spines

fruit

triangular corky knobs

SOUTHERN PRICKLY-ASH

COMPOUND LEAVES; SHRUBS WITHOUT SPINES

ELDERBERRY   **Flowers, berries, inner bark, leaves**
Sambucus canadensis L.   **C. Pl. 31**   Honeysuckle Family
Shrub; 3–12 ft. Stem with *white pith*. Leaves opposite (paired), compound, with *5–11* elliptical to lance-shaped leaflets; sharply toothed. Fragrant white flowers in flat, umbrella-like clusters; June–July. Fruits purplish black; July–Sept. **Where found:** Rich soils. N.S. to Ga.; Texas to Man.

 Uses: American Indians used inner-bark tea as diuretic, strong laxative, emetic; poulticed on cuts, sore or swollen limbs, newborn's navel, and boils to relieve pain and swelling; also for headaches. Leaves poulticed on bruises, and on cuts to stop bleeding. Bark tea was formerly used as a wash for eczema, old ulcers, skin eruptions. A tea with Peppermint (see p. 188) in water is a folk remedy for colds; induces sweating and nausea. Considered a mild stimulant, carminative, and diaphoretic. **Warning:** Bark, root, leaves, and unripe berries **toxic;** said to cause cyanide poisoning, severe diarrhea. Fruits edible when cooked. Flowers not thought to be toxic; eaten in pancakes and fritters.

YELLOWROOT   **Root**
Xanthorhiza simplicissima March.   Buttercup Family
Small shrub; 1–3 ft. Thick, deep-yellow root with yellowish bark. The erect, unbranched woody stem, usually 2–3 ft. high, bears leaves and flowers only on the upper portion, which is marked with the scars of the previous year's leaves. Leaves usually divided into *5 leaflets*, on long stalks; leaflets cleft, toothed. Flowers small, *brown-purple*, in drooping racemes; April–May. Petals 5; 2-lobed, with glandlike organs on a short claw. **Where found:** Moist woods, thickets, and stream banks. N.Y. to Fla.; Ala. to Ky.

Uses: American Indians used root tea for stomach ulcers, colds, jaundice, cramps, sore mouth or throat, menstrual disorders; blood tonic, astringent; externally for piles, cancer. A folk remedy used in the South for diabetes and hypertension. Contains berberine — anti-inflammatory, astringent, hemostatic, antimicrobial, anticonvulsant, immunostimulant, uterotonic; also produces a transient drop in blood pressure. Berberine stimulates the secretion of bile and bilirubin and may be useful in correcting high tyramine levels in patients with liver cirrhosis. Yellowroot was formerly used as an adulterant to or substitute for Goldenseal (p. 50), though 19th-century physicians believed its medicinal action was quite different than that of Goldenseal. **Warning:** Yellowroot is potentially **toxic,** especially in large doses.

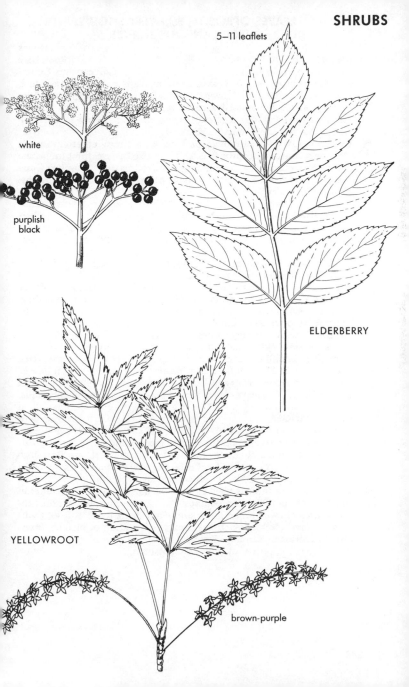

SHRUBS

5–11 leaflets

white

purplish
black

ELDERBERRY

YELLOWROOT

brown-purple

LEAVES OPPOSITE; FLOWERS SHOWY; MISCELLANEOUS SHRUBS

CAROLINA ALLSPICE   **Root, bark**
Calycanthus floridus L.   Calycanthus Family
Aromatic shrub; 3–9 ft. Leaves oval, opposite, entire (not toothed),
with *soft fuzz beneath*. Flowers terminal, maroon-brown, about 2 in.
across; on an urn-shaped receptacle, April–Aug. Flowers have a
strong, strawberry-like fragrance when crushed. **Where found:** Rich
woods. Va. to Fla.; Ala. to W. Va.

⚠ **Uses:** Cherokees used root or bark tea as a strong emetic, diuretic
for kidney and bladder ailments. Cold tea used as eye drops for failing
sight. Settlers used tea as a calming tonic for malaria. **Warning:** Grazing cattle have been reported to have a **toxic** reaction to eating this
plant.

BUTTONBUSH   **Bark**
Cephalanthus occidentalis L.   **C. Pl. 9**   Madder Family
Shrub; 9–20 ft. Leaves *oblong-ovate*; essentially smooth. *White*
flowers in a *globe-shaped cluster*; July–Aug. *Stamens strongly protruding*. **Where found:** Stream banks, moist soils. N.B., New England
to Fla. and Mexico; north to Wisc. and west to Calif.

⚠ **Uses:** American Indians chewed inner bark for toothaches; bark tea
used as a wash for eye inflammation; also emetic, stops bleeding.
Leaf tea was drunk to check menstrual flow. Thought to be tonic,
diuretic, astringent; promotes sweating. Leaf tea once used for fevers,
coughs, "gravel" (kidney stones), malaria, palsy, pleurisy, and toothaches. Interestingly, this plant, which superficially resembles a diminutive Cinchona bush (source of quinine), belongs to the same
plant family and has a folk reputation, as Dogwood does, for relieving
fever and malaria. **Warning:** Contains the glucosides cephalanthin
and cephalin. The leaves have caused **poisoning** in grazing animals.

WILD HYDRANGEA   **Root, bark**
Hydrangea arborescens L.   **C. Pl. 9**   Saxifrage Family
Shrub; to 9 ft. Leaves opposite, mostly ovate; toothed, pointed. Flow-
ers in flat to round clusters, often with *papery, white, sterile, petal-
like calyx lobes on outer edge*; June–Aug. **Where found:** Rich woods.
N.Y. to n. Fla., La.; Okla. to Ind., Ohio.

⚠ **Uses:** American Indians used root tea as diuretic, cathartic, emetic;
scraped bark poulticed on wounds, burns, sore muscles, sprains, tumors; bark chewed for stomach problems, heart trouble. Root traditionally used for kidney stones, mucous irritation of bladder, bronchial afflictions. **Warning:** Experimentally, causes bloody diarrhea,
painful gastroenteritis, cyanide-like **poisoning.**

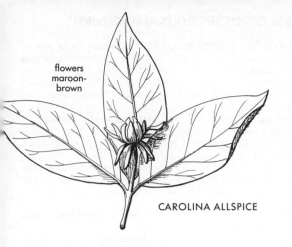

flowers
maroon-
brown

CAROLINA ALLSPICE

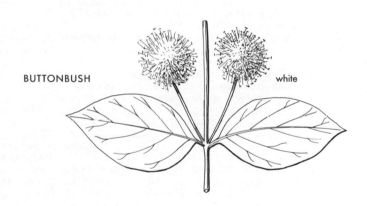

BUTTONBUSH

white

WILD HYDRANGEA

white

LEAVES OPPOSITE; FRUITS RED TO PURPLE

AMERICAN BEAUTY BUSH, FRENCH MULBERRY   **Leaves, roots, berries**
Callicarpa americana L.   **C. Pl. 39**   Verbena Family
Shrub; 3–6 ft. Leaves ovate-oblong, toothed; *woolly beneath.* Tiny, whitish blue flowers in whorl-like cymes; June–Aug. *Rich blue-violet berries* in clusters, in leaf axils; Oct.–Nov. **Where found:** Rich thickets. N. Md. to Fla.; north to Ark., Okla.
Uses: American Indians used root and leaf tea in sweat baths for rheumatism, fevers, and malaria. Root tea used for dysentery, stomachaches. Root and berry tea used for colic. Formerly used in the South for dropsy and as a "blood purifier" in skin diseases.
Related species: The Chinese use the leaves of a related *Callicarpa* species as a vulnerary (to stop bleeding of wounds). It is also used to treat flu in children and menstrual disorders.

STRAWBERRY BUSH   **Stem and root bark, seeds**
Euonymus americanus L.   Staff-tree Family
Erect or straggling, deciduous or nearly evergreen shrub; 3–6 ft. Stalks green, 4-angled. Leaves rather thick, lustrous, sessile; tips sharp-pointed. Flowers greenish purple; *petals stalked.* Flowers May–June. Fruits *scarlet, warty.* **Where found:** Rich woods. Se. N.Y., Pa. to Fla.; Texas, Okla. to Ill.
Uses: American Indians used root tea for uterine prolapse, vomiting of blood, stomachaches, painful urination; wash for swellings. Bark formerly used by physicians as tonic, laxative, diuretic, and expectorant. Tea used for malaria, indigestion, liver congestion, constipation, lung afflictions. Powdered bark applied to scalp was thought to eliminate dandruff. Seeds strongly laxative. **Warning:** Fruit, seeds, and bark may be **poisonous.** Do not ingest — fruits may cause vomiting, diarrhea, and unconsciousness.

WAHOO   **Stem and root bark, seeds**
Euonymus atropupureus Jacq.   **C. Pl. 8**   Staff-tree Family
Shrub or small tree; 6–25 ft. *Leaves hairy beneath;* oblong-oval, stalked. Flowers purplish; June–July. Fruits purplish, *smooth;* seeds covered with *scarlet* pulp. **Where found:** Rich woods. Ont. to Tenn., Ala.; Ark., Okla. to N.D.
Uses: Essentially the same as for *E. americanus* (see above). Historically, the bark was considered tonic, laxative, diuretic, and expectorant. Extracts, syrups, or tea were used for fevers, upset stomach, constipation, dropsy, lung ailments, liver congestion, and heart medicines. The seeds were considered emetic and strongly laxative. Bark and root contain digitalis-like compounds. **Warning:** Fruit, seeds, and bark are considered **poisonous.**

244

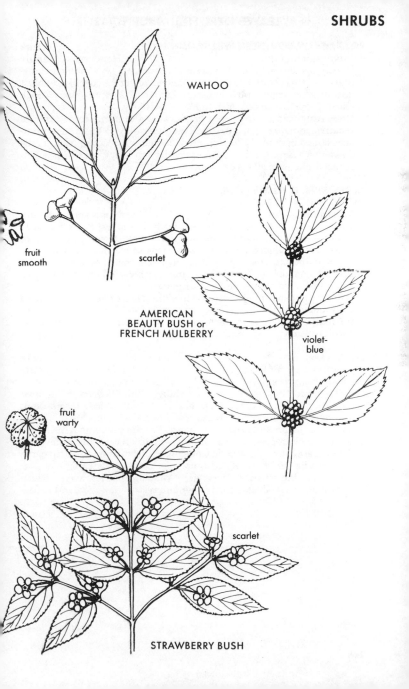

WAHOO

fruit
smooth

scarlet

AMERICAN
BEAUTY BUSH or
FRENCH MULBERRY

violet-
blue

fruit
warty

scarlet

STRAWBERRY BUSH

LEAVES OPPOSITE; VIBURNUMS

POSSUMHAW, SOUTHERN WILD-RAISIN
Bark

Viburnum nudum L.   Honeysuckle Family

Deciduous shrub; to 12 ft. Leaves *glossy, leathery;* oval, and wavy-edged or slightly toothed; those below flowers wedgelike, widest near middle. Small white flowers in flat clusters; April–June. **Where found:** Bogs, low woods. Md. to Fla.; Ark. to Ky.

Uses: American Indians used bark tea as a diuretic, tonic, uterine sedative, antispasmodic; for diabetes. According to Ed Croom, Lumbees boiled bark for 12 hours to reduce liquid to ⅓ original amount; a 1-ounce dose was taken 3 times per day for 4 days, then dosage was reduced to ½ ounce, taken twice a day.

CRAMPBARK, GUELDER ROSE, HIGHBUSH CRANBERRY
Bark

Viburnum opulus L.   Honeysuckle Family

Shrub; to 12 ft. Leaves maple-like, with 3–5 lobes; *hairy beneath.* Leaf stalks with a narrow groove, and a disk-shaped gland. White flowers in a rounded head, to 4 in. across; April–June. Berries red. **Where found:** Ornamental from Europe. Sometimes escaped.

Uses: In Europe bark tea has been used to relieve all types of spasms, including menstrual cramps; astringent, uterine sedative. Science confirms antispasmodic activity. In China, leaves and fruit are used as an emetic, laxative, and antiscorbutic. **Warning:** Berries are considered potentially **poisonous;** they contain chlorogenic acid, beta-sitosterol, and ursolic acid, at least when they are unripe.

BLACKHAW
Bark

Viburnum prunifolium L.   Honeysuckle Family

Large shrub to small tree; 6–30 ft. Leaves elliptic to ovate; finely toothed; mostly smooth, dull (not shiny). White flowers in flat clusters; March–May. Fruits black (bluish at first). **Where found:** Bogs, low woods. Conn. to Fla.; Texas to e. Kans.

Uses: Root- or stem-bark tea used by American Indians, then adopted by Europeans for painful menses, to prevent miscarriage, relieve spasms after childbirth. Considered uterine tonic, sedative, antispasmodic, and nervine. Also used for asthma. Research has confirmed uterine-sedative properties. **Warning:** Berries may produce nausea and other discomforting symptoms.

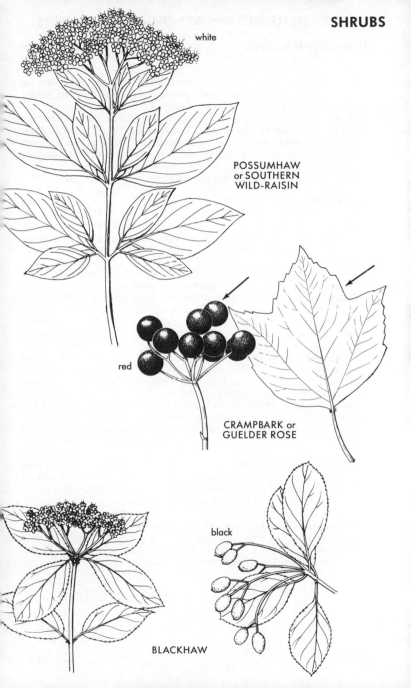

SHRUBS

white

POSSUMHAW
or SOUTHERN
WILD-RAISIN

red

CRAMPBARK or
GUELDER ROSE

black

BLACKHAW

MISCELLANEOUS SHRUBS WITH ALTERNATE LEAVES

NEW JERSEY TEA, RED ROOT   Leaves, root
Ceanothus americanus L.   **C. Pl. 38**   Buckthorn Family
Shrub; 1–2 ft. Leaves oval, toothed, to 2 in. long; with *3 prominent parallel veins*. White flowers in showy, puffy clusters on herbaceous *(non-woody) stems;* April–Sept. **Where found:** Dry, gravelly banks, open woods. Me. to Fla.; Okla. to Minn.
Uses: Leaf tea once a popular beverage. American Indians used root tea for colds, fevers, snakebites, stomachaches, lung ailments; laxative, blood tonic. Root strongly astringent (8 percent tannin content), expectorant, sedative. Root tea was once used for dysentery, asthma, sore throats, bronchitis, whooping cough, spleen inflammation or pain. Alkaloid in root mildly hypotensive (lowers blood pressure).

BLACK CURRANT   Root bark
Ribes americanum Mill.   Saxifrage Family
Thornless shrub; to 5 ft. Leaves maple-like; both sides with yellow *glandular dots* (use lens). Flowers large, tubular to bell-shaped, yellow-white, in a drooping raceme; April–June. Fruits black, smooth. **Where found:** Rich thickets. N.B. to W. Va., Md.; Mo. to Sask.
Uses: American Indians used root-bark tea to expel worms and for kidney ailments; poulticed root-bark for swelling.
Related species: Seeds of other *Ribes* species (*e.g.*, another Black Currant, *R. nigrum*) contain gamma-linolenic acid (see p. 92).

STEEPLEBUSH, HARDHACK   Leaves, flowers
Spiraea tomentosa L.   Rose Family
Small shrub; 2–4 ft. Stems woolly. Leaves *very white or tawny-woolly* beneath; oval-oblong, sawtoothed. Flowers rose (or white), in a *steeple-shaped* raceme; July–Sept. **Where found:** Fields, pastures. N.S. to N.C.; Ark. to Ont.
Uses: American Indians used leaf tea for diarrhea, dysentery; flower and leaf tea for morning sickness. Leaves and flowers were once used to stop bleeding; also for leukorrhea. Other spireas were used similarly.

LATE LOWBUSH BLUEBERRY   Leaves
Vaccinium angustifolium Ait.   Heath Family
Shrub; 3–24 in. Leaves narrowly *lance-shaped,* with tiny stiff teeth; green and hairless on both sides. Flowers white (or pink-tinged); urn-shaped, 5-lobed. Flowers May–June. Fruits (blueberries) Aug.–Sept. **Where found:** Sandy or acid soils. Nfld. to Md.; n. Iowa to Minn.
Uses: American Indians used leaf tea as a "blood purifier"; also used for colic, labor pains, and as a tonic after miscarriage; fumes of burning dried flowers were inhaled for madness.

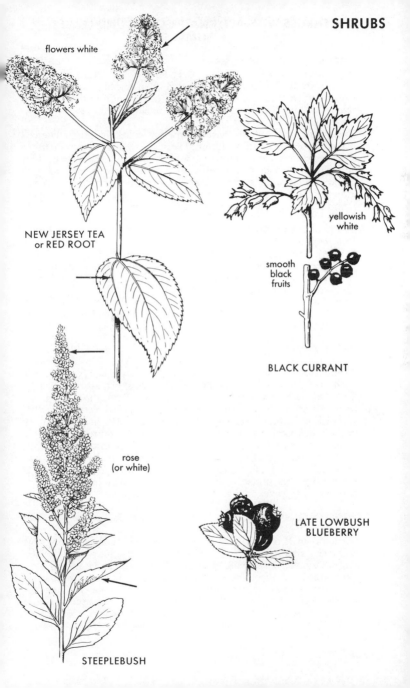

SHRUBS

flowers white

NEW JERSEY TEA
or RED ROOT

yellowish
white

smooth
black
fruits

BLACK CURRANT

rose
(or white)

LATE LOWBUSH
BLUEBERRY

STEEPLEBUSH

SHRUBS WITH ALTERNATE COMPOUND LEAVES;
SUMACS

FRAGRANT or STINKING SUMAC   All parts
Rhus aromatica Ait.   **C. Pl. 36**   Cashew Family
Bush or shrub; 2–7 ft. Leaves 3-parted, *fragrant*, blunt-toothed; end leaflet *not stalked*. Flowers small. Fruits *very oily to touch*; *hairy*, *red*; May–Aug. Highly variable. **Where found:** Dry soil. W. Vt. to nw. Fla.; Texas to S.D. and westward.
Uses: American Indians used leaves for colds, bleeding; chewed leaves for stomachaches; diuretic. Bark chewed for colds — patient slowly swallowed juice. Fruits chewed for toothaches, stomachaches, and grippe. Physicians formerly used astringent root bark to treat irritated urethra, leukorrhea, diarrhea, dysentery, bronchitis, laryngitis, and bed-wetting in children and elderly. Contraindicated if inflammation is present. **Warning:** May cause dermatitis.

WINGED or DWARF SUMAC   Berries, bark, leaves
Rhus copallina L.   Cashew Family
Shrub or small tree; to 30 ft. Leaves divided into 9–31 *shiny, mostly toothless* leaflets, with a prominent *wing* along midrib. Fruits red, short-hairy; Oct.–Nov. **Where found:** Dry woods, clearings. S. Me. to Fla.; e. Texas to n. Ill.
Uses: American Indians used bark tea to stimulate milk flow; wash for blisters. Berries chewed to treat bed-wetting and mouth sores. Root tea used for dysentery.

SMOOTH SUMAC   Fruits, bark, leaves
Rhus glabra L.   **C. Pl. 31**   Cashew Family
Shrub; 3–20 ft. Twigs and leafstalks *smooth, without hairs*. Leaves with 11–31 *toothed* leaflets. Fruits red, with short, appressed hairs; June–Oct. **Where found:** Fields and openings. Throughout our area.
Uses: American Indians used berries to stop bed-wetting. Leaves smoked for asthma; leaf tea used for asthma, diarrhea, stomatosis (mouth diseases), dysentery. Root tea emetic, diuretic. Bark tea formerly used for diarrhea, dysentery, fevers, scrofula, general debility from sweating; also for mouth or throat ulcers, leukorrhea, and anal and uterine prolapse; astringent, tonic, antiseptic. **Warning:** Do not confuse this sumac with Poison Sumac, which has white fruits and toothless leaves, and grows in or near swamps.

STAGHORN SUMAC   Leaves, berries, bark, root
Rhus typhina L.   Cashew Family
Shrub or small tree; 4–15 ft. Similar to *R. glabra* (above), but twigs and leaf stalks *strongly hairy*. Fruits long-hairy; June–Sept. **Where found:** Dry, rocky soil. N.S. to N.C., S.C., Ga.; Ill. to Minn.
Uses: Similar to those for *R. glabra*. American Indians used berries in cough syrups. Berry tea used for "female disorders," lung ailments. Gargled for sore throats, worms. Leaf tea used for sore throats, tonsillitis. Root or bark tea astringent; used for bleeding.

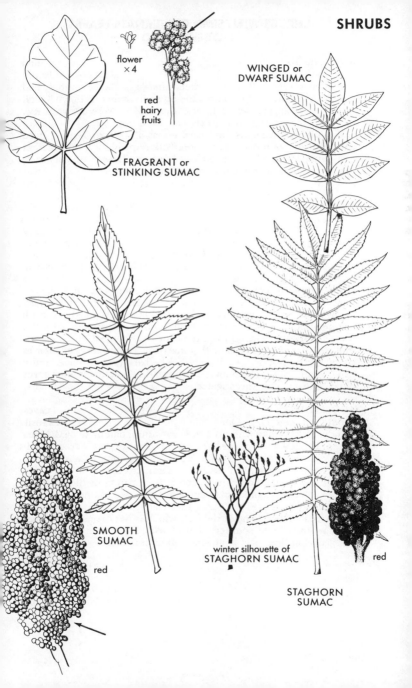

SHRUBS

flower
× 4

red
hairy
fruits

WINGED or
DWARF SUMAC

FRAGRANT or
STINKING SUMAC

SMOOTH
SUMAC

red

winter silhouette of
STAGHORN SUMAC

red

STAGHORN
SUMAC

SHRUBS WITH SIMPLE ALTERNATE LEAVES; NOT TOOTHED

LEATHERWOOD   Bark
Dirca palustris L.   Leatherwood Family
Branched shrub; 1–9 ft. Branchlets *pliable*, smooth, jointed; bark
very tough. Leaves oval to obovate, on short stalks. Yellowish, bell-
like flowers appear before leaves, April–May. **Where found:** Rich
woods, along streams. N.B. to Fla.; La. to Minn.
Uses: American Indians used bark tea as a laxative. Minute doses
cause burning of tongue, salivation. Folk remedy for toothaches, facial neuralgia, paralysis of tongue. **Warning: Poisonous.** Causes severe dermatitis, with redness, blistering, and sores.

SPICEBUSH   Leaves, bark, berries, twigs
Lindera benzoin (L.) Blume   **C. Pl. 8**   Laurel Family
Shrub; 4–15 ft. Leaves aromatic; ovate, without teeth. Tiny yellow
flowers in axillary clusters *appear before leaves*, March–April. Fruits
highly aromatic; glossy, scarlet, with a single large seed; Sept.–Nov.
Where found: Moist, rich soils; damp shady woods along stream
banks. Me. to Fla.; Texas to Mich.
Uses: American Indians used berry tea for coughs, cramps, delayed
menses, croup, measles; bark tea for sweating, "blood purifier,"
colds, rheumatism, anemia. Settlers used berries as an Allspice substitute. Medicinally, the berries were used as a carminative for flatulence and colic. The oil from the fruits was applied to bruises and
muscles or joints (for chronic rheumatism). Twig tea was popular for
colds, fevers, worms, gas, and colic. The bark tea was once used to
expel worms, for typhoid fevers, and as a diaphoretic for other forms
of fevers. Should be investigated.

STAGGERBUSH   Leaves
Lyonia mariana (L.) D. Don.   Heath Family
Slender, deciduous shrub; to 7 ft. Leaves thin, oblong to oval. White
or pinkish flowers in *umbel-like racemes, in clusters on old leafless
branches*; April–June. **Where found:** Sandy, acid pine thickets.
Southern R.I., Conn., N.Y. to Fla.; e. Texas to Ark.
Uses: Cherokees used leaf tea externally, for itching, ulcers. Benja-
min Smith Barton, in his classic *Essay Towards a Materia Medica of
the United States* (1801), wrote that leaf tea was used as wash for
"disagreeable ulceration of the feet, which is not uncommon among
the slave, &c., in the southern states." **Warning: Poisonous;** produces
"staggers" in livestock, hence the common name.

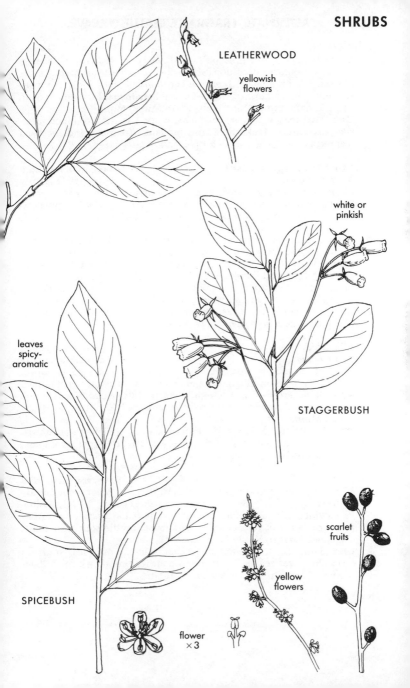

SHRUBS

LEATHERWOOD

yellowish flowers

white or pinkish

leaves spicy-aromatic

STAGGERBUSH

SPICEBUSH

yellow flowers

scarlet fruits

flower × 3

ALTERNATE, FRAGRANT, LEATHERY LEAVES

SWEETFERN
Leaves

Comptonia peregrina (L.) Coult. **C. Pl. 10** Wax-myrtle Family
Strongly aromatic, deciduous shrub; 2–5 ft. Leaves soft-hairy, lance-shaped; 3–6 in. long, with *prominent rounded teeth.* Flowers inconspicuous. Fruits *burlike;* Sept.–Oct. **Where found:** Dry soil. N.S. to Va., Ga. mountains; Ohio, Neb., Ill. to Minn., Man.
Uses: Leaf tea astringent; folk remedy for vomiting of blood, diarrhea, dysentery, leukorrhea, rheumatism. American Indians used leaf tea as a beverage; wash for poison-ivy rash, bleeding.

WAX-MYRTLE, CANDLEBERRY
Leaves, fruit, root bark

Myrica cerifera L. Wax-myrtle Family
Coarse shrub or small tree; to 26 ft. Young branchlets *waxy.* Leaves oblong to lance-shaped; leathery, evergreen, with waxy globules. Fruits ⅛ in. across; March–June. **Where found:** Swamp thickets. S. N.J. to Fla.; Texas to Ark.
Uses: Candle wax produced from fruits. Root bark formerly used in tea as an astringent and emetic for chronic gastritis, diarrhea, dysentery, leukorrhea, "catarrhal states of the alimentary tracts," jaundice, scrofula, and indolent (hard to heal) ulcers. Leaf tea was used for fevers, externally as a wash for itching. Powdered root bark was an ingredient in "composition powder," once a widely used home remedy for colds and chills. **Warning:** Wax is irritating. Constituents of the wax are reportedly carcinogenic.

SWEET GALE
Berries, root bark, leaves

Myrica gale L. Wax-myrtle Family
Fragrant deciduous shrub; 2–6 ft. Leaves gray; oblong to lance-shaped. Flowers in clusters, at ends of previous year's branchlets; April–June. Fruit with 2 winglike bracts; July–Aug. **Where found:** Swamps, shallow water. Nfld. to mountains of N.C.; Tenn. to Mich., Wisc., Minn.
Uses: Similar to those for *M. cerifera* (above). Branch tea once used as a diuretic for gonorrhea. **Warning:** Essential oil reportedly **toxic;** inhibits growth of various bacteria.

BAYBERRY
Leaves, bark, fruits

Myrica pensylvanica Loisel. **C. Pl. 10** Wax-myrtle Family
Stout shrub; 3–12 ft. *Branches grayish white.* Leaves elliptic to obovate (widened at tips). Flowers in clusters *below leafy tips;* April–July. Young fruits very hairy. **Where found:** Sterile soils near coast. Canadian coast to Va., N.C. (rare).
Uses: Same as for *M. cerifera* (above). Micmac used leaf snuff for headaches; leaf tea as a stimulant; poulticed root bark for inflammation. **Warning:** Wax is considered **toxic.**

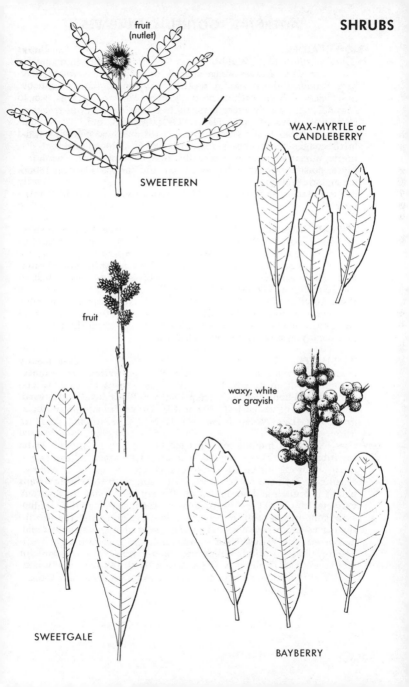

SHRUBS

fruit
(nutlet)

SWEETFERN

WAX-MYRTLE or
CANDLEBERRY

fruit

SWEETGALE

waxy; white
or grayish

BAYBERRY

ALTERNATE, TOOTHED, OVAL LEAVES

SMOOTH ALDER   **Stem bark**
Alnus serrulata (Ait.) Willd.   Hazelnut Family
Shrub; to 15 ft. Leaves wedge-shaped, or only slightly rounded at
base, *broadest above middle*; toothed, wavy-edged. Bark dark, *with
few speckles*. Male catkins *abruptly bent*. Flowers (catkins) Feb.–
May. "Cones" woody, erect, persistent. **Where found:** Forms thickets
along waterways. Me. to n. Fla.; se. Okla., Mo., Ill., Ind.
Uses: American Indians used bark tea for diarrhea, pain of childbirth, coughs, toothaches, sore mouth, and as a "blood purifier"; diuretic, purgative, emetic; externally, as an eye wash, and a wash for
hives, poison-ivy rash, piles, swellings, and sprains. Used in 1800s
for malaria and syphilis.
Related species: Indians across N. America used other alders similarly.

AMERICAN HAZELNUT   **Inner bark, twig hairs**
Corylus americana Walt.   Hazelnut Family
Shrub; to 10 ft. Stems and leafstalks with *stiff hairs*. Leaves *heart-
shaped, double-toothed*; to 5 in long. Flowers April–May. Fruits
with edible nuts encased in beaked, toothed bracts. **Where found:**
Thickets. Me. to Ga.; Mo., Okla. to Sask.
Uses: American Indians drank bark tea for hives, fevers; astringent.
Bark poultice used to close cuts and wounds, treat tumors, old sores,
and skin cancers. Twig hairs were used by American Indians and
historically by physicians to expel worms.

WITCH-HAZEL   **Bark, leaves**
Hamamelis virginiana L.   **C. Pl. 9**   Witch-hazel Family
Deciduous shrub or small tree; to 15 ft. Leaves obovate, wavy-
toothed; end buds distinctly scalpel-shaped. Flowers yellow, in axillary clusters; petals *very slender*, to 1 in. Flowers *bloom after leaves
drop*, Sept.–Dec. **Where found:** Woods. N.S., Que. to Fla.; Texas to
Minn.
Uses: American Indians took leaf tea for colds, sore throats. Twig
tea rubbed on athletes' legs to keep muscles limber, relieve lameness; tea drunk for bloody dysentery, cholera, cough, and asthma.
Astringent bark tea taken internally for lung ailments; used externally for bruises and sore muscles. Widely used today (in distilled
extracts, ointments, eye washes) as an astringent for piles, toning
skin, suppressing profuse menstrual flow, eye ailments. Tannins in
the leaves and bark are thought to be responsible for astringent and
hemostatic properties. Used commercially in preparations to treat
hemorrhoids, irritations, minor pain, and itching. Over-the-counter
products are available in every pharmacy. Bottled Witch-hazel water,
widely available, is a steam distillate that does not contain the astringent tannins of the shrub.

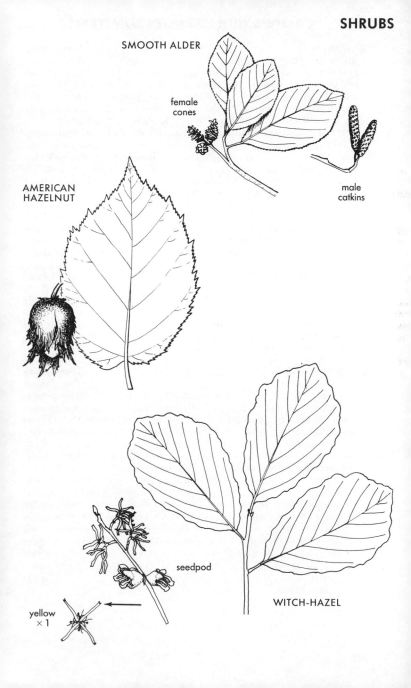

SHRUBS

SMOOTH ALDER

female cones

male catkins

AMERICAN HAZELNUT

seedpod

yellow ×1

WITCH-HAZEL

CONIFERS WITH FLAT NEEDLES IN SPRAYS

BALSAM FIR   Resin, leaves
Abies balsamea (L.) Mill.   Pine Family
Spire-shaped tree; to 60 ft. Flattish needles, to 1¼ in. long, in flat-tened sprays; stalkless. Needles *rounded at base,* each with *2 white lines beneath.* Cones 1–4 in. long, *erect;* purple to green; *scales mostly twice as long as broad.* Bark smooth, with numerous resin pockets. **Where found:** Moist woods. Canada, south through New England and along mountains to Va. and W. Va.; west through n. Ohio to ne. Iowa, Mich.
Uses: Canada Balsam, an oleoresin, is collected by cutting bark blisters or pockets in wood, July–Aug. Used as an antiseptic, and in creams and ointments for piles, and root-canal sealers. Diuretic (may irritate mucous membranes). American Indians applied resin as an analgesic for burns, sores, bruises, and wounds. Leaf tea used for colds, cough, and asthma. The oleoresin is pale yellow to greenish yellow; transparent and pleasantly scented. Its primary commercial application has been as a sealing agent for mounting microscope slides. **Warning:** Resin may cause dermatitis in some individuals.

FRASER FIR, SHE BALSAM   Resin
Abies fraseri (Pursh) Poiret   Pine Family
Similar to *A. balsamea* (above), but needles and cones are generally smaller; cone-scale *margins toothed or jagged.* **Where found:** Isolated to mountains. Va., N.C., Tenn.
Uses: Cherokees used resin for chest ailments, coughs, sore throat, urinary-tract infections, and wounds.

EASTERN HEMLOCK   Leaves, bark
Tsuga canadensis L.   Pine Family
Evergreen tree; 50–90 ft. Needles flat; ⁵⁄₁₆–⁹⁄₁₆ in. long, on short *slender stalks.* Needles bright green above, *silvery whitish beneath.* Cones drooping, to 1 in. long, with few scales; scales rounded. **Where found:** Hills in rocky woods. N.S. to Md., Ga. mountains; Ala. to Ky., Ind., e. Minn.
Uses: American Indians used tea made from leafy twig tips for kidney ailments, in steam baths for rheumatism, colds, and coughs, and to induce sweating. Inner-bark tea used for colds, fevers, diarrhea, coughs, "stomach troubles," and scurvy. Externally, used as a wash for rheumatism and to stop bleeding. Bark is very astringent; formerly used as poultice for bleeding wounds, and in tanning leathers. The oleoresin derived from the bark is dark reddish brown, opaque, and has a characteristic turpentine-like fragrance.

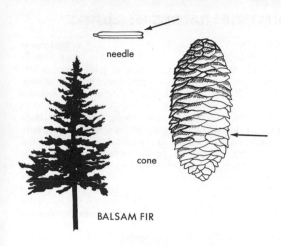

needle

cone

BALSAM FIR

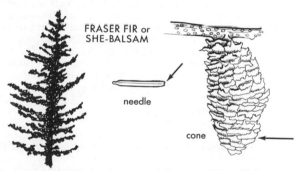

FRASER FIR or SHE-BALSAM

needle

cone

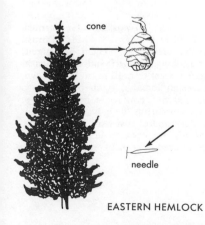

cone

needle

EASTERN HEMLOCK

NEEDLES OVER 1 IN. LONG, IN CLUSTERS

TAMARACK, BLACK LARCH   **Bark, gum**
Larix laricina (DuRoi) K. Koch   Pine Family
Coniferous tree; to 100 ft. *Deciduous* needles, to 1 in. long, in *circular clusters.* Cones oval, to ¾ in long; scales few, rounded. **Where found:** Swamps, wet soils. Lab. to W. Va., n. Ill.; across s. Canada to Alaska.

 Uses: Bark tea traditionally used as laxative, tonic, diuretic for jaundice, rheumatism, and skin ailments. Gargled for sore throats. Poulticed on sores, swellings, and burns. Leaf tea astringent; used for piles, diarrhea, dysentery, and dropsy; poulticed for burns and headaches. Gum chewed for indigestion. **Warning:** Sawdust can cause dermatitis.

SHORTLEAF PINE,
YELLOW or HARD PINE   **Inner bark, buds, pitch**
Pinus echinata Mill.   Pine Family
Straight evergreen tree; to 120 ft. Slender needles 3–5 in. long; in 2's or 3's. Cones oval; each *scale tipped with a short prickle.* **Where found:** Dry woods. Se. N.Y., Ohio to Fla.; Texas to s. Ill.
Uses: American Indians used inner bark in tea to induce vomiting. Cold tea of buds once used as a worm expellent. Pitch tea used as laxative and for tuberculosis; also for kidney ailments causing backaches. **Warning:** Wood, sawdust, balsam, and turpentine of various pines may cause dermatitis in sensitive individuals.

LONGLEAF PINE   **Pitch, turpentine**
Pinus palustris Mill.   Pine Family
Evergreen tree; to 90 ft. Needles in 3's; *very long* — 7–12 (occasionally 18) in. Cones cylindrical, 6–10 in. long; each scale with a *short, curved spine.* **Where found:** Sandy soil, coastal plain. Se. Va. to Fla.; Texas.
Uses: Turpentine, derived from sap, formerly used for colic, chronic diarrhea, worms; to arrest bleeding from tooth sockets; rubefacient (local irritant to skin); folk remedy for abdominal tumors. **Warning:** Considered potentially **toxic.**

WHITE PINE   **Twigs, bark, leaves, pitch**
Pinus strobus L.   **C. Pl. 47**   Pine Family
Evergreen tree; to at least 150 ft. Needles *in 5's;* slender, pale green, glaucous. Cones cylindrical; to 8 in. long. **Where found:** Common in East from Canada to Ga. mountains; west to n. Ill., cen. Iowa.
Uses: Used extensively by American Indians; pitch poulticed to "draw out" boils, abscesses; also used for rheumatism, broken bones, cuts, bruises, sores, felons, and inflammation. Twig tea used for kidney and lung ailments; emetic. Bark and/or leaf tea used for colds, coughs, grippe, sore throats, lung ailments; poulticed for headaches, backaches, etc. Inner bark formerly used in cough syrups.

TREES

TAMARACK or BLACK LARCH

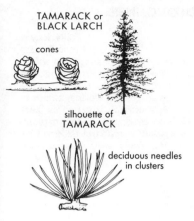

cones

silhouette of
TAMARACK

deciduous needles
in clusters

SHORTLEAF, YELLOW, or HARD PINE

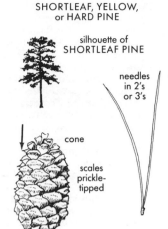

silhouette of
SHORTLEAF PINE

needles
in 2's
or 3's

cone

scales
prickle-
tipped

LONGLEAF PINE

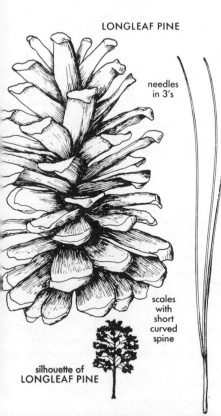

needles
in 3's

scales
with
short
curved
spine

silhouette of
LONGLEAF PINE

WHITE PINE

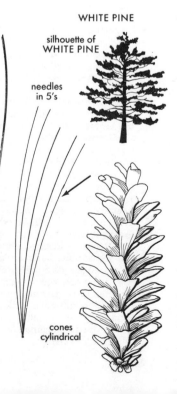

silhouette of
WHITE PINE

needles
in 5's

cones
cylindrical

MISCELLANEOUS CONIFERS

EASTERN RED CEDAR   **Fruits, leaves**
Juniperus virginiana L.   Pine Family
Spire-shaped; 10–50 ft. Leaves *scale-like, overlapping*; twigs *4-sided*.
Fruits hard, round, dry, blue-green. **Where found:** Infertile soils, old
pastures. Canada, Me. to Ga.; Texas to Minn., Mich.
Uses: American Indians used fruit tea for colds, worms, rheumatism, coughs, induce sweating. Chewed fruit for canker sores. Leaf
smoke or steam inhaled for colds, bronchitis, purification rituals,
rheumatism. Said to contain the antitumor compound podophyllotoxin, best known from Mayapple (p. 46). **Warning:** All parts may be
toxic.

BLACK SPRUCE (not shown)   **Inner bark, resin**
Picea mariana (Mill.) BSP   Pine Family
Evergreen tree; 10–90 ft. Needles stiff, crowded, 4-angled; dark-
green, *mostly glaucous*. Cones short-oval to rounded; dull gray-
brown. **Where found:** Woods. Canada to Pa., Va. mountains; Wisc.
Uses: American Indians poulticed inner bark on inflammations. Inner-bark tea a folk medicine for kidney stones, stomach problems,
rheumatism. Resin poulticed on sores to promote healing. Needles
used to make a beer that was drunk for scurvy. **Warning:** Sawdust,
balsam (resin), and even the needles may produce dermatitis.

RED SPRUCE   **Boughs, pitch**
Picea rubens Sarg.   Pine Family
Evergreen tree; to 100 ft., with hairy branchlets. Needles slender;
yellowish, *not glaucous*. Cones *elongate-oval; brown to red-tinged
brown*. **Where found:** Woods. Canada, New England to N.C., Tenn.,
Ohio.
Uses: American Indians used tea of boughs for colds and to "break
out" measles. Pitch formerly poulticed on rheumatic joints, chest,
and stomach to relieve congestion and pain. **Warning:** See under
Black Spruce (above).

NORTHERN WHITE CEDAR   **Leaves, inner bark, leaf oil**
Thuja occidentalis L.   Cypress Family
Evergreen tree; to 60 ft. Leaves in *flattened sprays*; small, *appressed,
overlapping*. Cones *bell-shaped*, with *loose scales*. **Where found:**
Swamps; cool, rocky woods. N.S. to Ga. mountains; n. Ill. to Minn.
Uses: American Indians used leaf tea for headaches, colds; also in
cough syrups; in steam baths for rheumatism, arthritis, colds,
congestion, headaches, gout; externally, as a wash for swollen feet,
and burns. Inner-bark tea used for consumption, coughs. Physicians
once used leaf tincture externally on warts, venereal warts, piles, ulcers, bed sores, and fungus infections. Internally, leaf tincture used
for bronchitis, asthma, pulmonary disease, enlarged prostate with
urinary incontinence. Folk cancer remedy. Experimentally, leaf oil is
antiseptic, expectorant, counterirritant; extracts have shown antiviral properties against *herpes simplex*. **Warning:** Leaf oil is **toxic,**
causing hypotension, convulsions. Fatalities have been reported.

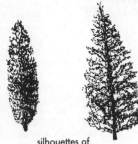

EASTERN
RED CEDAR

scales (leaves)
overlapping

silhouettes of
EASTERN
RED CEDAR

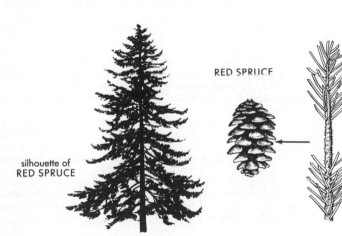

RED SPRUCE

silhouette of
RED SPRUCE

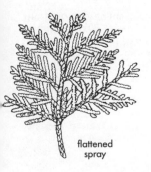

NORTHERN
WHITE CEDAR

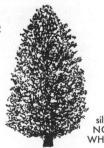

flattened
spray

silhouette of
NORTHERN
WHITE CEDAR

DECIDUOUS TREES WITH
OPPOSITE, COMPOUND LEAVES

OHIO BUCKEYE   Nuts
Aesculus glabra Willd.   **C. Pl. 44**   Horsechestnut Family
Small tree; 20–40 ft. Leaflets 5 (rarely 4–7); toothed, 4–15 in. long.
Twigs *foul-smelling* when broken. Buds not sticky; scales at tips
strongly ridged. Bark rough-scaly. Flowers yellow; April–May. Fruit
husk with *weak prickles;* Sept.–Oct. **Where found:** Rich, moist
woods. W. Pa., W. Va., e. Tenn., cen. Ala., cen. Okla. to Neb., Iowa.

 Uses: Traditionally, powdered nut (minute dose) used for spasmodic
cough, asthma (with tight chest), intestinal irritations. Externally,
tea or ointment used for rheumatism and piles. American Indians
put ground nuts in streams to stupefy fish, which floated to surface
for easy harvest. **Warning:** Nuts **toxic,** causing severe gastric irritation. Still, Indians made food from them after elaborate processing.

HORSECHESTNUT   Nuts, leaves, flowers, bark
Aesculus hippocastanum L.   Horsechestnut Family
To 100 ft. Leaflets 5–7; to 12 in. long; *without stalks,* toothed. Buds
large, *very sticky.* Broken twigs *not foul-smelling* as in Ohio Buckeye
(above). Flowers white (mottled red and yellow); May. Fruits *spiny or
warty;* Sept.–Oct. **Where found:** Planted in towns. Naturalized.
Uses: As in *A. glabra* (see above); also, peeled roasted nuts of this
tree were brewed for diarrhea, prostate ailments. Thought to increase
blood circulation. In Europe, preparations of the seeds are believed
to prevent thrombosis, and are used to treat varicose veins and hemorrhoids; thought to help strengthen weak veins and arteries. Also
used in gastritis and gastroenteritis. Leaf tea tonic; used for fevers.
Flower tincture used on rheumatic joints. Bark tea astringent; used
in malaria, dysentery; externally, for lupus and skin ulcers. **Warning:**
Outer husks **poisonous; all parts can be toxic.** Fatalities reported.
Seeds (nuts) contain 30–60 percent starch, but can be used as a food-
stuff only after the toxins have been removed.

WHITE or AMERICAN ASH   Bark, leaves
Fraxinus americana L.   Olive Family
To 100 ft. Twigs hairless. Leaves opposite, pinnate, with 5–9 leaflets;
oval, slightly toothed or entire; *white* or pale beneath. Flowers April–
June. Fruits narrow, winged; Oct.–Nov. **Where found:** Woods. N.S. to
Fla.; Texas, Neb. to Minn.
Uses: American Indians used inner-bark tea as an emetic or strong
laxative, to remove bile from intestines, as a "tonic" after childbirth,
and to relieve stomach cramps, fevers; diuretic, promotes sweating;
wash used for sores, itching, lice, snakebites. Inner bark chewed and
applied as a poultice to sores. Seeds thought to be aphrodisiac.

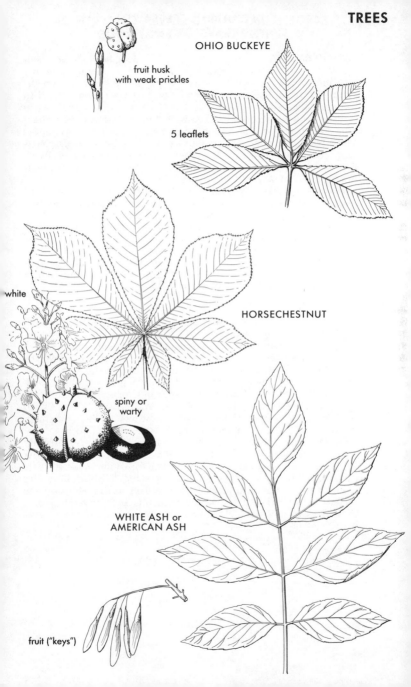

OHIO BUCKEYE

fruit husk
with weak prickles

5 leaflets

white

HORSECHESTNUT

spiny or
warty

WHITE ASH or
AMERICAN ASH

fruit ("keys")

LARGE, HEART-SHAPED LEAVES; OPPOSITE, OR WITH 3 LEAVES AT EACH NODE

COMMON CATALPA   **Bark, leaves, seeds, pods**
Catalpa bignonioides Walt.   **C. Pl. 44**   Bignonia Family
Ornamental tree; to 45 ft. Leaves opposite, or in 3's from each node; large — to 10 in. long and 7 in. wide; oval to heart-shaped, with an *abruptly pointed apex*; not toothed. Leaves foul-odored when bruised. Flowers whitish, marked with 2 orange stripes and numerous *purple spots* within; thimble-like, with 5 unequal, wavy-edged lobes. Flowers in large, upright, showy clusters; June–July. Seedpods long, cigar-shaped; seeds with 2 papery wings. **Where found:** Waste ground; street tree. Fla., Ala., Miss., La. Naturalized north to New England, N.Y., Ohio, and westward.
Uses: Bark tea formerly used as an antiseptic, snakebite antidote, laxative, sedative, worm expellent (a Chinese species is also used against worms). Leaves poulticed on wounds, abrasions. Seed tea used for asthma, bronchitis; externally, for wounds. Pods sedative; thought to possess cardioactive properties.
Related species: Northern or Hardy Catalpa (*Catalpa speciosa*, not shown) is a larger tree; leaves with a long-pointed tip, flowers with fewer spots. Original range is unclear; perhaps native from Ind. to e. Ark. Now commonly naturalized in se. U.S.

PRINCESS-TREE, PAULOWNIA   **All parts**
Paulownia tomentosa (Thunb.) Steud.   **C. Pl. 48**   Figwort Family
Medium-sized, thick-branched tree; 30–60 ft. Leaves *heart-shaped*, pointed at tip; large — to 12 in. long and broad (sometimes larger); velvety beneath; leafstalks to 8 in. long. Flowers fragrant, hairy, purple thimbles, to 2 in. long; with 5 flared, *unequal lobes*; in large, candelabra-like clusters; April–May. Fruits upright, hollow hulls filled with tiny winged seeds; hulls split in two, suggesting hickory fruits in shape; persist through winter. **Where found:** Occurs from N.Y. to Fla. and westward. Oriental alien; introduced as an ornamental in the U.S. by 1843. Widely escaped, especially in South.

Uses: In China, a wash of the leaves and capsules was used in daily applications to promote the growth of hair and prevent graying. Leaf tea was used as a foot bath for swollen feet. Inner-bark tincture (soaked in 2 parts whisky) given for fevers and delirium. Leaves or ground bark were fried in vinegar, poulticed on bruises. Flowers were mixed with other herbs to treat liver ailments. In Japan the leaf juice is used to treat warts. **Warning:** Contains potentially **toxic** compounds.

TREES

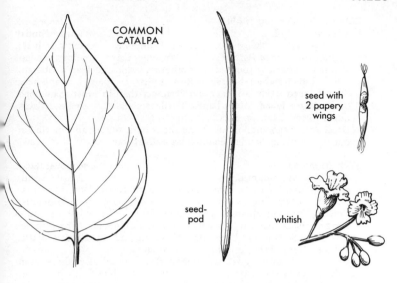

COMMON CATALPA

seed with 2 papery wings

seed-pod

whitish

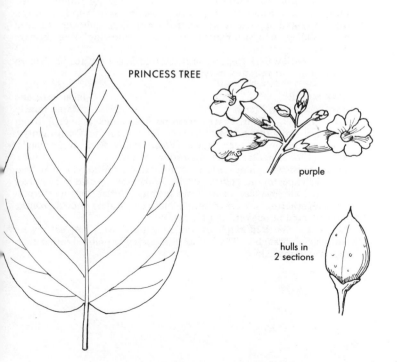

PRINCESS TREE

purple

hulls in 2 sections

BOX-ELDER, ASHLEAF MAPLE
Inner bark
Acer negundo L.   Maple Family
Tree; 40–70 ft. *Twigs glossy green.* Leaflets 3–5 (occasionally 7); *similar to those of Poison Ivy,* but Box-elder leaves are *opposite,* not alternate; coarsely toothed (or without teeth); end leaflet often 3-lobed, broader than lateral leaflets. Fruits are paired, maple-type "keys"; seed itself is longer and narrower than in most maple species. **Where found:** River banks, fertile woods. N.S. to Fla., Texas; north to cen. Man., s. Alta.; also in Calif.
Uses: American Indians used the inner-bark tea as an emetic (induces vomiting). Sap boiled down as a sugar source.

STRIPED MAPLE
Inner bark, leaves, twigs
Acer pensylvanicum L.   Maple Family
Slender tree; to 15 ft. *Bark greenish,* with *vertical white stripes.* Leaves 3-lobed, finely double-toothed; to 8 in. wide. Small, greenish flowers, in long clusters; May–June. Fruits ("keys") with paired winged seeds, usually set widely apart; June–Sept. **Where found:** Woods. N.S. and south through New England, mountains of Pa., Ohio to Tenn., N.C., n. Ga.; west to Mich.
Uses: American Indians used inner-bark tea for colds, coughs, bronchitis, kidney infections, gonorrhea, spitting of blood; wash used for swollen limbs. Inner-bark tea was used as a wash for paralysis. Historically, bark tea was used as a folk remedy for skin eruptions, taken internally and applied as an external wash. Leaf and twig tea used both to allay or induce nausea, and induce vomiting, depending on dosage.
Related species: Bark from a closely related Asian species has shown significant anti-inflammatory activity.

SUGAR MAPLE
Inner bark, sap
Acer saccharum Marsh.   Maple Family
Large tree; 60–130 ft. Leaves *green on both sides.* Leaves 5-lobed; *lobes not drooping, notches between lobes rounded.* Twigs glossy. Fruits paired, maple-type "keys." **Where found:** Rich, hilly woods, fields. Nfld. to n. Ga., e. Texas; north to Minn.
Uses: American Indians used inner bark in tea for coughs, diarrhea; diuretic, expectorant, "blood purifier." Maple syrup said to be a liver tonic and kidney cleanser, and used in cough syrups. During the maple sap-gathering process in spring, New Englanders once drank the sap collected in buckets as a spring tonic.
Related species: Red Maple (*A. rubrum,* not shown) has red flowers and reddish branches. The leaf lobes are sharply pointed rather than rounded. Range similar.

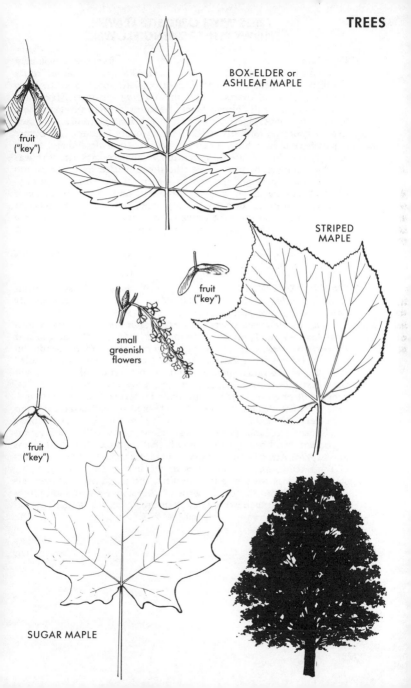

TREES

BOX-ELDER or ASHLEAF MAPLE

fruit ("key")

STRIPED MAPLE

fruit ("key")

small greenish flowers

fruit ("key")

SUGAR MAPLE

TREES WITH OPPOSITE LEAVES;
SHOWY WHITE SPRING FLOWERS

FRINGETREE   **Root bark, trunk bark**
Chionanthus virginica L.   **C. Pl. 45**   Olive Family
Shrub or small tree; 6–20 ft. Leaves opposite, oval, 3–8 in. long;
mostly smooth. Flowers white, *in drooping clusters*; May–June.
Petals slender. Fruits bluish black, resembling small olives. **Where
found:** Dry slopes. N.J. to Fla.; Texas, e. Okla. north to Mo., s. Ohio.
Uses: Physicians formerly used 10 drops (every 3 hours) of tincture
(1 part bark by weight in 5 parts 50 percent grain alcohol and water)
for jaundice. In the late 19th century Fringetree bark tincture was
widely employed by physicians who thought it relieved congestion
of glandular organs and the venous system. It was employed for hypertrophy of the liver, wounds, nephritis, and rheumatism. Once
considered diuretic, alterative, cholagogue, and tonic. American Indians used the root-bark tea to wash inflammations, sores, cuts, and
infections. **Warning:** Overdoses cause vomiting, frontal headaches,
slow pulse, etc.
Related species: Leaves of the Chinese species *C. retusus* have been
used in Asia as a tea substitute.

FLOWERING DOGWOOD   **Inner bark, berries, twigs**
Cornus florida L.   **C. Pl. 44**   Dogwood Family
Our most showy deciduous tree; 10–30 ft. Leaves ovate; *latex
threads appear at veins when leaves are split apart.* Flowers in clusters; April–May; *4 showy white (or pink) bracts surround the true
flowers.* Fruits scarlet, dry; inedible, very bitter. **Where found:** Un-
derstory tree of dry woods. Me. to Fla.; Texas to Kans. Widely cultivated in natural range and elsewhere as an ornamental.
Uses: Astringent root-bark tea or tincture widely used in South, especially during the Civil War, for malarial fevers (substitute for quinine); also for chronic diarrhea. Root bark also poulticed onto external ulcers. Scarlet berries soaked in brandy as a bitter digestive tonic
and for acid stomach. Twigs used as "chewing sticks" — forerunners
of modern toothbrushes. An 1830 herbal reported that the Indians
and captive Africans in Virginia were remarkable for the whiteness
of their teeth, and attributed it to the use of Dogwood chewing
sticks. Once chewed for a few minutes, the tough fibers at the ends
of twigs split into a fine soft "brush." **Warning:** As with hard toothbrushes, Dogwood chewing sticks can cause receding gums.

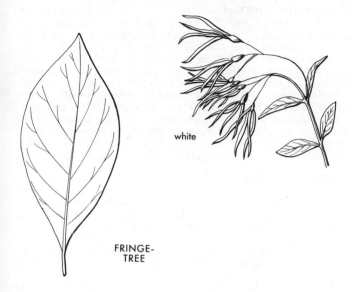

white

FRINGE-
TREE

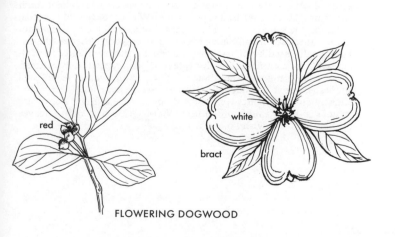

red

white

bract

FLOWERING DOGWOOD

MISCELLANEOUS TREES WITH COMPOUND LEAVES

TREE-OF-HEAVEN, STINKTREE   Bark, root bark
Ailanthus altissima (Mill.) Swingle   **C. Pl. 47**   Quassia Family
Smooth-barked tree; 20–100 ft. Leaves compound, similar to those
of sumacs; crushed leaves *smell like peanuts*. Each leaflet has *2 glan-
dular-tipped teeth at base* (on underside). Flowers small, yellow;
June–July. Male flowers *foul-smelling*. Fruits winged "keys," persist-
ing through winter. **Where found:** Waste places. Throughout our area.
Considered a weed tree in many American cities. Asian alien.

⚠ **Uses:** Two ounces bark infused in 1 quart water, given in teaspoon-
fuls for diarrhea, dysentery, leukorrhea, tapeworm; used in Traditional Chinese Medicine. Recently shown to contain at least
3 potent antimalarial compounds. **Warning:** Large doses potentially
poisonous. Gardeners who cut the tree may suffer from rashes.

KENTUCKY COFFEE-TREE   Bark, pods
Gymnocladus dioicus L.   Pea Family
To 50–60 ft. Compound leaves with 7–13 leaflets. Whitish flowers
in axillary wands; May–June. Hard, flat pods to 10 in. (2½ in. wide),
pulpy within; seeds large, hard. **Where found:** Rich woods. Cen. N.Y.
to Tenn.; Ark. to S.D.

⚠ **Uses:** Caramel-like pod pulp used by American Indians to treat "lu-
nacy." Leaf and pulp tea formerly employed for reflex troubles, and
as a laxative. Root-bark tea used for coughs due to inflamed mucous
membranes, diuretic, given to aid childbirth in protracted labor,
stops bleeding; used in enemas for constipation. **Warning: Toxic** to
grazing animals. Leaves are a fly poison. Seeds contain toxic saponins.

HOPTREE, WAFER ASH   Root bark, young leaves and shoots, fruits
Ptelea trifoliata L.   **C. Pl. 45**   Rue Family
Small tree; 10–20 ft. Leaves palmately divided into *3 parts or leaflets*, mostly without teeth; black-dotted (use lens). Flowers small,
greenish; May–July. Fruits round, 2-seeded "wafers"; July–Sept. Each
seed pair is surrounded by a papery wing. **Where found:** Rocky woods,
outcrops. Sw. Que., N.Y. to Fla.; Texas (Colo., N.M.) to n. Kans., Mo.
Uses: American Indians added root to strengthen other medicine.
Historically used by physicians as a tonic ("surpassed only by Goldenseal") for asthmatic breathing, fevers, poor appetite, gastroenteritis, irritated mucous membranes. A tea of the young leaves and
shoots was once considered useful as a worm expellent. The bitter,
slightly aromatic fruits were once thought to be a useful substitute
to hops in the manufacture of beer. **Warning:** Do not confuse leaves
of this small tree with Poison Ivy leaves.

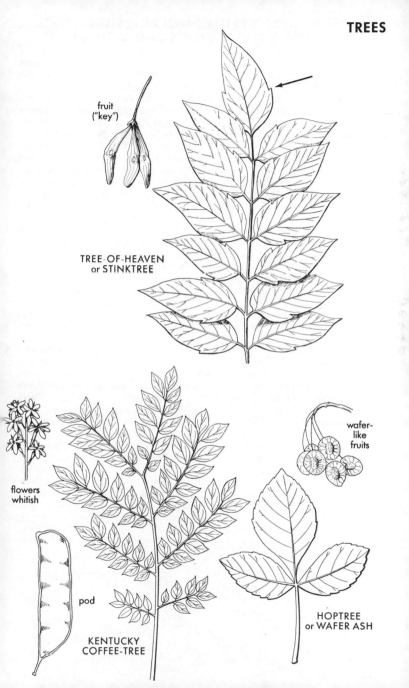

TREES

fruit ("key")

TREE-OF-HEAVEN
or STINKTREE

flowers
whitish

pod

KENTUCKY
COFFEE-TREE

wafer-
like
fruits

HOPTREE
or WAFER ASH

TREES WITH COMPOUND LEAVES;
TRUNK AND BRANCHES USUALLY THORNY

HONEY LOCUST   **Pods, inner bark**
Gleditsia triacanthos L.   **C. Pl. 48**   Pea Family
To 80 ft. This tree is usually armed with large, often compound
thorns (except in form *inermis*, which lacks thorns). Leaves feathery-
compound; leaflets lance-shaped to oblong, barely toothed. Flowers
greenish, clustered; May–July. Fruits flat, twisted pods; 8–18 in.
Where found: Dry woods, openings. N.S. to Fla.; Texas, w. Okla. to
S.D.

Uses: Pods formerly made into tea for indigestion, measles, catarrh
of lungs. Inner-bark tea (with Sycamore bark) was once used for
hoarseness, sore throats. Juice of pods antiseptic. Russian researchers
are studying compounds from leaves to retard certain types of cancer.
Related species: The seedpods of a Chinese species, *G. sinensis*, are
used in Chinese medicine for sore throats, asthmatic coughs, swellings, and stroke. Experimentally, seedpod causes the breakdown of
red blood cells, is strongly antibacterial, antifungal, and acts as an
expectorant, aiding in expelling phlegm and secretions of the respiratory tract. Minute amounts of the seeds are taken in powder for
constipation. The spines constitute another drug used in Traditional
Chinese Medicine; they are used as a wash to reduce swelling and
disperse toxic matter, in the treatment of carbuncles and lesions.
Early reports of cocaine in the plant have been discredited. **Warning:**
All plant parts of both species contain potentially **toxic** compounds.

BLACK LOCUST   **Root bark, flowers**
Robinia pseudo-acacia L.   Pea Family
To 70–90 ft.; armed with stout *paired thorns*, ½–1 in. long. Leaves
pinnately compound; 7–21 elliptic to oval leaflets. Fragrant white
flowers in racemes; May–June. Pods *smooth*, flat; 2–6 in. **Where
found:** Dry woods. Pa. to Ga.; La., Okla. to Iowa; planted elsewhere.
Uses: American Indians chewed root bark to induce vomiting; held
bark in mouth to allay toothaches. A folk tonic, purgative, emetic.
Flower tea used for rheumatism. In China the root bark is also considered purgative and emetic and the flowers are considered diuretic.
Flowers contain a glycoside, robinin, which is experimentally diuretic. **Warning:** All parts are **toxic** — even honey derived from flowers is said to be toxic. The strong odor of the flowers has been reported to cause nausea and headaches in some persons.

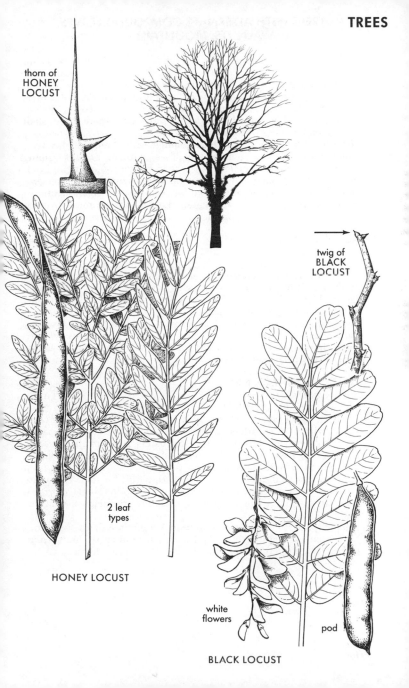

thorn of HONEY LOCUST

twig of BLACK LOCUST

2 leaf types

HONEY LOCUST

white flowers

pod

BLACK LOCUST

TREES WITH ALTERNATE COMPOUND LEAVES; WALNUTS, MOUNTAIN ASH

BUTTERNUT   **Inner bark, nut oil**
Juglans cinerea L.   Walnut Family
To 80 ft. Stem pith *dark brown*. Leaves pinnate, with 7–17 leaflets; leaflets *opposite, rounded at base*, with *minute clusters of downy hairs beneath*. Flowers April–June. Fruits egg-shaped; sticky on outer surface. Nuts rough and deeply furrowed. **Where found:** Rich woods. N.B. to Ga.; west to Ark., N.D.
Uses: Inner-bark tea or extract a popular early American laxative; thought to be effective in small doses, without causing griping (cramps). American Indians used bark in tea for rheumatism, headaches, toothaches; strong warm tea for wounds to stop bleeding, promote healing. Oil from nuts used for tapeworms, fungal infections. Juglone, a component, is antiseptic and herbicidal; some antitumor activity has also been reported.

BLACK WALNUT   **Inner bark, fruits, leaves**
Juglans nigra L.   **C. Pl. 47**   Walnut Family
To 120 ft. Stem pith *light brown*. Leaves pinnate, with 12–23 leaflets; leaflets *slightly alternate, heart-shaped* or *uneven at base*. Leaf stalks and leaf undersides slightly hairy; hairs solitary or in pairs, not in clusters. Fruits rounded; Oct.–Nov. **Where found:** Rich woods. W. Mass. to Fla.; Texas to Minn.
Uses: American Indians used inner-bark tea as an emetic, laxative; bark chewed for toothaches. Fruit-husk juice used on ringworm; husk chewed for colic, poulticed for inflammation. Leaf tea astringent, insecticidal against bedbugs.

AMERICAN MOUNTAIN ASH   **Fruits, bark**
Sorbus americana Marsh.   Rose family
[*Pyrus americana* (Marsh.) DC.]
Shrub or small tree; to 40 ft., with *red gummy* buds. Leaves compound with 11–17 leaflets; leaflets toothed, *long-pointed*, narrow — 3 times longer than broad. Flowers in clusters. Fruits in clusters; *red*, about ¼ in; Aug.–March. **Where found:** Woods, openings. Nfld. to N.C. mountains; Ill. to Man.
Uses: American Indians used tea from ripe fruit for scurvy, worms; tea made from inner bark or buds for colds, debility, boils, diarrhea, tonsillitis; also as a "blood purifier," appetite stimulant; astringent, tonic.
Related species: Fruits of the **European Mountain Ash** (*S. aucuparia*) have been used similarly, for piles, urinary difficulty, indigestion, gall bladder ailments, angina, and other coronary problems.

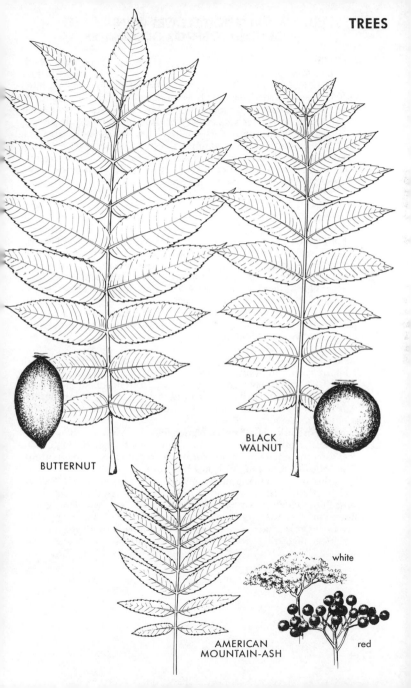

TREES

BUTTERNUT

BLACK
WALNUT

AMERICAN
MOUNTAIN-ASH

white

red

ALTERNATE LEAVES WITH
ROUNDED LOBES OR ODD SHAPES

TULIPTREE   **Bark, leaves, buds**
Liriodendron tulipifera L.   Magnolia Family
To 100 ft. Leaves *spicy; 4-lobed, apex notched.* Flowers to 2 in. long;
tulip-like, green to greenish yellow or yellow-orange. Flowers May–
June. **Where found:** Moist soil. Mass. to Fla.; La., e. Ark., Ill. to Mich.
Uses: American Indians used bark tea for indigestion, dysentery,
rheumatism, pinworms, fevers, and in cough syrups; externally, as a
wash on fractured limbs, wounds, boils, snakebites. Green bark
chewed as an aphrodisiac, stimulant. Bark tea a folk remedy for malaria, toothaches; ointment from buds used for burns, inflammation.
Crushed leaves poulticed for headaches.

WHITE OAK   **Bark**
Quercus alba L.   Beech Family
Tall tree, 60–120 ft. Bark light, flaky; flat-ridged. Leaves with *evenly
rounded lobes,* without bristle-tips; glabrous and whitened beneath
when mature. Bowl-shaped cup covers ⅓ or less of acorn. **Where
found:** Dry woods. Me. to n. Fla.; e. Texas to Minn.
Uses: Astringent inner-bark tea once used for chronic diarrhea, dysentery, chronic mucous discharge, bleeding, anal prolapse, piles; as
a gargle for sore throats and a wash for skin eruptions, poison-ivy
rash, burns; hemostatic. Folk cancer remedy. Contains tannins. Experimentally, tannic acid is antiviral, antiseptic, antitumor *and* carcinogenic. **Warning:** Tannic acid is potentially **toxic.**

SASSAFRAS   **Leaves, twig pith, root bark**
Sassafras albidum (Nutt.) Nees.   **C. Pl. 45**   Laurel Family
Tree; 10–100 ft. Leaves in *3 shapes: oval, mitten-lobed,* or *3-lobed;*
fragrant, mucilaginous. Yellow flowers in clusters; before leaves,
April–May. Fruits blue-black, 1-seeded. **Where found:** Poor soils. S.
Me. to Fla.; Texas to e. Kans.
Uses: Root-bark tea a famous spring blood tonic and "blood purifier"; also a folk remedy for stomachaches, gout, arthritis, high blood
pressure, rheumatism, kidney ailments, colds, fevers, skin eruptions.
The mucilaginous twig pith has been used as wash or poultice for
eye ailments; also taken internally, in tea, for chest, bowel, kidney,
and liver ailments. Leaves mucilaginous, once used to treat stomachaches; widely used as base for soup stocks. **Warning:** Safrole
(found in oil of Sassafras) reportedly is carcinogenic. Banned by FDA.
Yet the safrole in a 12-ounce can of old-fashioned root beer is not as
carcinogenic as the alcohol (ethanol) in a can of beer.

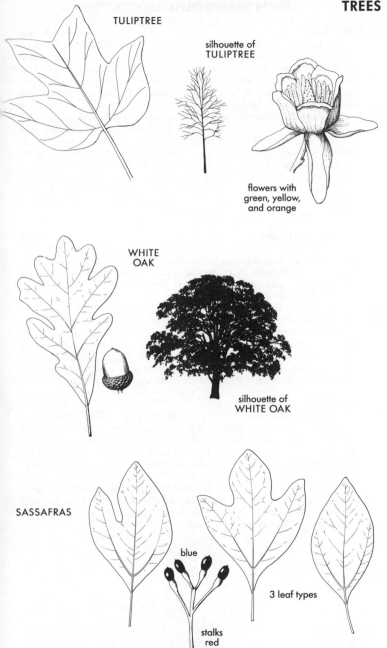

TREES

TULIPTREE

silhouette of
TULIPTREE

flowers with
green, yellow,
and orange

WHITE
OAK

silhouette of
WHITE OAK

SASSAFRAS

blue

3 leaf types

stalks
red

LEAVES SHARP-LOBED *AND* TOOTHED

SWEETGUM   **Inner bark, gum**
Liquidambar styraciflua L.   **C. Pl. 8**   Witch-hazel Family
Tree; to 125 ft. Outer branches often corky-winged. Leaves shiny, star-shaped or maple-like, with 5–7 lobes; lobes pointed, toothed; leaves pine-scented when rubbed or crushed. Fruits spherical (to 1½ in.), with projecting points. **Where found:** Moist woods, bottomland, along waterways. Often invasive in old fields or after logging. Se. Conn. to Fla., Mexico, Cen. America, and Texas; Mo. to Ill.
Uses: Gum or balsam (resin) was traditionally chewed for sore throats, coughs, colds, diarrhea, dysentery, ringworm; used externally for sores, skin ailments, wounds, piles. Ingredient in "compound tincture of benzoin," available from pharmacies. Considered expectorant, antiseptic, antimicrobial, anti-inflammatory. Children sometimes chew the gum in lieu of commercial chewing gum. The mildly astringent inner bark was used as a folk remedy, boiled in milk for diarrhea and cholera infantum.

NORTHERN RED OAK   **Inner bark**
Quercus rubra L.   Beech Family
To 60–120 ft. Bark dark, smoother than White Oak bark. Leaves *hairless, thin, dull,* with 7–11 *bristle-tipped* lobes; leaves 5–9 in. long, 3–6 in. wide. Cup covers ⅓ of acorn. **Where found:** Woods. N.S. to n. Ga.; se. Okla. to Minn.
Uses: Considered similar to but weaker than White Oak (p. 278). Astringent inner-bark tea once used for chronic diarrhea, dysentery, chronic mucous discharge, bleeding, anal prolapse, piles; gargle for sore throats; wash for skin eruptions, poison-ivy rash, burns; hemostatic. Folk cancer remedy. Contains tannins; experimentally, tannic acid has been shown to be antiviral, antiseptic, anticancer *and* carcinogenic. **Warning:** Tannic acid is potentially **toxic.**

SYCAMORE   **Inner bark**
Platanus occidentalis L.   **C. Pl. 46**   Plane-tree Family
Large tree; to 150 ft. Bark mottled, multi-colored, *peeling.* Leaves broadly oval, with 3–5 lobes; 5–8 in. long and wide, with round, shallow sinuses. Fruits globular; to 2 in. across. **Where found:** Moist soils, swamps, lake edges, and stream banks. S. New England to Fla.; Texas to N.M., north to cen. Iowa, Neb.
Uses: American Indians used inner-bark tea for dysentery, colds, lung ailments, measles, coughs; also as a "blood purifier" and emetic (to induce vomiting), laxative. Bark once suggested for rheumatism and scurvy. Efficacy unconfirmed.

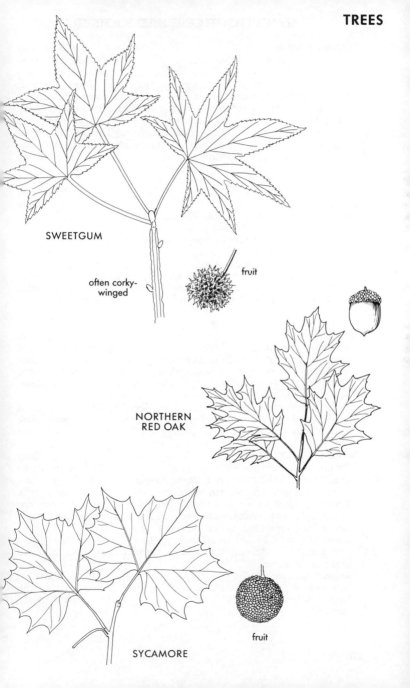

TREES

SWEETGUM

often corky-
winged

fruit

NORTHERN
RED OAK

SYCAMORE

fruit

LEAVES TOOTHLESS; INEDIBLE FRUIT

OSAGE-ORANGE   **Root, fruit**
Maclura pomifera (Raf.) Schneid.   Mulberry Family
Small tree; 30–60 ft. Branches armed with short spines. Leaves lustrous, oval or oblong to lance-shaped. Fruit large (to 6 in.), round, fleshy; surface *brain-like*. Fruits Oct.–Nov. **Where found:** Roadsides, clearings. Mostly spread from cultivation. Originally, Ark. to Texas.
Uses: American Indians used root tea as a wash for sore eyes. Fruit sections used in Md. and Pa. as a cockroach repellent. Inedible fruits contain anti-oxidant and fungicidal compounds. **Warning:** Milk (latex or sap) may cause dermatitis.

CUCUMBER MAGNOLIA   **Bark, fruits**
Magnolia acuminata L.   Magnolia Family
A *deciduous* magnolia; to 80 ft. Leaves large; oblong to lance-shaped. Greenish, cup-shaped flowers appear as leaves unfold, April–June. Fruits resemble small cucumbers. **Where found:** Rich woods. W. N.Y. to Ga.; Ala., Ark. to s. Ill., Ont.
Uses: Bark tea historically used in place of Cinchona (source of quinine) for malarial and typhoid fevers; also for indigestion, rheumatism, worms, toothaches. Bark chewed to break tobacco habit. Fruit tea a tonic for general debility; formerly esteemed for stomach ailments.

SWEETBAY   **Bark, leaves**
Magnolia virginiana L.   Magnolia Family
Small tree or shrub; to 30 ft. Leaves leathery, evergreen (deciduous in North); 3–6 in. long. Flowers white, cup-shaped, *very fragrant*; petals to 2 in. Flowers April–July. **Where found:** Low woods. Mass., Pa. to Fla.; Miss. north to Tenn.
Uses: American Indians used leaf tea to "warm blood," "cure" colds. Traditionally bark used like that of *M. acuminata* (see above). Bark also used for rheumatism, malaria, epilepsy.

CAROLINA BUCKTHORN   **Bark**
Rhamnus caroliniana Walt.   Buckthorn Family
Small tree; 10–30 ft. Leaves elliptic to oval, scarcely fine-toothed; usually smooth beneath when mature, but velvety in var. *mollis*. Flowers *perfect* (each one includes both male and female parts, and petals and sepals). Fruits black; 3-seeded, *not grooved on back*. **Where found:** Rich woods. Va. to Fla.; Texas to Neb.
Uses: American Indians used bark tea to induce vomiting; also a strong laxative. Still used for constipation with nervous or muscular atony of intestines.
Related species: The European species *R. cathartica* and the West Coast species *R. purshiana* (**Cascara Sagrada**) have been used similarly. **Warning:** Fruits and bark of all 3 species will cause diarrhea, vomiting.

TREES

branches spiny

OSAGE-
ORANGE

fruit
green

leaf

fruit

CUCUMBER
MAGNOLIA

greenish

black
fruits

CAROLINA
BUCKTHORN

fruit
("cone")

SWEETBAY

white

LEAVES TOOTHLESS; FRUITS EDIBLE OR A FLAT, INEDIBLE LEGUME

COMMON PAWPAW
Fruits, leaves, seeds

Asimina triloba (L.) Dunal.   **C. Pl. 46**   Custard-apple Family
Small tree or shrub; 9–30 ft. Leaves oblong to lance-shaped (wider above); *large* — to 1 ft. long. Flowers *dull-purple, drooping; petals curved backwards;* April–May. Fruits slightly curved, elongate; green to brown; edible (except seeds) — flavor and texture likened to that of bananas. Seeds toxic; *large, lima-beanlike.* **Where found:** Rich, moist woods. N.J. to Fla., Texas; se. Neb. to Mich.

Uses: Fruit edible, delicious; also a laxative. Leaves insecticidal, diuretic; applied to abscesses. Seeds emetic, narcotic (produce stupor). The powdered seeds, formerly applied to the heads of children to control lice, have insecticidal properties. **Warning:** Seeds **toxic.** Leaves may cause rash.

REDBUD
Bark, flowers

Cercis canadensis L.   **C. Pl. 44**   Pea Family
Small tree with a rounded crown; to 40 ft. Leaves heart-shaped, entire (toothless); 3–6 in. long and wide. Flowers red-purple, pea-like; on long stalks; *in showy clusters before leaves appear,* March–May. Fruit a flat, peapod-shaped, dry, inedible legume; Aug.–Nov. **Where found:** Rich woods, roadsides. S. Conn., s. N.Y. to Fla.; Texas to Wisc. Often planted as an ornamental.

Uses: Inner-bark tea highly astringent. An obscure medicinal agent once used for diarrhea and dysentery; also as a folk cancer remedy for leukemia. Flowers edible.

COMMON PERSIMMON
Bark, fruits

Diospyros virginiana L.   **C. Pl. 48**   Ebony Family
To 15–50 ft. Leaves shiny, elliptic; to 5 in. long. Flowers greenish yellow, thickish, lobed, urn-shaped; May–June. Fruits plumlike, 1–2 in. across; with 6–8 compressed seeds. **Where found:** Dry woods. S. New England to Fla.; Texas, e. Kans.

Uses: Inner-bark tea highly astringent. In folk use, gargled for sore throats and thrush. Bark tea once used as a folk remedy for stomachaches, heartburn, diarrhea, dysentery, and uterine hemorrhage. The bark tea was used as a wash or poulticed for warts and cancers. Fruits edible, but astringent before ripening; best after frost. Seed oil is suggestive of peanut oil in flavor. **Warning:** Contains tannins; potentially **toxic** in large amounts.

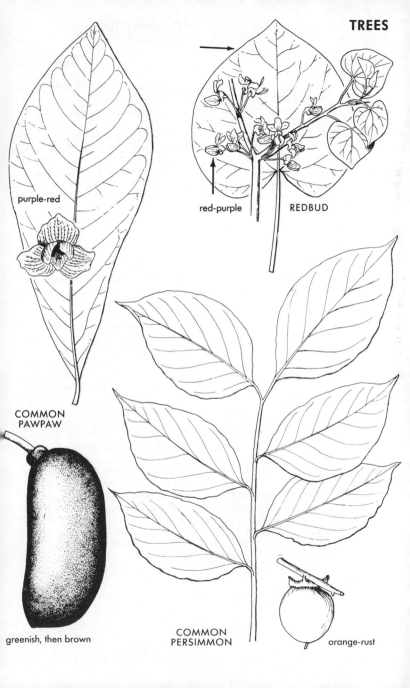

TREES

purple-red

red-purple   REDBUD

COMMON
PAWPAW

greenish, then brown

COMMON
PERSIMMON   orange-rust

MISCELLANEOUS TREES WITH
ALTERNATE, TOOTHED LEAVES

AMERICAN HOLLY   **Leaves, bark, berries**
Ilex opaca Ait.   Holly Family
Evergreen tree; to 90 ft. Leaves, smooth, leathery; with few to many
spine-tipped teeth. Fruits red or orange (rarely yellow); Sept.–Oct.
Sprigs a familiar Christmas decoration. **Where found:** Mixed woods.
E. Mass. to Fla.; Texas, Okla. to Ill.

Uses: American Indians chewed berries for colic, indigestion. Leaf
tea for measles, colds, flu, pneumonia; drops for sore eyes; externally, for sores, itching. Thick syrup of berries formerly used to treat
children's diarrhea. Chewing only 10–12 berries acts as strong laxative, emetic, and diuretic. Bark tea once used in malaria and epilepsy. **Warning:** Fruits considered **poisonous,** inducing violent vomiting.

SOURWOOD, SORREL-TREE   **Leaves, twigs**
Oxydendrum arboreum (L.) DC.   Heath Family
Deciduous tree; to 80 ft. Leaves finely toothed, wide, lance-shaped;
to 6 in. long. Leaf flavor acrid, sour — hence the common name.
Flowers white urns, resembling Lily-of-the-Valley flowers, in drooping panicles to 10 in. long; May–June. Fruits egg-shaped, *upturned;*
about ⅜ in. long. **Where found:** Rich woods. Pa. to Fla.; La. to s. Ind.,
Ohio. Cultivated as an ornamental elsewhere.
Uses: American Indians chewed bark for mouth ulcers. Leaf tea used
for "nerves," asthma, diarrhea, indigestion, and to check excessive
menstrual bleeding. Leaf tea a Kentucky folk remedy for kidney and
bladder ailments (diuretic), fevers, diarrhea, and dysentery. Flowers
yield the famous Sourwood honey.

WHITE WILLOW   **Bark**
Salix alba L.   Willow Family
To 90 ft. Branchlets pliable, *not brittle at base; silky.* Leaves lance-
shaped, mostly without stipules; *white-hairy above and beneath*
(use lens). **Where found:** Naturalized; in moist woods, along stream
edges. Alien (Europe).
Uses: The bark of this willow and other willows with very bitter
and astringent bark has traditionally been used for diarrhea, fevers,
pain, arthritis, rheumatism; poultice or wash used for corns, cuts,
cancers, ulcers, poison-ivy rash, etc. Salicylic acid, derived from salicin (found in bark), is a precursor to the most widely used semisynthetic drug, acetylsalicylic acid (aspirin), which reduces pain, inflammation, and fever. Aspirin reduces risk of heart disease in males;
experimentally, delays cataract formation.

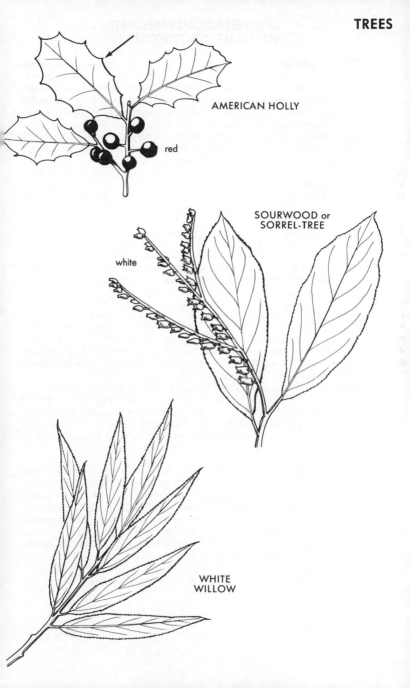

AMERICAN HOLLY

red

SOURWOOD or
SORREL-TREE

white

WHITE
WILLOW

MISCELLANEOUS TREES WITH ALTERNATE, TOOTHED LEAVES

AMERICAN BEECH   Nuts, bark, leaves
Fagus grandifolia Erh.   Beech Family
Large tree; to 80 ft. (occasionally 120 ft.). *Smooth gray bark.* Leaves
oval, *sharp-toothed*, yellow-green, persistent in winter; *veins silky
beneath.* Flowers April–May. Fruits edible *triangular nuts*; Sept.–
Oct. **Where found:** Rich woods. P.E.I. to Fla.; Texas to Ill., Ont.
Uses: American Indians chewed nuts as a worm expellent. Bark tea
used for lung ailments. Leaf tea a wash for burns, frostbite, poison-
ivy rash (1 ounce to 1 pint of salt water).

RED MULBERRY   Root, fruit
Morus rubra L.   Mulberry Family
Small tree; 20–60 ft. Leaves heart-shaped, toothed, often lobed;
sandpapery above, downy beneath. Flowers in tight, drooping clusters. Fruits like a thin blackberry; red, white, or black; June–July.
Where found: Rich woods. Sw. Vt., N.Y. to Fla.; Texas, Okla. to S.D.
Uses: American Indians drank root tea for weakness, difficult urination, dysentery, tapeworms; panacea; externally, sap used for ringworm. Nutritious fruits used for lowering fever. **Warning:** Large doses
cause vomiting.

WHITE MULBERRY (not shown)   Leaves, inner bark
Morus alba L.   Mulberry Family
Similar to Red Mulberry (above), but leaves are *less hairy* and
coarsely toothed, often with 3–5 lobes. Fruits whitish to purple.
Where found: Planted and naturalized in much of our range. Asian
alien; introduced for silkworm production.
Uses: In China, leaf tea used for headaches, hyperemia (congestion
of blood), thirst, coughs; "liver cleanser." Experimentally, leaf extracts are antibacterial. Young twig tea used for arthralgia, edema.
Fruits eaten for blood deficiency, to improve vision and circulation,
and for diabetes. Inner-bark tea used for lung ailments, asthma,
coughs, and edema.

AMERICAN BASSWOOD, LINDEN   Flowers, bark
Tilia americana L.   Basswood Family
Deciduous tree; 60–80 (occasionally 120) ft. Leaves *finely sharp-
toothed; heart-shaped,* base uneven; to 10 in. long. Flowers yellow,
fragrant; from an *unusual winged stalk;* June–Aug. **Where found:**
Rich woods. N.B. to Fla.; Texas to Man.
Uses: American Indians used inner-bark tea for lung ailments, heartburn, weak stomach; bark poultice to draw out boils. Leaves, flower
and bud tea, or tincture traditionally used for nervous headaches,
restlessness, painful digestion. **Warning:** Frequent consumption of
flower tea may cause heart damage.

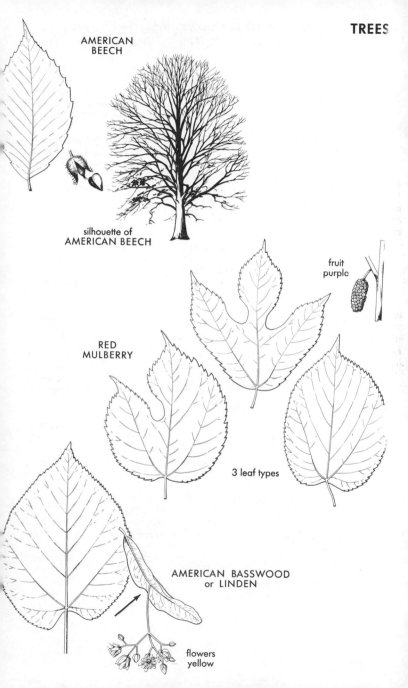

TREES

AMERICAN BEECH

silhouette of
AMERICAN BEECH

RED MULBERRY

fruit purple

3 leaf types

AMERICAN BASSWOOD
or LINDEN

flowers
yellow

TREES WITH ALTERNATE, TOOTHED LEAVES;
ROSE FAMILY: CHERRIES, SERVICEBERRY

SERVICEBERRY   **Root, bark**
Amelanchier canadensis (L.) Medic.   Rose Family
Small tree; to 24 ft. Leaves fine-toothed, oblong, tip rounded; *veins
in 10–15 main pairs, fading at edges.* Flowers white, in drooping
clusters; late March–June. Fruits black. **Where found:** In clumps.
Moist thickets. S. Que., Me. to Ga., Miss.
Uses: Chippewas used root-bark tea (with other herbs) as a tonic for
excessive menstrual bleeding, "female tonic," and to treat diarrhea.
Cherokees used in herb combinations as a digestive tonic. Bath of
bark tea used on children with worms.
Related species: American Indians and Chinese used bark tea of other
Amelanchier species to expel worms.

BLACK or WILD CHERRY   **Bark, fruits**
Prunus serotina Ehrh.   **C. Pl. 48**   Rose Family
Tree; 40–90 ft. Bark rough, dark; reddish beneath. Leaves oval to
lance-shaped, blunt-toothed; smooth above, pale beneath, with *whitish brown hairs on prominent midrib.* Flowers in drooping slender
racemes; April–June. Fruits nearly black cherries. **Where found:** Dry
woods. N.S. to Fla.; Texas to N.D.
Uses: *Aromatic* inner bark traditionally used in tea or syrup for
coughs, "blood tonic," fevers, colds, sore throats, diarrhea, lung ailments, bronchitis, pneumonia, inflammatory fever diseases, and dyspepsia. Useful for general debility with persistent cough, poor circulation, lack of appetite; mild sedative, expectorant. Fruits used as
"poor man's" cherry substitute. **Warning:** Bark, leaves, and seeds
contain a cyanide-like glycoside, prunasin, which converts (when di-
gested) to the **highly toxic** hydrocyanic acid. Toxins are most abundant in bark harvested in fall.

CHOKECHERRY   **Bark, fruits**
Prunus virginiana L.   Rose Family
Shrub or small tree; to 20 ft. Smaller than Black Cherry. Leaves oval,
sharp-toothed, midrib *hairless.* Flowers white, in a thicker raceme;
April–July. Fruits reddish. **Where found:** Thickets. Nfld. to N.C.;
Mo., Kans. to Sask.
Uses: *Non-aromatic* bark, similar to that of Black Cherry. Externally, used for wounds. Dried powdered berries once used to stimulate appetite, treat diarrhea, bloody discharge of bowels. **Warning:** As
with Black Cherry, seeds, bark, and leaves may cause cyanide poisoning.

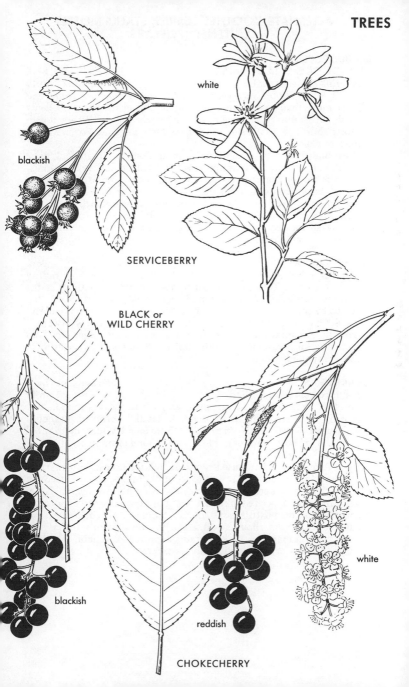

TREES

white

blackish

SERVICEBERRY

BLACK or
WILD CHERRY

blackish

white

reddish

CHOKECHERRY

ALTERNATE, TOOTHED LEAVES; STALKS MOSTLY FLATTENED; POPLARS

BALSAM POPLAR, BALM-OF-GILEAD, TACAMAHAC
Populus balsamifera L.

Leaf buds, root, bark
Willow Family

To 30–90 ft. Winter buds *yellowish, gummy, strongly fragrant;* end buds more than ½ in. long. Leaves broadly oval, with *fine wavy teeth;* leafstalks mostly *rounded* (rather than flat). **Where found:** Moist soils. Lab. to Alaska; south to n. New England, Wisc., Minn., Iowa to Colo.

Uses: Buds boiled to separate resin, then dissolved in alcohol, once used as preservative in ointments. Folk remedy (balm) used for sores; tincture for toothaches, rheumatism, diarrhea, wounds; tea used as a wash for inflammation, frostbite, sprains, and muscle strain. Internally, bud tea used for cough, lung ailments (expectorant). Inner-bark tea used for scurvy, also as an eye wash, "blood tonic." Root tea used as a wash for headaches. Probably contains salicin, explaining its aspirin-like qualities.

COTTONWOOD
Populus deltoides Marsh.

Bark
Willow Family

Large tree; to 150 ft. Leaves broadly oval, coarsely toothed; stalks *flattened* with *2–3 glands at top of each stalk* (use lens). Seeds dispersed by cottony "parachutes." **Where found:** Along streams and rivers. S. Que., w. New England to Fla.; Texas to Man. and westward.

Uses: Inner-bark tea used for scurvy, and as a female tonic. Tree held sacred by American Indians of the prairies. Bark contains the aspirin-like compound, salicin.

QUAKING ASPEN
Populus tremuloides Michx.

Root, bark, leaf buds
Willow Family

To 60 ft. Bark smooth, greenish to gray-white. Leaves roundish to broadly oval, smooth, *fine-toothed;* leafstalks *flattened.* Branches and leaves *sway restlessly in breeze.* **Where found:** Widely distributed in n. U.S.; absent south of n. Mo., Tenn.; found again in highlands of w. Texas, s. Calif.

Uses: American Indians used root-bark tea for excessive menstrual bleeding; poulticed root for cuts, wounds. Inner-bark tea used for stomach pain, venereal disease, urinary ailments, worms, colds, fevers, and as an appetite stimulant. Leaf buds used in a salve for colds, coughs, irritated nostrils. Bark tincture (contains salicin) a folk remedy used for fevers, rheumatism, arthritis, colds, worms, urinary infections, and diarrhea. Bark contains aspirin-like salicin, which is anti-inflammatory, analgesic; reduces fevers.

TREES

BALSAM POPLAR or
BALM-OF-GILEAD

buds
yellowish,
gummy

COTTONWOOD

seeds
with
cottony
parachutes

fruits

QUAKING ASPEN

flower
("catkin")

ALTERNATE, DOUBLE-TOOTHED LEAVES

SWEET or BLACK BIRCH   Bark, twigs, essential oil
Betula lenta L.   Birch Family
To 50–70 ft. Non-peeling, *sweet, aromatic, black bark*, often smooth, like that of our more familiar white birches, but black and not papery. Leaves oval, toothed; to 6 in. long. Buds and leaves *hairless*. Broken twigs and to a lesser extent, the leaves, have a strong *wintergreen fragrance*. Inconspicuous, separate male and female flowers in catkins; early spring. Fruits are oblong, upright; ¾–1¼ in. long. **Where found:** Rich woods. S. Que., sw. Me. to n. Ga., Ala.; north to e. Ohio.

⚠️ **Uses:** Our most fragrant birch was widely used by American Indians, in bark tea for fevers, stomachaches, lung ailments; twig tea for fever. Essential oil (methyl salicylate) distilled from bark was used for rheumatism, gout, scrofula, bladder infection, neuralgia; anti-inflammatory, analgesic. To alleviate pain or sore muscles, the oil has been applied as a counterirritant. Essential oil was formerly produced in Appalachia. But now, methyl salicylate is produced synthetically, using menthol as the precursor. **Warning:** Essential oil **toxic.** Easily absorbed through skin. Fatalities reported.

SLIPPERY ELM   Inner bark
Ulmus rubra Muhl.   Elm Family
[*U. fulva* Michx.]
To 40–60 ft., with large, *rust-hairy* buds. White, mildly scented, inner bark is very mucilaginous ("slippery"). Leaves oval; 3–7 in. long, to 3 in. wide; sides of base distinctly unequal. Leaves *sandpapery above*, soft-hairy below; *sharply double-toothed*. Papery, winged, yellowish green, 1-seeded fruits, about ½ in. wide, *without hairs on margins*; March–May. **Where found:** Moist woods. Me. to Fla.; Texas to N.D.
Uses: Three tablespoons of inner bark in a cup of hot water makes a thick, mucilaginous tea, traditionally used for sore throats, upset stomach, indigestion, digestive irritation, stomach ulcers, coughs, pleurisy; said to help in diarrhea and dysentery. Inner bark considered edible. Once used as a nutritive broth for children, the elderly, and convalescing patients who had difficulty consuming or digesting food. Externally, the thick tea, made from powdered inner bark, was applied to fresh wounds, ulcers, burns, scalds. Science confirms tea is soothing to mucous membranes and softens hardened tissue. Bark once used as an anti-oxidant to prevent rancidity of fat. Slivers of inner bark once used — dangerously — as a mechanical abortefacient.

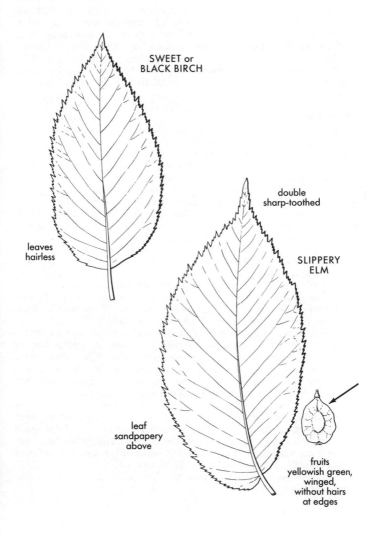

SWEET or
BLACK BIRCH

leaves
hairless

double
sharp-toothed

SLIPPERY
ELM

leaf
sandpapery
above

fruits
yellowish green,
winged,
without hairs
at edges

BARK GREEN; LEAVES SIMPLE, SHINY; VINES AND MISTLETOE

SUPPLEJACK, RATTAN VINE   **Leaf, bark**
Berchemia scandens (Hill) K. Koch.   Buckthorn Family
High-climbing, twining woody vine; stems *smooth, green*. Alternate, oval leaves with *conspicuous parallel veins*; no teeth. Tiny white flowers in panicles; May. Dark blue fruit in clusters; Sept.–Oct.
Where found: Moist woods, thickets. Se. Va. to Fla., Texas; north to s. Ill.
Uses: American Indians used bark or leaf tea as a "blood purifier" and to restore youthful vigor and sexual vitality. Tea of burned stems used for coughs.

MISTLETOE   **Leafy branches**
Phoradendron serotinum (Raf.) M.C. Johnston   Mistletoe Family
[*Phoradendron flavescens* (Pursh) Nutt.]
Parasitic, thick-branched perennial; semi-evergreen. Leaves oblong to obovate; to 3 in. long. Flowers small. Fruits *translucent white*.
Where found: On trees. N.J. to Fla.; Mo. north to Ohio, Minn.
Uses: American Indians used tea for epilepsy, "fits," headaches, hypertension, lung ailments, debility, paralysis; also as oral contraceptive. Formerly used to stop bleeding after childbirth. **Warning:** Often considered **poisonous.** Unconfirmed reports of deaths have been attributed to eating berries. May cause dermatitis.

SAWBRIER, WILD SARSAPARILLA   **Root**
Smilax glauca L.   Lily Family
Entangling, climbing shrub, with stiff prickles. Leaves with a *whitish film*; oval, base rounded or heart-shaped; *white beneath*. Flowers not showy. Berries blue to black; July–winter. **Where found:** Thickets. S. New England to Fla.; Texas to Okla., Ind.
Uses: American Indians rubbed stem prickles on skin as a counter-irritant to relieve localized pains, muscle cramps, twitching; leaf and stem tea used for rheumatism, stomach troubles. Wilted leaves poulticed on boils. Root tea taken to help expel afterbirth. We cannot confirm rumors that *Smilax* roots contain testosterone (male hormone); they may contain steroid precursors, however.

GREENBRIER, CATBRIER   **Leaves, stems, roots**
Smilax rotundifolia L.   **C. Pl. 32**   Lily Family
Green, stout-thorny, climbing shrub. Leaves leathery, round, shiny; base mostly heart-shaped. Fruits blue-black; July–Nov. **Where found:** Thickets. Weedy. N.S. to Fla.; e. Texas to s. Ill.
Uses: Same as for *S. glauca* (above). Most of our *Smilax* species are used similarly.

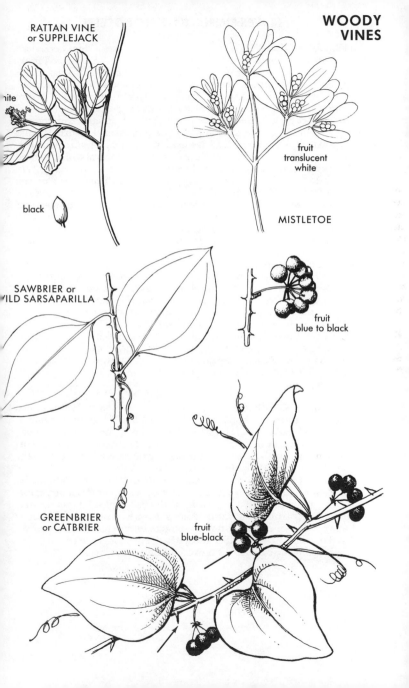

WOODY VINES

RATTAN VINE or SUPPLEJACK

white

black

MISTLETOE

fruit translucent white

SAWBRIER or WILD SARSAPARILLA

fruit blue to black

GREENBRIER or CATBRIER

fruit blue-black

LEAVES SIMPLE; BARK NOT GREEN

AMERICAN BITTERSWEET   **Root bark, fruits**
Celastrus scandens L.   Staff-tree Family
Climbing, twining shrub; to 50 ft. Leaves *ovate to oblong*, sharp-
pointed, fine-toothed. Flowers greenish, in clusters; May–June. Fruit
capsule scarlet to orange, *splitting*, to reveal *scarlet* seeds. **Where
found:** Rich thickets. Que. to Ga., Ala.; Okla. to N.D.

Uses: Root-bark tea induces sweating; diuretic, emetic. Folk remedy
for chronic liver and skin ailments, rheumatism, leukorrhea, suppressed menses. Externally, bark used in ointment for burns, scrapes,
skin eruptions. American Indians used this plant as above, also used
astringent leaf tea for diarrhea, dysentery. Root-bark tea used for pain
of childbirth. Bark extracts thought to be cardioactive. **Warning:**
Fruit **toxic. All parts potentially toxic.**
Related species: Oriental Bittersweet (*C. orbiculatus*), an Asian species naturalized in many areas, differs in that the flowers occur in
groups of 1–3, in axillary cymes. Uncommon, but a serious weed in
some areas. Uses in Asia similar to those for the American species.

YELLOW JESSAMINE   **Roots**
Gelsemium sempervirens (L.) Ait.   Logania Family
Twining, tangling evergreen shrub. Leaves lance-shaped to oval;
shiny. Flowers yellow, shaped like an open trumpet with *5 rounded
petal lobes* that are *notched at end*; sweetly fragrant. Feb.–June.
Where found: Dry or wet woods, thickets. Se. Va. to Fla.; Texas to Ark.
Uses: Root preparations were once used as a powerful CNS-depres-
sant, deadening pain, reducing spasms. Externally, a folk cancer rem-

edy. **Warning: Deadly poison.** Eating a single flower has resulted in
death. Can also cause contact dermatitis.

JAPANESE HONEYSUCKLE   **Bark, flowers, leaves**
Lonicera japonica Thunb.   **C. Pl. 32**   Honeysuckle Family
Evergreen trailing, twining vine. Leaves oval, entire (not toothed).
Flowers white or buff; lobes strongly spreading from throat, stamens
protruding; April–July. **Where found:** Noxious weed in much of the
South; north to Mass., Ind. Alien.
Uses: Leaves and flowers a beverage tea (Japan). Flowers traditionally
used (in e. Asia) in tea for bacterial dysentery, enteritis, laryngitis,
fevers, flu; externally, as a wash for rheumatism, sores, tumors (especially breast cancer), infected boils, scabies, swelling. Stem tea is
weaker. Experimentally, flower extracts lower cholesterol; also antiviral, antibacterial, tuberculostatic. This serious weed might be
managed by utilizing it for proven medicinal purposes.

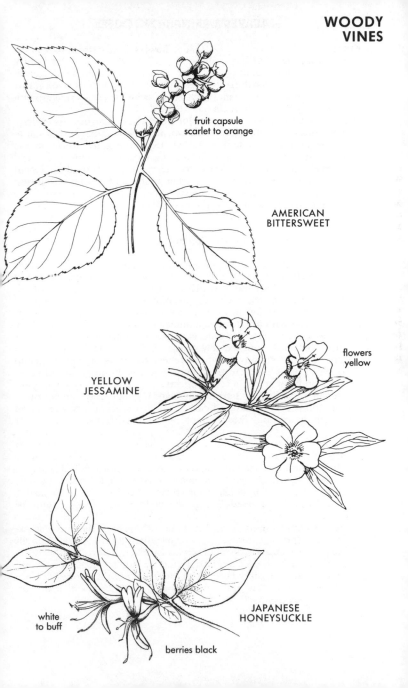

WOODY VINES

fruit capsule
scarlet to orange

AMERICAN
BITTERSWEET

YELLOW
JESSAMINE

flowers
yellow

white
to buff

JAPANESE
HONEYSUCKLE

berries black

LEAVES 3-PARTED OR LOBED

KUDZU
Root, flowers, seeds, stems, root starch

Pueraria lobata (Willd.) Owhi   **C. Pl. 32**   Pea Family

Noxious, robust, trailing, climbing vine. Leaves *palmate, 3-parted;* leaflets entire or palmately lobed. Flowers reddish purple, *grape-scented;* in a loose raceme; July–Sept. **Where found:** Waste ground. Pa. to Fla.; Texas to Kans. Asian alien.

Uses: In China, root tea used for headaches, diarrhea, dysentery, acute intestinal obstruction, gastroenteritis, deafness; to promote measle eruptions, induce sweating. Experimentally, lowers blood sugar and blood pressure. Flower tea used for stomach acidity, "awakens the spleen," "expels drunkenness." Seeds used for dysentery and to expel drunkenness. Stem poulticed for sores, swellings, mastitis; tea gargled for sore throats. Root starch (used to stimulate production of body fluids) eaten as food.

POISON IVY
Leaf preparations

Toxicodendron radicans (L.) Kuntze   Cashew Family
[*Rhus radicans* L.]   **C. Pl. 31**

Highly variable — trailing or climbing vine or erect shrub. Leaves on long, glossy to hairy stalks; 3 highly variable leaflets, outer one on a longer stalk. Flowers whitish; berries white. Fruits Aug.–Nov. **Where found:** Woods, thickets. Most of our area.

Uses: Once used by physicians for paralytic and liver disorders. Fighting fire with fire, American Indians rubbed leaves on poison-ivy rash as a treatment. Micro doses are used homeopathically to treat poison-ivy rash. Crushed Jewelweed, or Touch-me-not (p. 136), is also rubbed on skin to prevent or relieve outbreak of rash. **Warning:** Touching plant often causes severe dermatitis. Internal consumption of Poison Ivy may cause severe effects, necessitating steroid or other therapies. Smoke from burning plant and dried plant specimens more than 100 years old can still cause dermatitis. Ironically, the active ingredient, urushiol, inhibits prostaglandin synthesis.

FOX GRAPE
Leaves, berries

Vitis labrusca L.   Grape Family

A high-climbing liana vine. Leaves rounded in outline, heart-shaped at base; 3-lobed, toothed, with *dense whitish to reddish felt beneath.* Fruits about 20 purple-black (or amber white) grapes in a cluster; Sept.–Oct. **Where found:** Thickets, woods. S. Me. to Ga.; Tenn. to Mich.

Uses: American Indians used leaf tea for diarrhea, hepatitis, stomachaches, thrush; externally, poulticed wilted leaves for sore breasts; also poulticed leaves for rheumatism, headaches, fevers. Other *Vitis* species have been used similarly. Vines, when cut in summer, yield potable water, possibly purer than today's acid-rain water. **Warning:** Do not confuse this vine with Canada Moonseed, which is considered **toxic** (see p. 302).

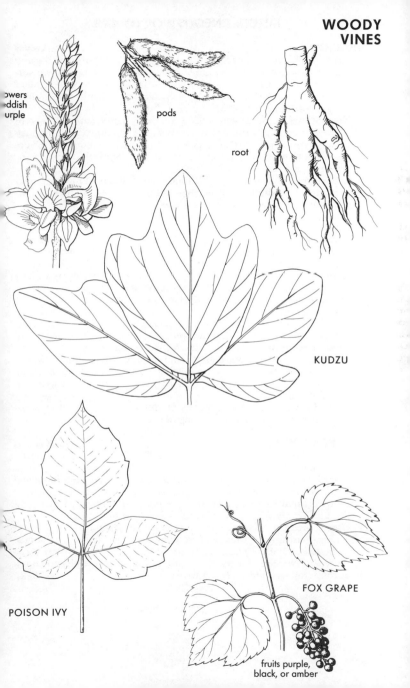

WOODY VINES

flowers
reddish
purple

pods

root

KUDZU

POISON IVY

FOX GRAPE

fruits purple,
black, or amber

MISCELLANEOUS WOODY VINES

DUTCHMAN'S-PIPE   **Leaves**
Aristolochia tomentosa Sims   Birthwort Family
Climbing woody vine. Leaves *heart-shaped*, blunt-tipped; lower surface *densely covered with soft white hairs*. Flowers *pipe-like*; calyx yellowish; May–June. **Where found:** Rich river banks. N.C., Fla., Texas; north to e. Kans., Mo., s. Ill., s. Ind.

 Uses: Similar to but much weaker in effect than Virginia Snakeroot (*A. serpentaria*, p. 224). Aromatic weak tea promotes sweating, appetite; expectorant. Used for fevers, stomachaches, indigestion, suppressed menses, snakebites. Little used. **Warning:** Potentially irritating in large doses.
Related species: *A. macrophylla* (not shown) differs in having nearly smooth, sharp-pointed leaves. Flowers brown-purple. Ironically, Virginia farmers spray *A. macrophylla* as a weed. It contains the antiseptic, antitumor compound aristolochic acid.

CANADA MOONSEED   **Leaves, root**
Menispermum canadense L.   Moonseed Family
Climbing woody vine; 8–12 ft. Root bright yellow within. Leaves smooth, with *3–7 angles or lobes; stalk attached above base.* Flowers small, whitish; in loose clusters; June–Aug. **Where found:** Rich, moist thickets. Que., w. New England south to Ga.; Ark., Okla.

 Uses: American Indians used root tea for indigestion, arthritis, bowel disorders; also as a "blood cleanser" and "female tonic"; externally, salve used for chronic sores. Historically, physicians used root (tincture) as a laxative, diuretic; for indigestion, rheumatism, arthritis, syphilis, general debility, and chronic skin infections. **Warning: Poisonous.** Fatalities have been reported from children eating seeds and fruits. Some people reportedly confuse this plant with edible wild grapes.
Related species: The Asian species *M. dahurica* has been used similarly; also for cervical and esophageal cancers.

VIRGINIA CREEPER   **Root, leaves**
Parthenocissus quinquefolia   **C. Pl. 32**   Grape Family
(L.) Planchon
Climbing (or creeping) vine with *adhesive disks on much-branched tendrils.* Leaves divided into *5 leaflets;* elliptical to oval, sharply toothed. Small flowers in terminal groups; June. **Where found:** Thickets, etc. Weedy. Me. to Fla.; Texas to Kans., Minn.

 Uses: American Indians used plant tea for jaundice; root tea for gonorrhea, diarrhea. Leaf tea used to wash swellings and poison-sumac rash; mixed with vinegar for wounds and lockjaw; astringent and diuretic. **Warning:** Berries reportedly **toxic.** Leaves **toxic;** touching autumn foliage may cause dermatitis.

302

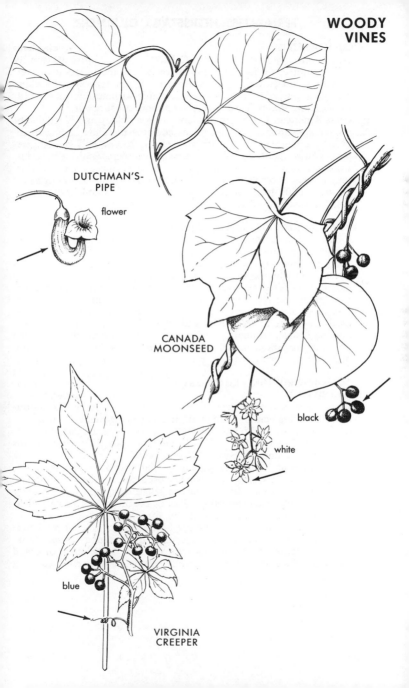

WOODY
VINES

DUTCHMAN'S-
PIPE

flower

CANADA
MOONSEED

black

white

VIRGINIA
CREEPER

blue

FERN ALLIES: HORSETAILS, CLUBMOSS

FIELD HORSETAIL
Whole plant

Equisetum arvense L.   **C. Pl. 7**   Horsetail Family

Stiff-stemmed, apparently leafless herb; to 1 ft. Internodes elongate; sheaths of nodes with 8–12 distinct teeth (the leaves). Branchlets *radiating upward from nodes*. Fertile stalks without branches; to 18 in. Variable. **Where found:** Damp sandy soil. Most of our area.

⚠️ **Uses:** American Indians used plant tea for kidney and bladder ailments, constipation. Asian Indians consider the Field Horsetail diuretic, hemostatic. Root given to teething babies. Folk remedy for bloody urine, gout, gonorrhea, stomach disorders. Poultice used for wounds. High silica content. Also once used in tea for tubercular lung lesions. Shown to be valuable against inflammation, though scientific validity in question. **Warning: Toxic** to livestock; questionable for humans — disturbs thiamine metabolism.

SCOURING RUSH, GREATER HORSETAIL
Whole plant

Equisetum hyemale L.   **C. Pl. 2**   Horsetail Family

Evergreen, hollow-stemmed, rough-surfaced, jointed herb; to 5 ft. Variable. **Where found:** Moist sandy soils. Most of our area.

⚠️ **Uses:** Essentially the same as for *E. arvense* (above), though this species is considered stronger by some authors. A folk remedy used throughout the Northern Hemisphere. Rough stems are used like sandpaper to give a very fine, satiny finish to wood. Early settlers used the stems to scour pots and pans. Homeopathically used for cystitis, bladder ailments, urinary incontinence, urethritis. **Warning: Toxic** to livestock; questionable for humans — disturbs thiamine metabolism.

COMMON or RUNNING CLUBMOSS, GROUND PINE
Leaves, spores

Lycopodium clavatum L.   Clubmoss Family

Mosslike evergreen; 3–15 in., with long, creeping runners. Tiny, linear leaves, *tipped with soft, hairlike bristles*. Spores on leafy-bracted stalk, with 1–6 strobiles. **Where found:** Dry woods. Canada south to N.Y., N.C. mountains; west to Wisc., Wash.

⚠️ **Uses:** American Indians used plant tea for postpartum pains, fever, weakness. In folk medicine, spores used for diarrhea, dysentery, rheumatism; also as diuretic, gastric sedative, aphrodisiac, styptic; externally, in powders for baby's chafing, tangled or matted hair with vermin, herpes, eczema, dermatitis in folds of skin, erysipelas. Spores, called "vegetable sulphur," formerly used to coat pills and suppositories. A related Chinese species in the clubmoss family is being researched as a potential treatment for Alzheimer's disease. **Warning:** This clubmoss (*L. clavatum*) contains a **toxic** alkaloid.

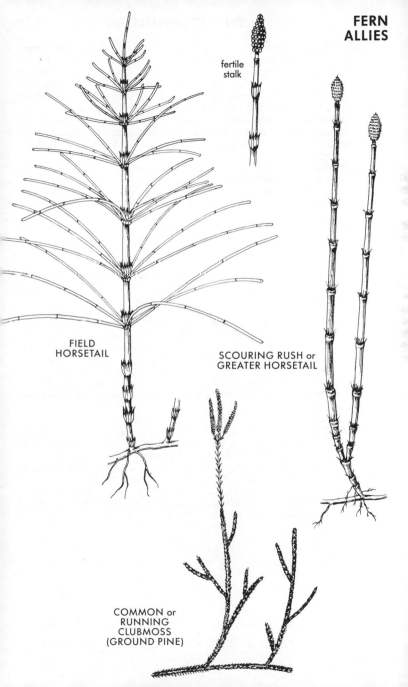

FERN ALLIES

fertile stalk

FIELD HORSETAIL

SCOURING RUSH or GREATER HORSETAIL

COMMON or RUNNING CLUBMOSS (GROUND PINE)

EVERGREEN FERNS

RESURRECTION FERN   **Leaves, stems**
Polypodium polypodioides (L.) D. Watt.   Fern Family
Small *evergreen* fern; to 8 in. Shrivels when dry; unfurls and turns green after rain. Leaves *leathery, blunt-lobed;* smooth above, densely scaly below. **Where found:** Shaded rocks, trees (epiphytic), stumps. N.J. to Fla., Texas, and Cen. America; north to Kans., Iowa.
Uses: American Indians used ointment of heated stem and leaves for sores, ulcers. Leaf tea used for headaches, dizziness, thrush, sore mouth, and bleeding gums.

COMMON POLYPODY   **Root, whole fern**
Polypodium virginianum L.   Fern Family
[*Polypodium vulgare* L.]
Vigorous, evergreen, mat-forming fern; to 12 in. Leaves leathery; deep green above, *smooth below;* 10–20 leaflet pairs; veins obvious, variable. **Where found:** Shaded, rich, shallow soils or among rocks. Nfld. to Ga. mountains; Ark. to e. S.D., Minn.

 Uses: American Indians used root tea for pleurisy, hives, sore throats, stomachaches; poulticed root for inflammations. Historically, root steeped in milk as laxative for children. Once considered valuable for lung ailments and liver disease. Tea or syrup of whole plant used for liver ailments, pleurisy, worms. Like Male Fern (p. 310), this fern was believed to be toxic to tapeworms. The root has a unique, rather unpleasant odor, and a sweet (cloying) flavor at first, but then quickly becomes nauseating. Root contains fructose, glucose, and sucrose, plus methyl salicylate (wintergreen flavor — see p. 26); it may also contain glycyrrhizin, the sweetener found in Licorice root (*Glycyrrhiza* species), but reports to that effect have not been confirmed. Root contains up to 2 percent insect-regulating "hormones." Resins active against worms. **Warning:** Of unknown toxicity.

CHRISTMAS FERN   **Root**
Polystichum acrostichoides (Michx.) Schott.   Fern Family
Shiny evergreen fern; 1–3 ft. Leaves lustrous, leathery, tapering; leaflets *bristle-tipped, strongly eared;* teeth incurved. **Where found:** Rich wooded slopes. N.B. to n. Fla.; e. Texas to Kans., Wisc.
Uses: American Indians used root tea for chills, fevers, stomachaches (to induce vomiting), pneumonia; poulticed root for rheumatism. **Warning:** Of unknown toxicity.

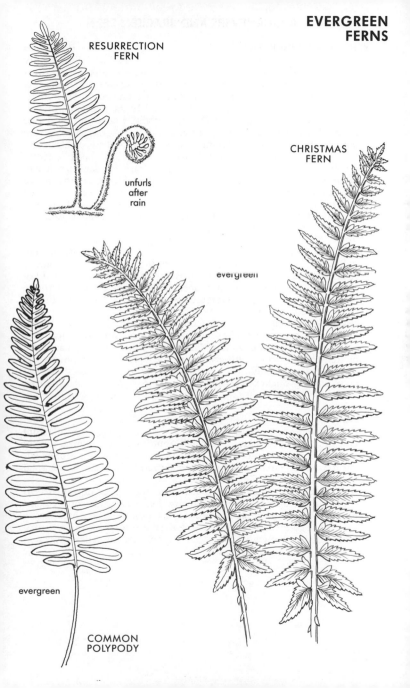

EVERGREEN FERNS

RESURRECTION FERN

unfurls after rain

CHRISTMAS FERN

evergreen

evergreen

COMMON POLYPODY

MAIDENHAIRS AND BRACKEN FERN

VENUS MAIDENHAIR FERN   **Whole fern**
Adiantum capillus-veneris L.   Fern Family
Fronds to 20 in.; oblong in outline, mostly twice-compound. Leaflets
very thin; wedge-shaped, lobed at apex. Stalk delicate, brittle; shiny,
dark, scaly at base. **Where found:** Wet limestone rocks, waterfalls,
bluffs; usually in shaded areas. Va. to Fla., Texas, and Calif.; north
through Utah, Colo. to Mo., S.D. Introduced as a curio farther north.
Found throughout many parts of the world.
Uses: In folk tradition, a handful of dried leaves are steeped to make
a tea drink as an expectorant, astringent, and tonic for coughs, throat
afflictions, and bronchitis. Used as a hair wash for dandruff and to
promote hair growth. In Traditional Chinese Medicine, the leaves
are similarly used for bronchial diseases and as an expectorant. This
fern has also been used as a worm expellent, an emetic, and an agent
to reduce fevers. Externally, it has been poulticed on snakebites, and
used as a treatment for impetigo.

MAIDENHAIR FERN   **Whole fern**
Adiantum pedatum L.   **C. Pl. 14**   Fern Family
A distinctive fern; to 1 ft. Flat, *horseshoe-like* fronds atop a *shiny
black* stalk. Leaflets long, fan-shaped, lobed on upper side; alternate.
Where found: Rich woods, moist limestone ravines. Me. south to Ga.,
La.; west to Okla.; north to Minn. and westward.
Uses: Considered expectorant, cooling, and antirheumatic. Tea or
syrup used for nasal congestion, asthma, sore throats, hoarseness,
colds, fevers, flu, and pleurisy. This fern was highly valued as a medicinal plant by some 19th-century medical practitioners, suggesting
that its efficacy should be investigated by science. Stems were used
by Indians throughout N. America as a hair wash to make their hair
shiny.

BRACKEN FERN   **Root**
Pteridium aquilinum (L.) Kuhn   Fern Family
Our most common fern; 3–6 ft. tall, forming large colonies. Leaves
triangular, divided into 3 parts; leaflets blunt-tipped; upper ones not
cut to midrib. Variable. **Where found:** Barren soils. Much of our area;
mostly absent from Great Plains.

Uses: American Indians used root tea for stomach cramps, diarrhea;
smoke for headaches; poulticed root for burns and sores, caked
breasts; wash to promote hair growth; astringent, tonic. Historically,
root tea used for worms. **Warning: Poisonous** in excess doses — disturbs thiamine metabolism. Recently reported to cause cancer in
grazing animals; contains at least 3 carcinogens.

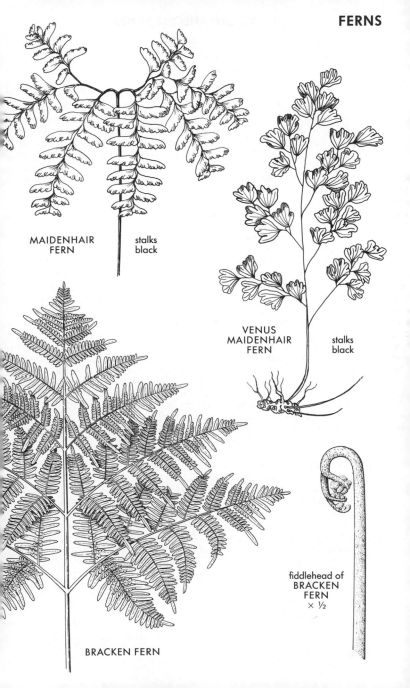

FERNS

MAIDENHAIR FERN

stalks black

VENUS MAIDENHAIR FERN

stalks black

fiddlehead of BRACKEN FERN × ½

BRACKEN FERN

MISCELLANEOUS FERNS

LADY FERN
Root (rhizome)

Athyrium filix-femina (L.) Roth. Fern Family

"Discouragingly variable" (*Gray's Manual*, 8th ed.). Fern; to 3 ft. Stems *smooth*, with a *few pale scales*. Grows in circular clumps from horizontal rootstock. Leaves (fronds) broad, lance-shaped; mostly twice-divided, lacy-cut; *tips drooping*. *Leaflets toothed*. **Where found:** Moist, shaded areas. Much of our area.

Uses: American Indians used root tea as a diuretic, to stop breast pains caused by childbirth, induce milk in caked breasts. Stem tea taken to ease labor. Like many ferns, this one was traditionally used to eliminate worms. Dried, powdered root used externally for sores.

Related species: Japanese researchers found anti-gout potential in the related fern *A. mersosorum*.

RATTLESNAKE FERN
Root

Botrychium virginianum (L.) Swartz Adder's-tongue Family

The largest *Botrychium* in our area. Delicate, lacy, nonleathery, broadly triangular leaf (sterile frond); to 10 in. long, 12 in. wide. Fertile frond on a much longer stalk, bearing bright yellow spores. **Where found:** Rich, moist or dry woods. P.E.I., Minn. to Fla.; Calif., B.C. Unfurls before other Botrychiums.

Uses: American Indians used root poultice or lotion for snakebites, bruises, cuts, sores. In folk medicine, root tea emetic, induces sweating; also an expectorant, used for lung ailments.

CRESTED WOOD FERN
Root

Dryopteris cristata (L.) Gray Fern Family

Ladderlike, blue-green fern. Leaves 30 in. long, to 5 in. wide (widest above middle), with 20 or so *horizontal* leaflet pairs. Spore-bearing areas (sori) kidney-shaped, halfway between margin and midvein (leaf underside). **Where found:** Damp woods. Nfld. to Tenn., n. La.; Neb. to N.D.

Uses: Root tea traditionally used to induce sweating, clear chest congestion, expel intestinal worms.

MALE FERN
Roots

Dryopteris filix-mas (L.) Schott Fern Family

Yellow-green, leathery, semi-evergreen fern; 7–20 in., with blackish, thick-wiry roots. Leaves divided into about 20 lance-shaped, pointed leaflets; leaflets narrow, oblong, cut nearly to midrib, with rounded lobes or subleaflets, or slightly toothed. **Where found:** Rocky woods. Me., Vt., N.Y. to Mich.

Uses: An oleoresin extracted from the roots has been used as a worm expellent. It is toxic to tapeworms. **Warning: Toxic** poison and skin irritant.

EVERGREEN FERNS

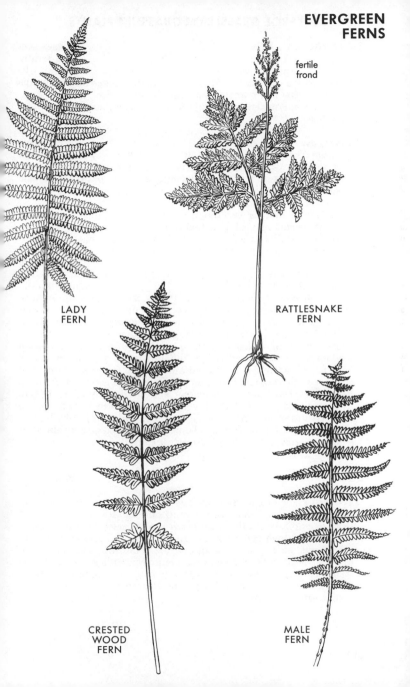

fertile frond

LADY FERN

RATTLESNAKE FERN

CRESTED WOOD FERN

MALE FERN

LARGE GRASSES OR GRASSLIKE PLANTS

SWEETFLAG, CALAMUS   **Rootstock**
Acorus americanus L.   **C. Pl. 5**   Arum Family
Strongly aromatic perennial; 1–4 ft. Root jointed. *Cattail-like leaves*, with a *vertical midrib*. Flowers tightly packed on a fingerlike spadix, jutting *at an angle* from leaflike stalk. Flowers May–Aug.
Where found: Pond edges, wet fields. Most of our area.
Uses: See p. 86.

GIANT CANE   **Root**
Arundinaria gigantea (Walt.) Muhl.   **C. Pl. 3**   Grass Family
Bamboo-like, woody-stemmed grass; to 10 ft. Lance-shaped leaves, in fanlike clusters. Flowers in racemes, on *leafy branches.* **Where found:** River and stream banks. Forms large thickets. S. Del. to Fla.; Texas to Ill.
Uses: Houma Indians used root decoction (see p. 7) to stimulate kidneys. **Warning:** Ergot, a highly toxic fungus, occasionally replaces the large seeds of Giant Cane. Do not collect or use any specimens from areas with diseased plants.

COMMON CATTAIL   **Root, seed down**
Typha latifolia L.   Cattail Family
Perennial; 4–8 ft., forming thick stands. Leaves *swordlike.* Stiff, erect flowering stalks, topped with yellow, pollen-laden *male flowers* above *hot dog–shaped, brown female flowerheads.* May–July. **Where found:** Fresh marshes, ponds. Throughout our area.
Uses: American Indians poulticed jelly-like pounded roots on wounds, sores, boils, carbuncles, inflammations, burns, and scalds. Fuzz from mature female flowerheads applied to scalds, burns, and to prevent chafing in babies. Young flowerheads eaten for diarrhea. Root infused in milk, for dysentery and diarrhea. Anthers, pollen, rhizomes, and shoots have all served as human food. Pulp can be converted to rayon. **Warning:** Though it is widely eaten by human foragers, Cattail is suspected of being **poisonous** to grazing animals. **Related species:** Root tea of **Narrowleaf Cattail** (*T. angustifolia,* not shown) has been used for "gravel" (kidney stones).

CORN   **Whole plant**
Zea mays L.   **C. Pl. 28**   Grass Family
Too well known to describe. Introduced to the U.S. by American Indians centuries ago; cultivated throughout our area.
Uses: Seed oil (corn oil) recommended as a health food for arteriosclerosis and high cholesterol. Corn "silk," a well-known herbal diuretic, was once used in tea for cystitis, gonorrhea, gout, and rheumatism; seeds contain a cell-proliferant, wound-healing substance, allantoin (best known from Comfrey, p. 180). Science has confirmed diuretic, hypoglycemic, and hypotensive activity in animal experiments with corn extracts.

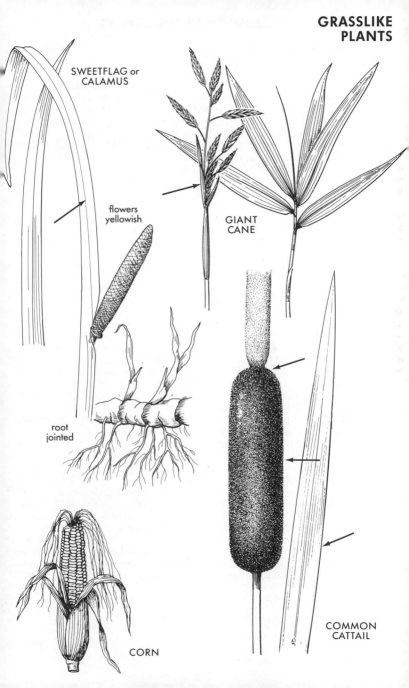

GRASSLIKE PLANTS

SWEETFLAG or CALAMUS

flowers yellowish

GIANT CANE

root jointed

CORN

COMMON CATTAIL

MISCELLANEOUS GRASSES

QUACK GRASS
Whole plant

Agropyron repens (L.) Beauvois
Grass Family

Grass; to 3 ft. Spreads on creeping *yellow* rhizomes. Leaves soft, flat, somewhat drooping; *crowded with fine ribs.* Flower spike *not square* as in most *Agropyron* species. 2–9 flowered spikelets; bract below spikelets not stiff, with slender keel and ribs. **Where found:** Fields, gardens. Troublesome weed throughout our area. Eurasian alien.

Uses: American Indians used tea as a diuretic for "gravel" (kidney stones) and urinary incontinence; worm expellent; wash for swollen limbs. In famines, rhizomes have served to make breadstuffs; also scorched as a coffee substitute. Roots sometimes chewed like licorice. Considered an antidote to arrow poisons in Africa.

BIG BLUESTEM GRASS
Root, leaves

Andropogon gerardii Vitm.
Grass Family

Coarse grass; 4–7 ft. Large clumps. Stem bluish. Flowers in a purplish or bronze-green raceme. Bristle-like awn projects from stalkless flowers — *stiff, sharply bent, to ¾ in. long.* Awn absent on stalked flowers. **Where found:** Prairies, open ground. Que., Me. to Fla., Texas; north to Minn., Wyo., Sask., Man.

Uses: Diuretic, analgesic. Chippewas used root decoction for stomachaches, gas. Omahas used leaf tea as an external wash to relieve fevers, general debility.

BROOMSEDGE
Leaves

Andropogon virginicus L.
Grass Family

Highly variable grass; 28–55 in. Bluish or green stem. Leaf sheath *overlapping, keeled,* and *strongly compressed.* Small flowers emerge from envelopes that are *not inflated;* racemes usually in pairs, with *silvery white* hairs. **Where found:** Dry soil, open woods. Mass., N.Y. south to Fla.; west to Texas, Kans.; north to Ill., Ind., Ohio.

Uses: Catawbas used root decoction for backaches. Cherokees used leaf tea for diarrhea; externally, as a wash for frostbite, sores, and itching. Also used for piles and poison-ivy rash.

SWEET GRASS
Leaves

Hierochloe odorata L.
Grass Family

Vanilla-scented grass; 10–24 in. Spreads on slender, creeping rhizomes. Leaf clumps arise from dead foliage of previous year and wither soon after flowering. Flowers in pyramid-shaped clusters. **Where found:** Meadows. N.S. to Pa., Ohio, Iowa, S.D.

Uses: American Indians widely used it as incense for ceremonies. Tea used for coughs, sore throats, chafing, venereal infections; also to stop vaginal bleeding, expel afterbirth. **Warning:** Roots contain a coumarin, sometimes considered carcinogenic.

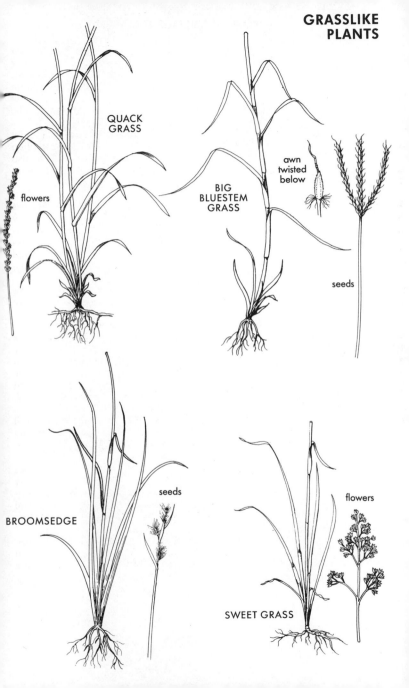

GRASSLIKE PLANTS

QUACK GRASS

flowers

BIG BLUESTEM GRASS

awn twisted below

seeds

BROOMSEDGE

seeds

SWEET GRASS

flowers

GLOSSARY
BIBLIOGRAPHY
INDEX

GLOSSARY

Medicinal Terms

Adaptogenic: Helping the human organism adapt to stressful conditions.

Alkaloid: A large, varied group of complex nitrogen-containing compounds, usually alkaline, that react with acids to form soluble salts, many of which have physiological effects on humans. Includes nicotine, cocaine, caffeine, etc.

Alterative: A medicinal substance that gradually restores health.

Analgesic: A pain-relieving medicine.

Anodyne: A pain-relieving medicine, milder than analgesic.

Anti-allergenic: Reducing or relieving allergies.

Anti-aphrodisiac: Suppressing sexual desire.

Antibiotic: An agent that inhibits the growth or multiplication of, or kills, a living organism; usually used in reference to bacteria or other microorganisms.

Anticonvulsant: Reducing or relieving convulsions or cramps.

Antifungal: An agent that inhibits the growth or multiplication of fungi, or kills them outright.

Antihistaminic: Neutralizing the effect or inhibiting production of histamine.

Anti-inflammatory: Reducing or neutralizing inflammation.

Antimicrobial: An agent that inhibits the growth or multiplication of microorganisms, or kills them.

Anti-oxidant: Preventing oxidation; a preservative.

Antiscorbutic: An agent effective against scurvy.

Antiseptic: Preventing sepsis, decay, putrification; also, an agent that kills germs, microbes.

Antispasmodic: Preventing or relieving spasms or cramps.

Antitumor: Preventing or effective against tumors (cancers).

Antitussive: Preventing or relieving cough.

Antiviral: An agent that inhibits growth or multiplication of viruses, or kills them.

Aphrodisiac: Increasing or exciting sexual desire.

Astringent: An agent that causes tissue to contract.

Bactericidal: An agent that kills bacteria.

Calmative: An agent with mild sedative or calming effects.

Cardioactive: Affecting the heart.

Carminative: An agent that relieves and removes gas from the digestive system.

Cathartic: A powerful purgative or laxative, causing severe evacuation, with or without pain.

Cholagogue: An agent that increases bile flow to the intestines.

CNS: The central nervous system.

Counterirritant: An agent that produces inflammation or irritation when applied locally to affect another, usually irritated surface to stimulate circulation. (Example: a mustard plaster or liniment.)

Cytotoxic: An agent that is toxic to certain organs, tissues, or cells.

Decoction: A preparation made by boiling a plant part in water. Compare with **infusion** (see also p. 6).

Demulcent: An agent that is locally soothing and softening.

Diaphoretic: An agent that induces sweating.

Digestive: An agent that promotes digestion.

Diuretic: An agent that induces urination.

Emetic: An agent that induces vomiting.

Emollient: An agent that softens and soothes the skin when applied locally.

Estrogenic: A substance that induces female hormonal activity.

Expectorant: An agent that induces the removal (coughing-up) of mucous secretions from the lungs.

Fungicidal: An agent that kills fungi.

Hemostatic: An agent that checks bleeding.

Homeopathic: Relating to homeopathy, a system of medicine founded in the late 1700s by Samuel Hahnemann. The system is based on the principle that "like cures like." Practitioners believe that a substance that produces a set of symptoms in a well person will, in minute, "potentized" doses, cure those same symptoms in a diseased individual.

Hypertensive: Causing or marking a rise in blood pressure.

Hypoglycemic: Causing a deficiency of blood sugar.

Hypotensive: Causing or marking a lowering of blood pressure.

Immunostimulant: Stimulating various functions or activities of the immune system.

Infusion: A preparation made by soaking a plant part in hot water (or cold water, for a cold infusion); in essence, a "tea." Compare with **decoction.**

Laxative: A mild purgative.

Mitogenic: An agent that affects cell division.

Moxa: A dried herb substance burned on or above the skin to stimulate an acupuncture point or serve as a counterirritant. A famous technique of Traditional Chinese Medicine, using dried, pressed leaves of Mugwort (*Artemisia vulgaris*).

Mucilaginous: Pertaining to or resembling or containing mucilage; slimy.

Nervine: An agent that affects, strengthens, or calms the nerves.

Panacea: An agent good for what ails you, or what doesn't ail you. A "cure-all."

Poultice: A moist, usually warm or hot mass of plant material applied to the skin, or with cloth between the skin and plant material, to effect a medicinal action.

Purgative: An agent that causes cleansing or watery evacuation of the bowels, usually with griping (painful cramps).

Rubefacient: An agent that causes reddening or irritation when applied to the skin.

Saponin: A glycoside compound common in plants, which, when shaken with water, has a foaming or "soapy" action.

Spasmolytic: Checking spasms or cramps.

Stimulant: An agent that causes increased activity of another agent, cell, tissue, organ, or organism.

Styptic: Checking bleeding by contracting blood vessels.

Tincture: A diluted alcohol solution of plant parts (see p. 7).

Teratogen: A substance that can cause the deformity of a fetus.

Tonic: An ambiguous term referring to a substance thought to have an overall positive medicinal effect of an unspecified nature (see **adaptogenic**).

Tuberculostatic: Arresting the tubercle bacillus (the "germ" responsible for causing tuberculosis).

Uterotonic: Having a positive effect of an unspecified nature on the uterus.

Vasoconstrictor: An agent that causes blood vessels to constrict.

Vasodilator: An agent that causes blood vessels to dilate.

Vermicidal: Having worm-killing properties; an agent that kills worms; a vermifuge.

Vulnerary: An agent used for healing wounds.

Botanical Terms

Basal rosette: Leaves radiating directly from the crown of the root.

Bracts: The leaflike structures of a grouping or arrangement of flowers (inflorescence).

Calyx: The sepals collectively; the external floral envelope.

Decompound: Divided several or many times; compound with further subdivisions.

Floret: A very small flower, especially one of the disk flowers of plants in the composite family.

Glaucous: Covered with a fine, white, often waxy film, which rubs off.

Herbaceous: Non-woody.

Liana: A vigorous woody vine (usually refers to tropical vines).

Obovate: Oval, but broader toward the apex; refers to leaf shape.

Ovate: Oval, but broader toward the base; egg-shaped.

Palmate: With 3 or more leaflets, nerves, or lobes radiating from a central point.

Panicle: A branching flower grouping, with branches that are usually **racemes** (see p. 322).

Perfect (flower): A flower that has a full complement of male and female parts as well as floral envelopes (petals *and* sepals).

Perfoliate: A leaf that appears to be perforated by the stem.

Pinnate: A featherlike arrangement; usually refers to a compound leaf with leaflets arranged on each side of a central axis.

Raceme: An unbranched, elongated flower grouping, with individual flowers on distinct stalks.

Rays (ray flowers): The straplike, often sterile flowers (commonly called "petals") surrounding the flowerhead (disk) of a plant in the composite family. (Examples: the yellow rays of sunflowers, or the purple rays surrounding the cone of Purple Coneflower).

Rhizome: A creeping underground stem.

Rosette (basal): Leaves radiating directly from the crown of the root.

Saprophytic: A plant (usually lacking chlorophyll) that lives on dead organic matter.

Sepals: The individual divisions of the calyx (outer floral envelope).

Sessile: Lacking a stalk; such as a leaf or flower with no obvious stalk.

Silique: A term applied to the peculiar seedpod structure of plants in the mustard family.

Spadix: A thick, fleshy flower spike (usually enveloped by a spathe), as in members of the arum family (Skunk Cabbage, Jack-in-the-Pulpit, Dragon Arum, etc.).

Spathe: A modified, leaflike structure surrounding a spadix, as in members of the Arum family (Skunk Cabbage, Jack-in-the-Pulpit, Dragon Arum, etc.).

Spike (flower): An unbranched, elongated flower grouping in which the individual flowers are sessile (attached without stalks).

Stamens: The pollen-bearing anthers with attached filaments (sometimes without filaments).

Stipules: Appendages (resembling small or minute leaves) at the base of leaves of certain plants.

Subshrub: Somewhat or slightly shrublike; usually a plant with a stem that is woody at the base, but mostly herbaceous.

Tendrils: A modified leaf or branch structure, often coiled like a spring, used for clinging in plants that climb.

Umbels: A flower grouping with individual flower stalks or floral groupings radiating from a central axis; often flat-topped and umbrella-like.

BIBLIOGRAPHY

Technical Manuals

Bailey, Liberty Hyde, and Ethel Zoe Bailey. Revision by L.H. Bailey Hortorium Staff. 1976. *Hortus Third,* New York: Macmillan.

Barkley, T.M., ed. 1986. *Flora of the Great Plains.* Lawrence: University Press of Kansas.

Fernald, Merritt Lyndon. 1950. *Gray's Manual of Botany.* 8th ed. New York: Van Nostrand.

Gleason, Henry A., and Arthur Cronquist. 1963. *Manual of Vascular Plants of Northeastern United States and Adjacent Canada.* New York: Van Nostrand.

Radford, Albert E., Harry E. Ahles, and C. Ritchie Bell. 1968. *Manual of the Vascular Flora of the Carolinas.* Chapel Hill: University of North Carolina Press.

Popular Guides

Cobb, Boughton. 1963. *A Field Guide to the Ferns.* Boston: Houghton Mifflin.

Dobells, Inge N., ed. 1986. *Magic and Medicine of Plants.* Pleasantville, N.Y.: The Reader's Digest Association.

Duke, James A. 1986. *Handbook of Northeastern Indian Medicinal Plants.* Lincoln, Mass.: Quarterman Publications.

Foster, Steven. 1984. *Herbal Bounty — The Gentle Art of Herb Culture.* Layton, Utah: Gibbs M., Smith, Inc.

Grieve, Maude. 1931. *A Modern Herbal.* 2 vols. Reprint ed. 1971. New York: Dover.

Kowalchik, Claire, and William H. Hylton, ed. 1987. *Rodale's Illustrated Encyclopedia of Herbs.* Emmaus, Pa.: Rodale Press.

Krochmal, Arnold, Russell S. Walters, and Richard M. Doughty. 1971. *A Guide to Medicinal Plants of Appalachia.* Agricultural Handbook No. 400, Forest Service, U.S.D.A. Washington, D.C.: U.S. Government Printing Office.

Millspaugh, Charles F. *American Medicinal Plants.* 1892. Reprint ed. 1974. New York: Dover.

Moerman, Daniel E. 1982. *Geraniums for the Iroquois: A Field Guide to American Indian Medicinal Plants.* Algonac, Mich.: Reference Publications.

Peterson, Lee Allen. 1977. *A Field Guide to Edible Wild Plants.* Boston: Houghton Mifflin.

Peterson, Roger Tory, and Margaret McKinney. 1968. *A Field Guide to Wildflowers.* Boston: Houghton Mifflin.

Petrides, George A. 1972. *A Field Guide to Trees and Shrubs.* 2nd ed. Boston: Houghton Mifflin.

Tyler, Varro E. 1987. *The New Honest Herbal.* Philadelphia: George F. Stickley.

Scholarly Works

DerMarderosian, A., and Lawrence Liberti. 1988. *Natural Products Medicine: A Scientific Guide to Foods, Drugs, Cosmetics.* Philadelphia: George F. Stickley.

Duke, James A. 1986. *Handbook of Medicinal Herbs.* Boca Raton, Florida: CRC Press.

Felter, Harvey Wickes, and John Uri Lloyd. 1901. *King's American Dispensatory* 18th ed. 2 vols. Reprint ed. 1983. Portland, Oregon: Eclectic Medical Publications.

Hardin, James W., and Jay M. Arena. 1974. *Human Poisoning from Native and Cultivated Plants.* 2nd ed. Durham: Duke University Press.

Leung, Albert Y. 1980. *Encyclopedia of Common Natural Ingredients Used in Foods, Drugs, and Cosmetics.* New York: Wiley-Interscience.

Lewis, Walter and Memory Elvin-Lewis. 1977. *Medical Botany — Plants Affecting Man's Health.* New York: Wiley-Interscience.

Moerman, Daniel E. 1986. *Medicinal Plants of Native America.* 2 vols. Ann Arbor: University of Michigan, Museum of Anthropology.

Tyler, Varro E., Lynn R. Brady, and James E. Robbers. 1988. *Pharmacognosy.* 9th ed. Philadelphia: Lea & Febiger.

Weiss, Rudolf Fritz. 1988. *Herbal Medicine* (translated from 6th German ed. of *Lehrbuch der Phytotherepie* by A. R. Meuss). Beaconsfield, England: Beaconsfield Publishers, Ltd.

INDEX TO PLANTS

Wormseed, American. *See
    under* Mexican Tea, 216.
Wormwood, 220
    Annual, 222, **Pl. 27**
    Tall, 222

Xanthium strumarium, 212
Xanthorhiza simplicissima, 240
*Xanthoxylum. See
    Zanthoxylum,* 238.
Xyris caroliniana, 86

Yam, Wild, 204, **Pl. 15**
Yarrow, 64, **Pl. 26**
Yaupon Holly, 232
Yellow Dock, 214, **Pl. 25**
Yellow Giant Hyssop, 112
Yellow Jessamine, 298

Yellow Jewelweed, 106
Yellow Pine. *See* Shortleaf Pine,
    260.
Yellow Pond Lily. *See*
    Spatterdock, 88.
Yellow Sweet-clover, 116, **Pl. 22**
Yellow-eyed Grass, 86
Yellowroot, 240
Yew, American, 226
Yucca filamentosa, 18, 228
    glauca, 18, 228, **Pl. 39**
Yucca, 18, 228, **Pl. 39**

Zanthoxylum americanum, 238
    clava-herculis, 238, **Pl. 46**
Zea mays, 312, **Pl. 28**
Zizia aurea, 110

INDEX TO MEDICAL TOPICS

Caution: This field guide is a guide to the recognition of plants, not a prescriptor. Only your doctor or other health-care professional who is licensed to do so can prescribe medications for you. We cannot and do not prescribe herbal medication. This index simply serves as a guide to the listings of medicinal usage of the plants treated in this book. Qualified medical diagnosis is essential to the treatment of disease. See your health-care professional rather than attempting self-diagnosis, which may be unreliable or incorrect.

LIFE LIST

WHITE

- PRICKLY POPPY, 12, Pl. 39 _____ to _____
- TURTLEHEAD, 12, Pl. 2 _____ to _____
- LILY-OF-THE-VALLEY, 12, Pl. 24 _____ to _____
- DUTCHMAN'S-BREECHES, 12, Pl. 18 _____ to _____
- WILD CALLA, 14 _____ to _____
- BUCKBEAN, 14 _____ to _____
- FRAGRANT WATER-LILY, 14, Pl. 1 _____ to _____
- LIZARD'S-TAIL, 14 _____ to _____
- WATER-PLANTAIN, 16 _____ to _____
- BROAD-LEAVED ARROWHEAD, 16, Pl. 1 _____ to _____
- RATTLESNAKE-MASTER, 18 _____ to _____
- YUCCA *(Y. filamentosa)*, 18, 228 _____ to _____
- YUCCA *(Y. glauca)*, 18, 228, Pl. 39 _____ to _____
- FIELD BINDWEED, 20 _____ to _____
- HEDGE BINDWEED, 20 _____ to _____
- JIMSONWEED, 20, Pl. 33 _____ to _____
- WILD POTATO-VINE, 20 _____ to _____
- VIRGIN'S BOWER, 22 _____ to _____
- WILD CUCUMBER, 22 _____ to _____
- PASSION-FLOWER, 22 _____ to _____
- DOWNY RATTLESNAKE-PLANTAIN, 24, Pl. 18 _____ to _____
- NODDING LADIES' TRESSES, 24 _____ to _____
- PINK LADY'S-SLIPPER, 24, Pl. 19 _____ to _____
- BEARBERRY, 26, 232, Pl. 10 _____ to _____
- TRAILING ARBUTUS, 26 _____ to _____
- WINTERGREEN, 26, 232, Pl. 29 _____ to _____
- PARTRIDGEBERRY, 26, 232, Pl. 11 _____ to _____
- ROUND-LEAVED SUNDEW, 28, Pl. 4 _____ to _____
- INDIAN-PIPE, 28, Pl. 18 _____ to _____
- GIANT BIRD'S NEST, 28 _____ to _____
- WILD LEEK, 30 _____ to _____
- GARLIC, 30 _____ to _____
- FALSE SOLOMON'S-SEAL, 32 _____ to _____
- SOLOMON'S-SEAL, 32, Pl. 14 _____ to _____
- FALSE LILY-OF-THE-VALLEY, 32 _____ to _____
- COLIC-ROOT, 32 _____ to _____
- SHEPHERD'S PURSE, 34 _____ to _____

_____SWEET JOE-PYE-WEED, 164 _____to_____
_____GREAT BURDOCK, 166 _____to_____
_____COMMON BURDOCK, 166 _____to_____
_____CANADA THISTLE, 166 _____to_____

BLUE/VIOLET
_____CRESTED DWARF IRIS, 168, Pl. 15 _____to_____
_____BLUE FLAG, 168 _____to_____
_____SPIDERWORT, 168, Pl. 42 _____to_____
_____ASIATIC DAYFLOWER, 168, Pl. 6 _____to_____
_____PASSION-FLOWER, 170, Pl. 32 _____to_____
_____KUDZU, 170, 300, Pl. 32 _____to_____
_____TALL BELLFLOWER, 172 _____to_____
_____FOXGLOVE, 172, Pl. 28 _____to_____
_____BLUE VERVAIN, 172, Pl. 34 _____to_____
_____BLUETS, 174, Pl. 21 _____to_____
_____COMMON SPEEDWELL, 174, Pl. 21 _____to_____
_____THYME-LEAVED SPEEDWELL, 174 _____to_____
_____JOHNNY-JUMP-UP, 174 _____to_____
_____BLUE-EYED GRASS, 176 _____to_____
_____STIFF GENTIAN, 178 _____to_____
_____FLAX, 178 _____to_____
_____GREEK VALERIAN, 178, Pl. 17 _____to_____
_____HOUND'S TONGUE, 180 _____to_____
_____WILD COMFREY, 180 _____to_____
_____VIPER'S BUGLOSS, 180 _____to_____
_____COMFREY, 180, Pl. 28 _____to_____
_____HORSE-NETTLE, 182, Pl. 33 _____to_____
_____WOODY NIGHTSHADE, 182, Pl. 33 _____to_____
_____LOBELIA, 184, Pl. 42 _____to_____
_____GREAT LOBELIA, 184, Pl. 2 _____to_____
_____PALE-SPIKE LOBELIA, 184 _____to_____
_____WILD BERGAMOT, 186, Pl. 42 _____to_____
_____PERILLA, 186, Pl. 7 _____to_____
_____MAD-DOG SKULLCAP, 186 _____to_____
_____WATERMINT, 188 _____to_____
_____PEPPERMINT, 188, Pl. 30 _____to_____
_____SPEARMINT, 188, Pl. 30 _____to_____
_____BLUE GIANT HYSSOP, 190, Pl. 29 _____to_____
_____AMERICAN PENNYROYAL, 190 _____to_____
_____HYSSOP, 190, Pl. 30 _____to_____
_____CALAMINT, 190, Pl. 37 _____to_____
_____DOWNY WOODMINT, 192 _____to_____
_____GROUND IVY, 192, Pl. 30 _____to_____
_____HEAL-ALL, 192, Pl. 23 _____to_____
_____LYRE-LEAVED SAGE, 192, Pl. 38 _____to_____
_____ALFALFA, 194 _____to_____
_____BLUE FALSE INDIGO, 194, Pl. 36 _____to_____
_____WILD LUPINE, 194 _____to_____
_____ROUGH BLAZING-STAR, 196, Pl. 41 _____to_____
_____DEER'S TONGUE, 196 _____to_____
_____IRONWEED, 196 _____to_____
_____NEW ENGLAND ASTER, 198 _____to_____
_____MILK THISTLE, 198, Pl. 26 _____to_____
_____NARROW-LEAVED PURPLE CONEFLOWER, _____to_____
200, Pl. 40

____PALE PURPLE CONEFLOWER, 200, Pl. 40   _____ to _____
____PURPLE CONEFLOWER, 200, Pl. 40   _____ to _____

GREEN
____DRAGON ARUM, 202, Pl. 16   _____ to _____
____JACK-IN-THE-PULPIT, 202, Pl. 16   _____ to _____
____SKUNK CABBAGE, 202, 224, Pl. 11   _____ to _____
____WILD YAM, 204, Pl. 15   _____ to _____
____HOPS, 204, Pl. 32   _____ to _____
____MARIJUANA, 206, Pl. 28   _____ to _____
____BLUE COHOSH, 206, Pl. 17   _____ to _____
____WILD IPECAC, 206   _____ to _____
____CASTOR-OIL-PLANT, 208, Pl. 33   _____ to _____
____ALUMROOT, 210   _____ to _____
____DITCH STONECROP, 210   _____ to _____
____FIGWORT, 210   _____ to _____
____STINGING NETTLE, 212, Pl. 6   _____ to _____
____COCKLEBUR, 212   _____ to _____
____COMMON SMARTWEED, 214   _____ to _____
____SHEEP-SORREL, 214   _____ to _____
____YELLOW DOCK, 214, Pl 25   _____ to _____
____SMOOTH PIGWEED, 216   _____ to _____
____GREEN AMARANTH, 216   _____ to _____
____LAMB'S-QUARTERS, 216   _____ to _____
____MEXICAN TEA, 216   _____ to _____
____COMMON RAGWEED, 218   _____ to _____
____GIANT RAGWEED, 218   _____ to _____
____WORMWOOD, 220   _____ to _____
____MUGWORT, 220   _____ to _____
____ANNUAL WORMWOOD, 222, Pl. 27   _____ to _____
____TALL WORMWOOD, 222   _____ to _____
____WILD TARRAGON, 222   _____ to _____

GREEN/BROWN
____VIRGINIA SNAKEROOT, 224   _____ to _____
____DUTCHMAN'S-PIPE, 224, 302   _____ to _____
____BEECH-DROPS, 224   _____ to _____

SHRUBS
____COMMON JUNIPER, 226, Pl. 43   _____ to _____
____AMERICAN YEW, 226   _____ to _____
____SAW PALMETTO, 228   _____ to _____
____SHEEP LAUREL, 230, Pl. 43   _____ to _____
____MOUNTAIN LAUREL, 230   _____ to _____
____LABRADOR TEA, 230, Pl. 4   _____ to _____
____GREAT RHODODENDRON, 230, Pl. 44   _____ to _____
____YAUPON HOLLY, 232   _____ to _____
____CREEPING THYME, 232, Pl. 30   _____ to _____
____NINEBARK, 234, Pl. 9   _____ to _____
____LARGE-HIP ROSE, 234, Pl. 10   _____ to _____
____RED RASPBERRY, 234   _____ to _____
____BLACK RASPBERRY, 234, Pl. 31   _____ to _____
____AMERICAN BARBERRY, 236   _____ to _____
____COMMON BARBERRY, 236, Pl. 47   _____ to _____
____HAWTHORNS, 236   _____ to _____
____DEVIL'S WALKING-STICK, 238, Pl. 46   _____ to _____

___MAIDENHAIR FERN, 308 _____ to _____
___BRACKEN FERN, 308 _____ to _____
___LADY FERN, 310 _____ to _____
___RATTLESNAKE FERN, 310 _____ to _____
___CRESTED WOOD FERN, 310 _____ to _____
___MALE FERN, 310 _____ to _____

GRASSES or GRASSLIKE PLANTS
___GIANT CANE, 312, Pl. 3 _____ to _____
___COMMON CATTAIL, 312 _____ to _____
___CORN, 312, Pl. 28 _____ to _____
___QUACK GRASS, 314 _____ to _____
___BIG BLUESTEM GRASS, 314 _____ to _____
___BROOMSEDGE, 314 _____ to _____
___SWEET GRASS, 314 _____ to _____